Contents

T.

Practical Chemotherapy

A multidisciplinary guide

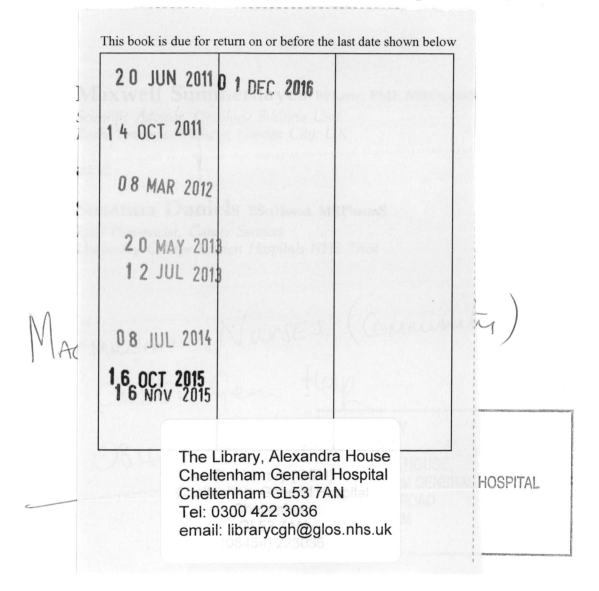

Radcliffe Medical Press

Radcliffe Medical Press Ltd
18 Marcham Road
Abingdon
Oxon OX14 1AA
United Kingdom

www.radcliffe-oxford.com
The Radcliffe Medical Press electronic catalogue and online ordering facility.
Direct sales to anywhere in the world.

Every effort has been made to ensure the accuracy of this text, and that the best information available has been used. This does not diminish the requirement to exercise clinical judgement, and neither the publishers nor the authors can accept any responsibility for its use in practice.

British Library Cataloguing in Publication Data

A catalogue record for this book is available from the British Library.

ISBN 1 85775 965 6

Typeset by Aarontype Limited, Easton, Bristol
Printed and bound by Biddles Ltd, Guildford and King's Lynn

About the authors

Max Summerhayes graduated in pharmacy from the London School of Pharmacy in 1981 and, after completing a pre-registration year at Guy's Hospital, returned to the School of Pharmacy to undertake research on the pharmacology of brain dopamine systems, for which he was awarded a PhD in 1985. After 18 months as a post-doctoral researcher at the Institute of Cancer Research in London, investigating the use of monoclonal antibodies as vehicles for drug delivery, he returned to work as a hospital pharmacist at Guy's. Two years later he took over responsibility for the satellite oncology pharmacy unit there. This was one of the first of its kind in the UK. By the time of his departure in 2002 he was responsible for about 15 staff in three units. In the same year, he decided on a career change and joined the oncology medical team at Roche Products.

Max was the founding chairman of the British Oncology Pharmacy Association and has had more than 25 peer-reviewed articles published, as well as a large number of other commissioned articles. He is a clinical pharmacology examiner for the Royal College of Radiologists and serves on the editorial board of the *Journal of Oncology Pharmacy Practice*.

Susanna Daniels studied at Aston University and then completed her pre-registration training at Guy's Hospital. Her basic training continued at UCLH where she developed an interest in oncology. After completing the rotational training, Susanna was appointed Haematology Pharmacist at the Royal London Hospital, managing the cytotoxic unit. Susanna then moved to a position at St Thomas' Hospital which involved managing the busy cytotoxic unit. During this time, she increased her role with the Drug and Therapeutics Committee and in training. A promotion led to a new role as Clinical Governance Pharmacist for Oncology for the Trust, which involved the production of various guidelines. Susanna has also gained valuable experience developing the website for the Drug Development Program at Princess Margaret Hospital in Toronto, Canada, during a one-year sabbatical. In addition, she co-ordinated the pharmacy training programme during this period.

Susanna is now Lead Pharmacist, Cancer Services, at University College London Hospitals NHS Trust.

List of abbreviations

AIC	5-amino-imidazole-4-carboxamide
ALT	alanine transaminase
AST	aspartate transaminase
AUC	area under plasma concentration–time curve
BBB	blood–brain barrier
BSA	body surface area
CNS	central nervous system
CrCl	creatinine clearance
dFdU	2′-deoxy-2′,2′-difluorouridine
DPD	dihydropyrimidine dehydrogenase
ECOG	Eastern Cooperative Oncology Group
EDTA	ethylene diamine tetra-acetic acid
FBC	full blood count
G-CSF	granulocyte colony-stimulating factor
GFR	glomerular filtration rate
GM-CSF	granulocyte-macrophage colony-stimulating factor
GTN	glyceryl trinitrate
h	hour
INR	international normalised ratio
IP	inpatient
IU	International Unit
IV	intravenous
kg	kilogram
L	litre
LFT	liver function test
MAO	monoamine oxidase
MAOI	monoamine oxidase inhibitor
mg	milligram
min	minute
MUGA	multiple gated acquisition test of cardiac output
NCIC	National Cancer Institute of Canada
NICE	National Institute for Clinical Excellence
NSCLC	non-small-cell lung cancer
od	once daily
PICC	peripherally inserted central catheter
PO	by mouth
PT	prothrombin time
s	second
SC	subcutaneous

SPC	summary of product characteristics
TTO	'to take out' medication
ULN	upper limit of normal
WBC	white blood count

Acknowledgements

Max Summerhayes would like to thank Dr Stephen Houston for critically reading an earlier draft of some of the monographs in this book, his staff for tolerating his neglect while he was working on this and other projects, his wife Bev for her constant support, and his parents for starting him on the road to where he is now.

Susanna Daniels would like to thank Stephen for his continual support – he has grown used to seeing her surrounded by reams of paper and red pens! She would also like to thank her family for their ongoing encouragement.

Both authors would like to acknowledge the work of Steven Wanklyn on the pharmacy patient record sheet in Appendix 3.

We would like to dedicate this book to Roger Horne and Tony West — two very different people, although they are equally good managers — for whom we have had the privilege of working at Guy's and St Thomas' Hospitals.

Introduction

The first thing that we would like you as a potential reader of this volume to know is what this book is *not*. This will save you from wasting your time looking for something that isn't here, and us from appearing to have failed in our task (even though we have doubtless failed in other ways).

This book is *not* a general discourse on cancer chemotherapy – it will give you no guidance on selection of the most appropriate chemotherapy regimen for use in a particular setting. It follows that we are not endorsing any of the regimens in this book as being the gold standard. A regimen is included if we have experience of it and believe it to have significant use in current UK practice. We are aware that current clinical practice is constantly changing and that our experience, based as it is on one institution, is limited.

Neither is this book a reference source that will enable the user to deal with any situation that arises during the use of the chemotherapy regimens described within it. For example, it does not describe many of the rarer drug-induced adverse effects that have been reported. Instead, it concentrates on those that are common, and those where knowledge can help either to prevent them or to facilitate an appropriate response when they do occur.

Having dealt with what this book is not, it is incumbent upon us to state what it does aspire to be, which is perhaps best done by explaining how it came into being. Oncology pharmacy in the UK is a relatively new discipline, and its growth in recent years has mirrored the increase in the use of cytotoxic drugs for the management of cancer. One of us (MS) is old enough to have experienced this change at first hand. When he first started working as an oncology pharmacist a decade and a half ago, chemotherapy was only routinely given for haematological malignancies, testicular cancers and metastatic breast cancer – virtually every other use was experimental. Since then, the introduction of first-, second- and, in some cases, third- and fourth-line chemotherapy for most solid tumours, as well as the introduction of adjuvant and primary chemotherapy, have led to a dramatic increase in the amount of chemotherapy being given. Therefore there has of necessity been a corresponding increase in the number of people involved in its prescription, preparation and administration. The pharmacy team of MS has increased in size from two to almost 15 during this time.

It follows that an area of treatment which was once the preserve of a few specialists, who had been involved in this field for many years and who had acquired an in-depth knowledge of the subject during that time, is now drawing in ever increasing numbers of less experienced practitioners.

These newcomers are required to 'hit the ground running' without the luxury of years of learning on the job. This is a particular problem in an area such as this, where learning by one's mistakes can have a very high price.

Clearly, newcomers need to learn fast, and they can do this by reading textbooks and by paying attention to more experienced team members. In an ideal world such approaches would ensure that no member of the chemotherapy team would be asked to do anything until they were fully conversant with the job to be done and understood everything that might go wrong.

In practice, we do not live in an ideal world — people forget what they have been told, their mentor is not around when he or she is needed, or their state of ignorance is such that they do not recognise that they are straying into an area where they need help.

To try to help with this problem at a local level, MS drew up some 'Chemo-therapy Guidance Notes' for use by the three main professional groups involved in cytotoxic chemotherapy. Taking an optimistic view, the intention was that these would act as an *aide-mémoire*, reminding newer staff to check things and do tasks that they were aware should be done, but which they might otherwise forget to do because of pressure of work or inexperience. Taking a slightly less optimistic view — that not everyone is as well trained as they should be, so there may be gaps in people's knowledge — these notes were intended to stop the majority of serious chemotherapy errors. For example, it was hoped that they would prevent patients with renal impairment from receiving treatment with nephrotoxic drugs, and neutropenic patients from being given myelosuppressive chemotherapy.

The notes were also intended to oil the machinery of chemotherapy administration and make everyone's life a little easier. For example, they reminded the harassed junior doctor, whose general experience was that patients receive chemotherapy every three weeks, that some regimens require interim appointments for additional treatment. Points such as this may seem obvious, and of course they flow directly from the dose regimen that is being used. All we can say is that all of the information included in the original notes, and in this book, is based on our experience of what goes wrong in practice, and we *have* seen patients return to start their second cycle of BEP without receiving their day 8 and day 15 bleomycin doses!

The 'Guidance Notes' were well received by staff working at Guy's and St Thomas' hospitals, and more regimens have been added over the years. The production of these guidance notes inspired SD to produce guidelines for cytotoxic drug use in patients with hepatic and renal impairment (*see* Appendices 1 and 2). These were originally produced for local use, but were also well received by members of the British Oncology Pharmacy Association (BOPA).

By 2001 it was obvious not only that more new 'Guidance Notes' were needed, but also that the existing monographs required substantial revision. In particular, in view of the current drive towards evidence-based medicine, we felt that the regimens should be referenced to literature reports of their use.

Since much work needed to be done, it seemed to us that others outside Guy's and St Thomas' should be able to benefit in the way that we believe our local colleagues have done on occasions. We therefore developed the guidance notes into this book, which we hope will be useful to all those who are involved in the practical aspects of giving chemotherapy, but especially those who are new to the area. Its primary aim is to make the prescribing, dispensing and administering of cytotoxic treatment a little safer and easier.

Of course, no work of this kind can foresee every problem that might arise. This is because each patient is a unique individual, and also because the ability of human beings to make inexplicable errors is almost unlimited. This book cannot be a substitute for good training and experience.

We would urge you to consult the first chapter, entitled 'What's in the monographs and how to use them'. Not only will this enable you to get more out of the book, but also it will alert you to the limitations of the book and prevent you from relying on it inappropriately.

We have tried very hard to prevent errors or misleading material from creeping into the text, but we cannot take responsibility for the way in which the book's content is applied in practice. Furthermore, we would urge any of you working in this high-risk area not to rely on one book or one person's view. If for any reason you are uneasy about a patient or their treatment, seek more information and the counsel of someone experienced whom you trust.

Finally, we hope that you gain something of value from our work, and we would welcome your comments − positive or negative, but hopefully constructive − on any aspect of it.

Maxwell Summerhayes
Susanna Daniels
January 2003

What's in the monographs and how to use them

This book consists of a series of monographs, each of which deals with a specific chemotherapy regimen or, in a very few cases, with two very closely related regimens (e.g. weekly and 3-weekly paclitaxel). All of the monographs have the same format and begin with nine core sections (usual indication, doses, administration, anti-emetics, cycle length, number of cycles, side-effects, blood nadir and TTOs required) with which we believe anyone involved in prescribing, preparing or administering chemotherapy should be familiar. There then follow three longer sections consisting of notes for prescribers, nurses and pharmacists, respectively.

We hope that those using this book will read through the introductory sections of the relevant monograph and the notes specific to their profession each time they are about to use a chemotherapy regimen with which they are not completely familiar. Of course, there is nothing to stop the reader consulting the sections designed for their professional colleagues – indeed this will probably become increasingly necessary as the previously rigid boundaries between the professions are eroded.

We certainly would not expect anyone to read this book from cover to cover – its layout and writing style would not make for a gripping read!

It will not have escaped your notice that we, the authors, are both pharmacists, and you may be wondering how we decided what each professional group needs to know. For pharmacists, we included anything that we felt any of our staff should be aware of if involved with chemotherapy. For the other disciplines we drew on our experience both of questions that we are often asked by doctors and nurses and of things that we have seen go wrong because a test was not performed, a question was not asked, or a prescription was incorrectly written. In addition, we have revised the text on the basis of feedback from professional colleagues who used earlier versions of some of these monographs.

The more observant among you will also notice that there is some overlap between the core introductory sections of each monograph and the discipline-specific sections that follow, and between the specialist text intended for the different professional groups. We make no apology for this. Our aim was to convey in as few words as possible what people need to know when dealing with a typical patient. By presenting the information separately for nurses, doctors and pharmacists, we were able to remove from each section information that was more relevant to other disciplines, thereby reducing the volume of text that each professional has to read, even though this increases the overall length of each monograph by duplicating some key information several times. By keeping the notes for each profession as short as possible, we hope that we will encourage the reader at least to consult the whole of the section relevant to them. The overlap between the initial core sections of each monograph and the profession-specific parts is also deliberate and its aim is to emphasise particularly important points.

Within the sections targeted at different professional groups the bullet points are not arranged in any particular order. This is because the original monographs were written in a piecemeal way without reference to a rigid template. When revising the text for publication we decided to adhere to this slightly haphazard arrangement in the hope that it would encourage the reader to consult the whole of the relevant section and not just skim through it for specific pieces of information. We can only hope that this plan works and does not cause too much irritation!

The format of the monographs that follow is outlined below, with an explanation of the content of each section, how to interpret that content and its limitations. We hope that you will take the time to read it (even if it seems tedious), as we believe you will gain more from the book if you do so.

REGIMEN

We have used what we believe to be the most widely used name or acronym first, followed by any alternatives of which we are aware, and a full list of the drugs included in the regimen, with their approved names. It should be noted that as well as some regimens having several names, some of the acronyms used may also be employed outside this book to describe different treatment protocols. Always ensure that you know exactly what treatment is intended before reading further.

The regimens we have included are those with which we are familiar and which we believe have relatively widespread use in the UK. We have included all of those that have been the subject of completed or ongoing appraisal by the National Institute for Clinical Excellence (NICE) at the time of writing. We have specifically excluded the regimens used for acute leukaemias (these are often rolling programmes of treatment that do not lend themselves to the format of this book) and for myelo-ablation prior to stem-cell transplantation. These very intensive regimens, like those for the acute leukaemias, are much more difficult to view in isolation from the comprehensive treatment programme that is used during transplantation, and are also of limited interest to those working outside transplant centres.

USUAL INDICATION

Although this is self-explanatory, it must be reiterated that the inclusion of a regimen does not indicate that it is recommended for this purpose, but merely that it has been used. Similarly, it should not be assumed that a regimen with a particular 'usual indication' cannot, on occasion, be appropriately used for other conditions.

DOSES

In general we have used doses that can be traced to a research report included in the citations at the end of the monograph. There are a few regimens — mostly those that have been used for many years — for which we could not find any publication that could be said to describe the 'original' or 'classic' version. In such cases, we have described local practice within our own hospital and we hope that we have made this clear. It is also true that, for some regimens, there are many variants in use. These have evolved locally, within research groups and nationally. In such cases we have generally opted for the version that has been best characterised by use in large, published clinical trials. However, this does not necessarily mean that other variants are inferior or incorrect. Above all, make sure that you know what regimen is intended for a particular patient. *The regimens that are used in your hospital should be part of a local treatment strategy, which should be clearly documented.* However, beware of patients who are enrolled in clinical trials, where the intended treatment may be subtly different to that which is usually used in your hospital.

Most chemotherapy doses are based on the patient's body surface area. A few drugs are dosed in other ways (e.g. flat dosing, doses based on body weight or capped doses), and we have tried to emphasise such deviations from the norm, but you should be alert to such possibilities when looking at unfamiliar regimens.

ADMINISTRATION

We have tried to indicate key features that need to be considered (e.g. the need for hydration, the need for slow infusion, incompatibility of some drugs with certain infusion fluids, etc.). In this book it is not practicable for us to give detailed instructions on how each regimen should be delivered.

We would strongly advise the use of computerised prescribing systems, or at least pre-printed pro formas bearing all of the details of the drugs, fluids, anti-emetics and other concomitant medications to be given, which only require the addition of individual patient details to turn them into a high-quality, legible prescription. We use this approach in our hospital and it makes life both easier and, we believe, safer for all concerned, but *only* when clinicians complete all of the sections of the pro forma in full and do not 'adapt' standard prescriptions for other regimens. This practice frequently leads to errors and is to be avoided at all costs.

One issue that frequently causes controversy is the degree of hydration that is required with cisplatin chemotherapy. In these monographs, we describe current practice within our own hospital, where many regimens are now administered on an outpatient basis with relatively little fluid. In others, where patients are treated as inpatients (perhaps because of the need for multiple-day therapy), more fluid is administered, possibly unnecessarily in some cases. In other words, with cisplatin hydration, as with other administration details, we describe here what has worked for us. This is not to say that other regimens do not exist that would be as safe and efficacious. If you feel confident enough to argue for an alternative, you probably do not need this book! We also highlight drugs that are particularly hazardous when extravasated. Virtually all cytotoxic drugs are capable of causing unpleasant tissue damage when accidentally infused/injected into perivascular tissue. However, those highlighted are particularly likely to cause severe pain and tissue damage. In all cases of extravasation we would refer you to your local hospital policy for dealing with this problem. Because of its important medico-legal implications, it is important that you follow local procedures in such cases. Therefore, it is important that you are familiar with the policy in your hospital, and we would urge you to read this before giving any chemotherapy. If you are interested in learning more about this subject, it is well reviewed in the most recent (2002) edition of the *The Cytotoxics Handbook*.[1]

We have deliberately avoided regimens that involve intrathecal drug administration. This has been the subject of recent guidance from the Chief Medical

Officer,[2] which requires all UK centres where such treatment is administered to have in place robust local procedures covering all aspects of the prescribing, preparative and administration processes, and to compile registers of those nurses, doctors and pharmacists who are competent to participate in these activities. It is vital that non-accredited professionals do not take part in this activity, and that those who are accredited follow local protocols. Therefore we do not wish to complicate matters by providing any advice that might conflict with local guidance.

ANTI-EMETICS

Any unit that is using cytotoxic chemotherapy to treat cancer should have a policy for the optimal use of anti-emetics to control treatment-induced nausea and vomiting. The fundamental principles of drawing up such a policy were laid down by the American Society of Clinical Oncology several years ago.[3] A good policy recognises that it is important to match the anti-emetic prophylaxis given to the emetogenic potential of the chemotherapy regimen in use. To this end, regimens are usually divided into those that are weakly, moderately and highly emetogenic, with anti-emetic policies specifying anti-emetics that are suitable for each group. We have followed this general approach and described regimens as requiring anti-emetics appropriate to weakly, moderately or highly emetogenic chemotherapy. However, we have labelled as highly emetogenic some regimens that under other classification systems are ranked as only moderately emetogenic. This is deliberate. Since the key to good long-term control of chemotherapy-induced nausea and vomiting is good short-term control, we feel that it is better to over-treat rather than under-treat. As a consequence of this, more patients will receive 5-HT_3 anti-emetics than would otherwise be the case. We believe that this is justified, even though these agents are rather expensive, if it means that more patients will not suffer the distress of uncontrollable nausea and vomiting. Moreover, this extra expenditure will be more than offset if professionals refrain from using these drugs to treat delayed emesis in the days following chemotherapy, when other drugs are generally more effective and much cheaper.

It cannot be emphasised too strongly that prophylaxis of nausea and vomiting is much more likely to succeed than intervention after its onset – any patient receiving anything but the most weakly emetogenic treatment should receive prophylactic anti-emetics. It is important to be familiar with the local policy in this area and apply it.

CYCLE LENGTH

This is the time between giving a dose of chemotherapy and giving the same drug at the start of the next identical cycle (e.g. for a combination of drugs given on 5 consecutive days every 3 weeks, the cycle is 21 days, and cycle 2 starts 21 days after the first day of cycle 1; if a drug is given weekly for 3 weeks in every 5 weeks, the cycle length is 5 weeks, not 7 days).

Don't forget that although many chemotherapy regimens are given every 3 weeks, quite a few are not, so check if you are not sure. Similarly, although most regimens consist of the same group of drugs administered at regular intervals, some involve alternating cycles of different treatments, so do not *assume* that a patient's treatment will be the same as it was the last time they were treated.

NUMBER OF CYCLES

This is a guide to the duration of treatment in patients who are responding to treatment and tolerating it well. Chemotherapy should always be stopped or changed in patients whose tumours continue to grow during treatment.

SIDE-EFFECTS

Lists of side-effects are not exhaustive. In general, those listed are either common or important because they may be mistaken for signs and symptoms of disease and ignored at a point where treatment modification may prevent further morbidity. Rare idiosyncratic reactions are not usually listed. Treatment-related adverse effects should be considered as a possibility in any patient who develops new and otherwise inexplicable symptoms during chemotherapy.

BLOOD NADIR

Measurement of nadir blood counts is of limited value in most circumstances. The main reasons for wanting to know the timing of the nadir blood count are listed below.

- Any patient who develops symptoms of infection near the time of their projected white blood count nadir should be investigated swiftly and thoroughly and, if necessary, treated 'blind' to prevent the development of neutropenic sepsis.
- There can be confidence that any pretreatment blood count has been taken after the nadir resulting from any previous cycle. This ensures that the patient's blood count is stable or rising, but not falling, when further chemotherapy is given.

TTOS ('TO TAKE OUT' MEDICATIONS) REQUIRED

This section lists any items of medication that, as a matter of routine, should be supplied to patients to take home after chemotherapy. The list is restricted to those medications that would usually be considered essential, and does not include those that may be required by specific patients in particular circumstances.

NOTES FOR PRESCRIBERS

Blood counts

It is essential to perform an FBC before administering cytotoxic chemotherapy. A low neutrophil count is often the limiting factor with regard to giving chemotherapy on time, low platelet counts being a less common problem. The absolute levels at which it is acceptable to treat vary depending on the planned regimen (is it going to lower the count a great deal more or is it relatively mild?) and the therapeutic intent (maintaining treatment intensity is important in patients who are being treated with curative intent, whereas the avoidance of excessive toxicity is paramount during palliative chemotherapy). However, it can be stated that cytotoxic treatment is seldom contraindicated if the neutrophil count is $>1.5 \times 10^9$/L and the platelet count is $>100 \times 10^9$/L. In the absence of a local protocol, an experienced prescriber should generally be consulted if pretreatment counts are below these levels.

Where possible we have included details of dose modifications made for haematological toxicity in key clinical trials involving the regimens in question. However, there are several problems in this area.

- Many trials were published a number of years ago when prescribers were often more conservative, modifying doses for blood counts that now appear quite acceptable.
- The aim of the protocol-mandated dose reductions was to try to prevent excessive toxicity, but they did not necessarily achieve this.
- Some trials were conducted in countries, notably the USA, where higher levels of toxicity seem to be acceptable than in the UK.

We have commented on these issues where appropriate, but consider that the information is still worth including. We have also included, where it is available, information from the summaries of product characteristics (SPCs) of agents used within their licensed indications. Some of these appear quite cautious, but for medico-legal reasons it is important to be aware of their content, even if it is not acted upon.

Use of haematopoietic growth factors

Although these agents undoubtedly raise neutrophil counts, direct evidence that they have a positive impact on important clinical outcomes during standard chemotherapy is very limited. They are also very expensive. Therefore they should not be used indiscriminately to manage or prevent low blood counts, although their use may be justified to enable chemotherapy dose intensity to be maintained in curable cancers. In any case, all cancer treatment units should have a growth factor policy, the contents of which should reflect the American Society of Clinical Oncology guidelines in this area,[4] and this policy should be adhered to.

Liver and renal function

Because several cytotoxic drugs are toxic to the liver and kidneys, and most have a narrow therapeutic index and are excreted by one or the other of these organ systems, it is often important to check renal and hepatic function prior to treatment. Guidance on suitable dose adjustments for impaired hepatic and renal function is given in Appendices 1 and 2. These deal with degrees of impairment that are commonly encountered. It should not be assumed that where no dose reductions are suggested, treatment can be given without modification even at extreme levels of dysfunction. If a patient has very severe renal or hepatic impairment, a check should always be made on their suitability for chemotherapy before prescribing takes place.

For most patients, calculation of renal function using the Cockcroft–Gault equation is adequate, with isotopic clearance tests reserved for patients with either borderline renal function or serum creatinine levels that are unlikely to reflect their renal function (e.g. those in catabolic states).

Oral treatments

Quite a few regimens include short courses of oral steroids and cytotoxic drugs. It cannot be overemphasised how dangerous the inadvertent continuation of such short courses can be – it has resulted in fatalities. Take time to explain the treatment to patients, and convey this information clearly on any prescription and in letters to other clinicians, especially the patient's GP. It is vital that patients do not seek and receive further supplies once they have finished the short course of treatment that they are due.

Hair loss

This is a problem that may be of little concern to some patients but very important to others. In most of the monographs we have tried to give some idea of the likely extent of the problem with particular regimens, although of course there can be no guarantees that particular patients will keep or lose their hair. If a patient is anxious about hair loss, and there is a fair chance that it will be severe, consideration should be given to referring the patient to a wig-fitter. As this may take a little time, liaise with whoever organises this (often the nursing staff) at the start of treatment, so that the wig is available when hair loss first occurs.

Liaison with other professionals

Several monographs, such as those for regimens that require ambulatory infusion therapy, call for early liaison with other professional groups. Although it should not be necessary to point this out, it is sometimes forgotten. Good teamwork in this area will result in a safer and more effective service for patients. Remember that it may only take two minutes to write a prescription, but it takes considerably longer to dispense and administer it.

NOTES FOR NURSES

Blood counts

It is essential to perform an FBC before administering cytotoxic chemotherapy. A low neutrophil count is often the limiting factor with regard to giving chemotherapy on time, low platelet counts being a less common problem. The absolute levels at which it is acceptable to treat vary depending on the regimen planned (is the treatment going to lower the count a great deal more or is it relatively mild?) and the therapeutic intent (maintaining treatment intensity is important in patients who are being treated with curative intent, whereas the avoidance of excessive toxicity is paramount during palliative chemotherapy). However, it can be stated that cytotoxic treatment is seldom contraindicated if the neutrophil count is $>1.5 \times 10^9/L$ and the platelet count is $>100 \times 10^9/L$. In the absence of a local protocol, it is generally appropriate to seek confirmation of any prescription for a patient with blood counts below these levels. It is strongly recommended that the pharmacy department does not release chemotherapy for patients until they have evidence of a satisfactory blood count. However, if this is done in your institution, robust procedures need to be in place to prevent administration prior to confirmation of a satisfactory blood count.

Use of haematopoietic growth factors

See Notes for prescribers above for comments on the use of haematopoietic growth factors to maintain neutrophil numbers.

Oral treatments

Quite a few regimens include short courses of oral steroids and cytotoxic drugs. It cannot be overemphasised how dangerous the inadvertent continuation of such short courses can be – it has resulted in fatalities. Take time to explain the treatment to patients – if this prevents them seeking inappropriate continuation supplies via their GP you could save them much discomfort or worse.

Hair loss

This is a problem that may be of little concern to some patients but very important to others. In most of the monographs we have tried to give some idea of the likely extent of the problem with particular regimens, although of course there can be no guarantees that particular patients will keep or lose their hair. If a patient is anxious about hair loss, and there is a fair chance that it will be severe, consideration should be given to referring the patient to a wig-fitter. This should be done at the start of treatment, so that the wig is available when hair loss first occurs.

Hair loss due to some drugs can be minimised by the use of scalp cooling, although this is only appropriate for drugs with a short circulation time, where scalp cooling can be maintained for the time period over which appreciable blood levels of the drug remain. Again we have tried to give some indication of regimens where scalp cooling may be of value.

Extravasation

We have attempted to identify regimens that are associated with a particular extravasation hazard in this section as well as in the Administration section, since most chemotherapy is now administered by nurses and this information is therefore of most use to them. For further information about extravasation, *see* Administration section above.

NOTES FOR PHARMACISTS

Blood counts

It is essential to perform an FBC before administering cytotoxic chemotherapy. A low neutrophil count is often the limiting factor with regard to giving chemotherapy on time, low platelet counts being a less common problem. The absolute levels at which it is acceptable to treat vary depending on the planned regimen (is it going to lower the count a great deal more or is it relatively mild?) and the therapeutic intent (maintaining treatment intensity is important in patients who are being treated with curative intent, whereas the avoidance of excessive toxicity is paramount during palliative chemotherapy). However, it can be stated that cytotoxic treatment is seldom contraindicated if the neutrophil count is $>1.5 \times 10^9$/L and the platelet count is $>100 \times 10^9$/L. In the absence of a local protocol, it is generally appropriate to seek confirmation of any prescription for a patient with blood counts below these levels. It is strongly recommended that the pharmacy department does not release chemotherapy for patients until they have evidence of a satisfactory blood count. However, if this is to be done, robust procedures need to be in place to prevent administration prior to confirmation of a satisfactory blood count.

Where possible we have included in the 'Notes for prescribers' details of dose modifications made for haematological toxicity in key clinical trials involving the regimens in question. However, there are several problems in this area.

- Many trials were published a number of years ago when prescribers were often more conservative, modifying doses for blood counts that now appear quite acceptable.
- The aim of the protocol-mandated dose reductions was to try to prevent excessive toxicity, but they did not necessarily achieve this.
- Some trials were conducted in countries, notably the USA, where higher levels of toxicity seem to be acceptable than in the UK.

We have commented on these issues where appropriate, but consider that the information is still worth including. We have also included, where it is available, information from the summaries of product characteristics (SPCs) of agents used within their licensed indications. Some of these appear quite cautious, but for medico-legal reasons it is important to be aware of their content, even if it is not acted upon.

Liver and renal function

Because several cytotoxic drugs are toxic to the liver and kidneys, and most have a narrow therapeutic index and are excreted by one or the other of these organ systems, it is often important to check renal and hepatic function prior to treatment. Guidance on suitable dose adjustments for impaired hepatic and renal function is given in Appendices 1 and 2. These deal with levels of impairment that are commonly encountered. It should not be assumed that where no dose reductions are suggested, treatment can be given without modification even at extreme levels of dysfunction. If a patient has very severe renal or hepatic impairment, a check should always be made on their suitability for chemotherapy at the time of dispensing.

For most patients, calculation of renal function using the Cockcroft–Gault equation is adequate, with isotopic clearance tests reserved for patients with either borderline renal function or serum creatinine levels that are unlikely to reflect their renal function (e.g. those in catabolic states). The Cockcroft–Gault equation is reproduced in each relevant monograph, in the 'Notes for prescribers' section. It is our experience that most pharmacists, but not many doctors, know this formula by heart. However, if you don't, you now know where to look for it.

Oral treatments

Quite a few regimens include short courses of oral steroids and cytotoxic drugs. It cannot be overemphasised how dangerous the inadvertent continuation of these short courses can be – it has resulted in fatalities. If you are counselling patients, make sure that they understand which tablets they should be taking long term and which are for short courses only. If you are checking a prescription to be dispensed by others, make sure that there is no ambiguity with regard to the way in which it is written (just because you understand the treatment, don't assume that everyone else does), and make sure that packs of tablets or capsules are clearly labelled with start and stop dates or the duration of treatment.

Pharmacy record keeping

In many monographs we make reference to pharmacy patient records, an example of which can be found in Appendix 3. We believe that it is vital for pharmacists to keep good records of chemotherapy treatments prepared and dispensed, checks that were made at the time of dispensing, reasons for dose reduction or treatment change, etc. As well as reminding future users of patient characteristics that may have an important bearing on clinical decisions with regard to dosing, etc., these records are also a professional safeguard for the pharmacist who can demonstrate that they took proper steps to ensure patient safety, should they ever be called upon to do so.

CITED REFERENCES AND SOURCE MATERIAL

This apparently straightforward section probably caused us more problems than any other. We did not wish to include more than one or two references per regimen, and we wanted those that were included to:

- give credit to the originators of the regimen
- provide a basis for the doses currently in use
- give some useful information about the regimen's clinical efficacy.

The problem is that, particularly for older regimens, the first reports of their use were often uninformative abstracts in the proceedings of obscure meetings. In addition, early studies frequently used doses that differed somewhat from those routinely employed today. This is especially true of some very widely used regimens which appear to have evolved along several parallel paths with no obvious common starting point.

Ultimately we have had to compromise, and we have generally used the first report that gives useful clinical information with a dosage regimen close or identical to that in clinical use today. We have also, where possible, selected references that give some credit to the originators of the regimen, and we would like to apologise for those cases where we have not achieved this.

REFERENCES

1 Allwood M, Stanley A and Wright P (eds) (2002) *The Cytotoxics Handbook* (4e). Radcliffe Medical Press, Oxford.
2 Department of Health (2001) *HSC 2001/02 National Guidance on the Safe Administration of Intrathecal Chemotherapy*. Department of Health, London (also available at http://www. doh.gov.uk/publications/coinh.html)
3 Gralla RJ, Osoba D, Kris MG *et al.* (1999) Recommendations for the use of antiemetics: evidence-based clinical practice guidelines. *J Clin Oncol.* **17**: 2971–94 (also available at http://www.asco.org/prof/pp/html/guidelines/antiemetics.htm)
4. Ozer H, Armitage JO, Bennett CL *et al.* (2000) Update of recommendations for the use of hematopoietic colony-stimulating factors: evidence-based, clinical practice guidelines; http://www.asco.org/prof/pp/html/guide/color/m_colorintro.htm.

5-Fluorouracil (5FU) continuous infusion (single-agent)

USUAL INDICATION

Adjuvant and palliative treatment of cholangiocarcinoma and colorectal cancer.

DOSES

200–300 mg/m^2/day. Most patients will tolerate 200 mg/m^2/day, but many will experience toxicity problems at 300 mg/m^2/day. Even if one is aiming for the higher dose, it may be prudent to start at the lower dose and increase in increments of 50, then 25 and then 25 mg/m^2/day, over a period of several weeks, until the target dose or the maximum tolerated dose is reached.

Note: Some patients are deficient in the 5-FU-catabolising enzyme dihydropyrimidine dehydrogenase (DPD) and will only tolerate much smaller doses of 5-FU.

ADMINISTRATION

By continuous IV infusion via a permanently implanted IV access (e.g Hickman or Groschong line) or a peripherally inserted central catheter (PICC line).

ANTI-EMETICS

Not necessary, as nausea and vomiting are almost unheard of with this regimen.

CYCLE LENGTH

Continuous, but logistically patients need to return to the treatment centre regularly both for assessment and for resupply and pump maintenance, unless a home-care service is in place. Liaison between nursing, medical and pharmacy staff is important to ensure continuity of care and drug supplies.

NUMBER OF CYCLES

Usually 6 months (adjuvant) or for as long as the regimen is still benefiting the patient (palliative).

SIDE-EFFECTS

This treatment is minimally emetogenic, and causes minimal hair loss and little bone-marrow suppression. The main problems are mucositis, diarrhoea and palmar-plantar erythrodysasthesia ('hand-and-foot' syndrome).

BLOOD NADIR

Not relevant.

TTOS REQUIRED

- Anti-emetics are *not* required.
- Unless it is contraindicated, low-dose warfarin therapy (1 mg/day) should be considered once a central venous line (but not a PICC line) is *in situ*, in order to prevent line thrombosis.

NOTES FOR PRESCRIBERS

When considering treatment options

- Ask yourself *'Will this patient really be able to cope with the demands of looking after an infusion pump?'*. This is important. Home infusion therapy, particularly where an electromechanical infusion pump is used, requires patients or their immediate carers to take an active role in their treatment. If they are unwilling or unable to do so, other treatment options should be explored. Normally they should also have access to a telephone in case problems arise out of hours.

Note: Not all community nursing and medical staff are familiar with home chemotherapy. It cannot be assumed that they will take on responsibility for looking after the patient's pump at home. If this is intended, contact must be made and consent obtained for such an approach at an early stage.

- If your department has a finite number of infusion pumps available, liaise with whoever looks after them to ascertain whether there is a free infusion pump *before* you promise the patient treatment.
- Liaise in advance with those responsible for setting up the pumps and educating the patient about his or her treatment. Both processes can be time consuming, and in a busy department they need to be scheduled in advance.

At the time of first prescription

- Prescribe supplies for a suitable period depending on local arrangements. However long this is, it is recommended that patients are seen 10–14 days after starting treatment to check whether there are any problems. Subsequently, they should be seen by an oncologist at least every 3–4 weeks to check on progress and toxicity (*see also* note in Cycle length section above about resupply arrangements).

- If the patient is prescribed low-dose warfarin (*see* TTO section above), ensure that arrangements are made for either the GP or the hospital to check the INR about 1 week after starting, and to stop treatment if the patient is hypersensitive (i.e. if the INR is significantly elevated). Communicate to the GP that this dose of warfarin is not intended to alter the INR significantly and should not be increased.
- Check LFTs and renal function. Consideration should be given to dose adjustment in patients with severe renal or hepatic impairment (*see* Appendices 1 and 2).

Subsequently

- This treatment should be low in toxicity. Toxicity that is causing more than mild discomfort is an indication for a dose reduction. Grade III/IV toxicities are an indication for a treatment break. 'Hand-and-foot' syndrome, mucositis and diarrhoea all resolve very rapidly (5–7 days) after stopping treatment. Empirical dose reductions should be of the order of 25–30% to be worthwhile.
- Pyridoxine, 50 mg three times a day, is sometimes used to treat 'hand-and-foot' syndrome and mucositis, but its value is dubious and it should not be relied upon as the sole measure.

NOTES FOR NURSES

- Patients with home infusion pumps will need support at home, including advice on problems with their treatment, their pump and venous access. They are also likely to need practical help with the dressing of venous line insertion sites, changing of infusion reservoirs and flushing of unused lumens on the venous line in accordance with local policies.

  Local arrangements for this support must be formalised and robust. District and practice nurses may be unfamiliar with this type of treatment, and it should not be assumed that they will be willing to support patients. Liaise with them first.
- Detailed descriptions of setting up pumps, etc., are beyond the scope of this book. If this activity is being undertaken by nursing staff, it should be the subject of robust and formal local procedures.
- If the patient's dose has been adjusted, ensure as far as is possible that the infusion rate on any variable-rate infusion pump (if the dose is governed by the infusion rate) is reset to deliver the correct dose.

NOTES FOR PHARMACISTS

- Detailed descriptions of setting up pumps, etc., are beyond the scope of this book. If this activity is being undertaken by pharmacy staff, it should be the subject of robust and formal local procedures.
- If the patient is not prescribed low-dose warfarin at the start of treatment, check whether this is needed (*see* TTO section above). If it is contraindicated, make sure this is marked clearly on any pharmacy notes system (*see* Appendix 3 for an example) to prevent future prescribing.

- If pharmacy staff set up infusion pumps and if the patient's dose has been adjusted, ensure as far as is possible that the infusion rate on any variable-rate infusion pump (if the dose is governed by the infusion rate) is reset to deliver the correct dose.
- Remember, if calculating 5-FU requirements for a given period of time, to allow enough overage to ensure that the patient will not run out before their next supply is due. The overage necessary will depend on the type of pump that is used.
- Check the LFTs and renal function. Consideration should be given to dose adjustment in patients with severe renal or hepatic impairment (*see* Appendices 1 and 2).

SOURCE MATERIAL

- Lokich JJ, Ahlgren JD, Gullo JJ *et al.* (1989) A prospective randomized comparison of continuous-infusion fluorouracil with a conventional bolus schedule in metastatic colorectal carcinoma: a Mid-Atlantic Oncology Program study. *J Clin Oncol.* **7**: 1419–26.

ABVD (doxorubicin ['Adriamycin'], bleomycin, vinblastine, dacarbazine)

Hodgkin's disease.

DOSES

Doxorubicin ('Adriamycin') 25 mg/m^2 IV on days 1 and 15
Bleomycin 10 000 units/m^2 (equivalent to 10 old units or 10 mg/m^2) IV
    on days 1 and 15
Vinblastine 6 mg/m^2 IV on days 1 and 15
Dacarbazine 375 mg/m^2 IV on days 1 and 15

The cumulative dose of doxorubicin should not exceed 450 mg/m^2 without further consultation, because the risk of anthracycline-induced cardiomyopathy increases rapidly beyond this point.

ADMINISTRATION

Doxorubicin and vinblastine

By slow IV injection into the side-arm of a free-running saline drip.

Doxorubicin and vinblastine are powerful vesicants and should be administered with appropriate precautions to prevent extravasation. If there is any possibility that extravasation has occurred, contact a senior member of the medical team immediately and follow local guidance on dealing with cytotoxic extravasation.

Bleomycin

By slow IV bolus injection or short infusion in 100 mL of 0.9% sodium chloride.

Dacarbazine

Dacarbazine is administered by IV infusion, normally in 500 mL of 0.9% sodium chloride over 30 min. However, it can cause venous pain during infusion, which can sometimes be reduced by administering in a larger volume of saline. It is reasonable to administer in 1 L of 0.9% sodium chloride and/or to increase the infusion time to 60–120 min.

ANTI-EMETICS

High emetogenic potential (apply local policy).

CYCLE LENGTH

28 days.

NUMBER OF CYCLES

Usually 6 courses (i.e. 12 treatments).

SIDE-EFFECTS

Bone-marrow suppression, alopecia, nausea and vomiting, mucositis, cardiac arrhythmias, dilated cardiomyopathy (especially at cumulative doxorubicin doses in excess of $450\,mg/m^2$), peripheral neuropathy (from vinblastine), lung fibrosis (from bleomycin), rigors (from bleomycin).

BLOOD NADIR

10 days.

TTOs REQUIRED

- Anti-emetics appropriate to highly emetogenic chemotherapy (see local protocol).
- Allopurinol 300 mg each morning to prevent tumour lysis syndrome, especially early in treatment when there is a large tumour bulk.

NOTES FOR PRESCRIBERS

- Patients over 60 years of age or with a history of heart disease must have an echocardiogram or MUGA scan prior to initial treatment to ensure that there is adequate left ventricular function.
- Check full blood count prior to giving the go-ahead for chemotherapy, and seek advice if the neutrophil count is $<1.5 \times 10^9/L$ or the platelet count is $<100 \times 10^9/L$. Note that because treatment is being given with curative intent, it may proceed with a count lower than would be acceptable for palliative regimens. In the original description of this regimen,[1] the following somewhat complex

[1] Bonadonna G, Zucali R, Monfardini S *et al.* (1975) Combination chemotherapy of Hodgkin's disease with Adriamycin, bleomycin, vinblastine and imidazole carboxamide (ABVD) vs. MOPP. *Cancer.* **36**: 252–9.

scheme was used to modify doses according to blood count at the start of each cycle. However, the suggested dose modifications appear somewhat conservative by today's standards.

WBC count ($\times 10^9/L$)	Platelet count ($\times 10^9/L$)	Dose adjustments
>4.0	>130	None required
3.00–3.99	100–129	50% reduction in doxorubicin and vinblastine
2.00–2.99	80–99	50% reduction in dacarbazine, 75% reduction in doxorubicin and vinblastine
1.5–1.99	50–79	75% reduction in dacarbazine; withhold other drugs
<1.5	<50	Withhold all treatment

- Check liver function tests. If these show serious impairment, then a reduction in doxorubicin and possibly also vinblastine and dacarbazine doses may be required. Further advice is given in Appendix 1.
- Renal function should be formally assessed at the start of treatment. Estimation from the serum creatinine concentration using the Cockcroft–Gault equation is acceptable if the patient has stable creatinine levels and no confounding factors (e.g. catabolic states):

CrCl (mL/min)

$$= \frac{1.04 \text{ (females) or } 1.23 \text{ (males)} \times (140 - \text{age in years}) \times \text{weight in kg}}{\text{serum creatinine concentration } (\mu\text{mol/L})}.$$

Consideration should be given to reducing dacarbazine doses in patients with a CrCl of <60 mL/min and bleomycin doses in patients with a CrCl of <50 mL/min (see Appendix 2).

- This is a potentially curative treatment, and it is important to maintain dose intensity. Dose delays should be avoided if at all possible. Therefore this is one regimen where the use of haematopoietic growth factors (G-CSF or GM-CSF) can be justified to support neutrophil numbers. The dosage should be in accordance with local guidelines.
- Vinblastine can cause peripheral neuropathy. Patients should be questioned about abnormal sensations, jaw pain or constipation, any of which may be indicative of neuropathy. Discuss such symptoms with an experienced member of the medical team with a view to dose modification.
- Enquire about symptoms of breathlessness when prescribing repeat courses, as such symptoms may indicate bleomycin-induced lung damage. Discuss the symptoms with a senior member of the medical team, as they may be an indication for formal testing of respiratory function (transfer factor).
- Prior to treatment, hair loss should be discussed with the patient. Scalp cooling is of limited benefit in preventing hair loss with ABVD, because of the prolonged half-life of some of the drugs that are included in this regimen. Liaise with nurses with regard to referral to a wig-fitter at the start of treatment and before alopecia is evident if this is appropriate.

- If administering treatment, *see* Administration section above for notes on the vesicant nature of doxorubicin and vinblastine.
- If venous pain is a problem during dacarbazine administration, try slowing down the infusion (give the drug over a period of 60–120 min) and request preparation in a larger volume of saline for the next course. If these measures fail, it is worth trying a GTN patch downstream of the infusion site to counteract any vasospastic component of the pain.
- Lymphomas are very sensitive to chemotherapy, and massive tumour lysis is likely to occur at the start of chemotherapy. This can result in the generation of large amounts of insoluble uric acid which is capable of precipitating in the kidneys, causing renal damage. To prevent this, allopurinol 300 mg once daily should be commenced the day before starting cytotoxic therapy and continued for as long as there is a significant tumour burden.

NOTES FOR NURSES

- Prior to treatment, hair loss should be discussed with the patient. Scalp cooling is unlikely to be of much benefit because of the prolonged circulation of some of the drugs involved. If appropriate, referral to a wig-fitter should be made at the start of treatment and before alopecia is evident.
- If administering treatment, *see* Administration section above for notes on the vesicant nature of doxorubicin and vinblastine.
- The administration time and volume for dacarbazine are not critical. Therefore if venous pain during infusion is a problem, slowing down the infusion (to 60–90 min) may help, as may diluting the drug in a larger volume of saline (request the pharmacy to prepare the next dose in 1 L of saline).

NOTES FOR PHARMACISTS

- Check that a full blood count has been determined and is within acceptable limits before making up the chemotherapy. Because this is a potentially curative treatment, it is reasonable to treat on a somewhat lower neutrophil/platelet count than would be considered acceptable for a palliative regimen.
- This is a potentially curative treatment, and it is important to maintain dose intensity. Dose delays should be avoided if at all possible. Therefore this is one regimen where the use of haematopoietic growth factors (G-CSF or GM-CSF) to support neutrophil numbers can be justified. These should be used in accordance with the local policy.
- Check that renal function has been measured/calculated at the start of treatment. Record the CrCl and the corresponding creatinine concentration on any pharmacy patient record (*see* Appendix 3 for an example). Recalculate the CrCl if the creatinine concentration changes. A dacarbazine dose reduction is needed if the CrCl drops below 60 mL/min, and a bleomycin dose reduction should also be considered if the CrCl is below 50 mL/min (*see* Appendix 2 for further guidance).
- Check liver function tests. If these show serious impairment, then a reduction in doxorubicin, vinblastine and possibly dacarbazine may be required. Further advice is given in Appendix 1.

- Check that anti-emetics appropriate to highly emetogenic chemotherapy have been prescribed according to protocol.
- Keep a close eye on the cumulative dose of doxorubicin, and alert the prescriber if it exceeds 450 mg/m^2. It is especially important when a patient starts a course of treatment to check your records and their notes to see whether they have received prior anthracycline therapy in your hospital or elsewhere. If so, calculate the previous cumulative doxorubicin dose and add this information to any pharmacy patient record (*see* Appendix 3 for an example). Take into consideration the cumulative doses of other anthracyclines (e.g. epirubicin, daunorubicin, idarubicin) that have been received by the patient.
- The administration time and volume for dacarbazine are not critical. Therefore if venous pain is a problem during infusion, slowing down the infusion to run over a period of 60–90 min may help, as may diluting the drug in a larger volume of saline (i.e. 1 L). If this fails to solve the problem, a GTN patch downstream of the infusion site is worth trying, as this will counteract any vasospastic component of the pain.
- Lymphomas are very sensitive to chemotherapy, and massive tumour lysis is likely to occur at the start of chemotherapy. This can result in the generation of large amounts of insoluble uric acid, which is capable of precipitating in the kidneys, causing renal damage. To prevent this, allopurinol 300 mg once daily should be commenced the day before starting cytotoxic therapy and continued for as long as there is a significant tumour burden.

SOURCE MATERIAL

- Bonadonna G, Zucali R, Monfardini S *et al.* (1975) Combination chemotherapy of Hodgkin's disease with Adriamycin, bleomycin, vinblastine and imidazole carboxamide (ABVD) vs. MOPP. *Cancer.* **36**: 252–9.

BCD (carmustine [BCNU], cisplatin, dacarbazine; the 'Dartmouth' regimen)

USUAL INDICATION

Metastatic malignant melanoma.

DOSES

Dacarbazine 220 mg/m^2 IV on days 1-3
Cisplatin 25 mg/m^2 IV on days 1-3
Carmustine 150 mg/m^2 IV on day 2 on *alternate courses only*
Tamoxifen 20 mg PO daily continuously

ADMINISTRATION

Cisplatin

All three drugs are given as IV infusions in saline. Relatively large volumes of fluid are included in this regimen. This is necessary because cisplatin is nephrotoxic, and hydration is mandatory to dilute the drug as it is excreted via the kidneys, thus minimising renal toxicity. The aim of hydration is to maintain a urine output of 100 mL/h during and for 6-8 h after cisplatin administration. Typically 1 L of saline is given over 2 h as pre-hydration (the dacarbazine infusion can be used as part of the pre-hydration), followed by 1 L of saline containing cisplatin and a further 2 L of saline as post-hydration. Mannitol is also often given to ensure that fluid output is brisk. Electrolytes are added to compensate for cisplatin-induced electrolyte loss. To facilitate outpatient treatment, post-hydration can be reduced to 1 L, in which case the patient should be advised to drink 3 L of fluid in the 24 h following the completion of IV hydration.

Dacarbazine

Dacarbazine may cause venous pain during infusion, which can sometimes be reduced by administering the drug in a larger volume of saline. It is reasonable to administer it in volumes of up to 1 L.

Carmustine

Carmustine can also cause venous pain. Unfortunately, slowing down the infusion is not an option in this case. Carmustine has very limited stability after preparation, so it must be administered as scheduled and immediately after preparation. This will require liaison between pharmacy staff and those administering the drug.

ANTI-EMETICS

High emetogenic potential (see standard policy).

CYCLE LENGTH

21 days, but note that carmustine is only administered every 42 days.

NUMBER OF CYCLES

Usually 6.

SIDE-EFFECTS

Nephrotoxicity (dose limiting, due to cisplatin), bone-marrow suppression (all blood components affected), alopecia (often total), nausea and vomiting (may be severe), sensory and motor neuropathy (sometimes irreversible, due to cisplatin) including significant potential for ototoxicity, mucositis (not usually serious), lung fibrosis and/or infiltrates (carmustine induced).

TTOS REQUIRED

- Anti-emetics appropriate to highly emetogenic chemotherapy (apply local policy), plus tamoxifen 20 mg once daily continuously.

NOTES FOR PRESCRIBERS

Before each course

- Check FBC before giving the go-ahead for chemotherapy. Seek advice if the neutrophil count is $<1.5 \times 10^9$/L or the platelet count is $<100 \times 10^9$/L at the time of treatment. Both dacarbazine and carmustine are highly myelosuppressive and produce a prolonged decrease in cellular blood components.
- Renal function should be formally assessed at the start of treatment. Ideally this should be done by measurement of EDTA clearance, but estimation of CrCl using the Cockcroft–Gault equation is acceptable if the patient has a stable creatinine concentration and no confounding factors (e.g. catabolic states):

CrCl (mL/min)

$$= \frac{1.04 \text{ (females) or } 1.23 \text{ (males)} \times (140 - \text{age in years}) \times \text{weight in kg}}{\text{serum creatinine concentration } (\mu\text{mol/L})}.$$

On subsequent cycles renal function should be reassessed. Cisplatin doses *must be reduced* if creatinine clearance drops below 60 mL/min, and consideration should be given to reducing carmustine doses (*see* Appendix 2 for further guidance).

- Check blood biochemistry for cisplatin-induced renal electrolyte wasting, especially of magnesium, calcium and potassium. Additional supplementation may be required.
- Seek further advice if the patient reports symptoms indicative of neurotoxicity (parasthesias, difficulty with motor control) or ototoxicity (tinnitus, deafness).
- Do not forget that carmustine should only be prescribed on each *alternate* course.
- Do not forget to add tamoxifen to TTOs.
- If venous pain is a problem during carmustine or dacarbazine infusion, try increasing the fluid volume for dacarbazine and/or using a GTN patch downstream of the infusion site for either drug. Further dilution of carmustine is difficult, since it still has to be infused within 2 h of preparation (the limit of its stability).
- Carmustine is very unstable and has to be administered as soon as it has been prepared by pharmacy. Therefore do not chart it to be given outside normal pharmacy working hours. There is no reason to believe that scheduling is particularly critical in this regimen, so carmustine can be moved around within days and on to day 1 or 3 if this facilitates treatment.
- Dacarbazine is also of limited stability. Do not schedule its administration over weekends without prior discussion with pharmacy.

On the day after each cisplatin dose

- Check the fluid balance/body weight (if the patient is in hospital or visiting the day-case unit). In general, if the patient gains 1.5 L/kg or more during chemotherapy, extra diuresis will be required.

NOTES FOR NURSES

- The aim of hydration is to ensure an average urine output of 100 mL/h or more during and for 6–8 h post cisplatin. Any patient who is being treated as an inpatient should be on a fluid-balance chart and daily weights should be recorded. Contact the prescriber if the patient's urine output is inadequate or their body weight increases by 1.5 kg from baseline.

  For outpatients, efforts should be made to ensure that urine output is adequate (e.g. by ensuring that the patient has passed 500 mL of urine between the start of IV hydration and the commencement of cisplatin infusion).

  Outpatients should also be encouraged to drink 3 L of fluid in the 24 h following each period of IV hydration, and to contact the hospital if this is impossible because of nausea/vomiting or other problems.
- Liaise with pharmacy staff about the timing of carmustine administration. This drug is very unstable and needs to be given immediately after preparation. Therefore you need to be sure that you will be in a position to administer the drug immediately after it has been prepared.
- Patients on this regimen start long-term tamoxifen therapy. When giving patients their TTOs, explain to them that they may need to obtain more

tamoxifen from their GP in order to continue therapy, but that oral anti-emetics are short-term treatments which should not be routinely continued.

NOTES FOR PHARMACISTS

Day of prescribing

- Check that an FBC has been determined and is within acceptable limits before issuing chemotherapy.
- Check that renal function has been measured/calculated at the start of treatment. Record CrCl and the corresponding creatinine concentration on any patient pharmacy record. Recalculate CrCl if the creatinine concentration changes. Cisplatin dose reduction is *essential* if CrCl drops below 60 mL/min, and consideration should be given to reducing the carmustine dose. Further advice can be found in Appendix 2.
- On the first course, block out the carmustine column of any pharmacy record sheet (*see* Appendix 3 for an example) for each alternate course in order to prevent accidental administration on two consecutive courses.
- Liaise with the nurse who is administering chemotherapy before preparing carmustine. It is very unstable and needs to be given immediately after preparation, so you need to be sure that the nurse will be in a position to administer the drug once it is prepared.
- Check that anti-emetics appropriate to highly emetogenic chemotherapy have been prescribed according to local policy.
- Check that oral tamoxifen has been prescribed on TTOs on the first course, and on subsequent courses if the patient does not have his or her own supply. If the opportunity arises, counsel the patient about the need to continue tamoxifen once the supply issued by the hospital has been used up.

Subsequent days

- When visiting the treatment area, check that the patient has not gained more than 1.5 L/kg since the start of treatment. If they have, discuss additional diuresis with the prescriber (if such a measure has not already been instituted).

SOURCE MATERIAL

- DelPrete SA, Maurer LH, O'Donnell J *et al.* (1984) Combination chemotherapy with cisplatin, carmustine, dacarbazine and tamoxifen in metastatic melanoma. *Cancer Treat Rep.* **68**: 1403–5.

BEP (3 day) and BEP (5 day)
(bleomycin, etoposide, cisplatin)

Note: There are several variants on these regimens that use slightly different doses, especially of etoposide. BEP may also be combined with another regimen, such as EP (etoposide plus cisplatin), to make a hybrid regimen. Make sure that you know which BEP regimen is required and the number of cycles intended.

USUAL INDICATION

Germ-cell tumours.

DOSES

There are many variations on this protocol, but the most commonly used ones are listed below.

3-day BEP

Etoposide 165 mg/m^2 IV on days 1, 2 and 3
Cisplatin 50 mg/m^2 IV on days 1 and 2
Bleomycin 30 000 IU (equivalent to 30 old units or 30 mg) IV on days 2,
    8 and 15

5-day BEP

Etoposide 100 mg/m^2 IV on days 1, 2, 3, 4 and 5
Cisplatin 20 mg/m^2 IV on days 1, 2, 3, 4 and 5
Bleomycin 30 000 IU (equivalent to 30 old units or 30 mg) IV on days 2,
    8 and 15

ADMINISTRATION

Bleomycin

Can be given as an IV bolus or short IV infusion.

Etoposide

Must be infused in saline over a period of at least 1 h. More rapid infusion can result in hypotensive reactions. Usually it is administered as part of the pre-hydration that is required before cisplatin treatment.

Cisplatin

Cisplatin is nephrotoxic, and hydration is mandatory to dilute the drug as it is excreted via the kidneys in order to minimise toxicity. The aim of hydration is to maintain a urine output of 100 mL/h during and for 6–8 h after cisplatin administration. Mannitol is also given to ensure that urine output is brisk. Electrolytes are added to compensate for cisplatin-induced renal electrolyte wasting. Typically, hydration will consist of 1 L of saline over 2 h prior to cisplatin, 1 L of saline with cisplatin over 2–4 h followed by a further 2 L over 8–12 h. However, post-hydration is sometimes reduced to 1 L to facilitate outpatient treatment. In this case, patients should be instructed to drink a further 3 L of fluid in the 24 h following completion of each day's IV hydration.

ANTI-EMETICS

- High emetogenic potential (apply local policy).

CYCLE LENGTH

21 days.

NUMBER OF CYCLES

Variable, depending on the diagnosis and disease stage and, in some cases, the trial protocol. Sometimes treatment is started with BEP and ended with EP (i.e. bleomycin is omitted from later cycle(s) to reduce lung toxicity). If you are in any doubt, check with the appropriate trial protocol or consultant.

SIDE-EFFECTS

Nephrotoxicity (dose limiting, cisplatin induced), bone-marrow suppression (all blood components affected), alopecia (often total), nausea and vomiting (may be severe), sensory, motor and occasionally autonomic neuropathy (sometimes irreversible, caused by cisplatin) including significant potential for ototoxicity, mucositis (not usually serious), lung fibrosis (bleomycin induced), rigors (bleomycin induced).

TTOS REQUIRED

- Anti-emetics appropriate to highly emetogenic chemotherapy (see local protocol).
- Germ-cell tumours can be very sensitive to cytotoxic chemotherapy, resulting in massive tumour lysis at the start of treatment. This may give rise to the release of large quantities of poorly soluble uric acid, which can precipitate in the renal tubules, causing renal failure. Consideration should be given to prescribing allopurinol (300 mg PO once daily, reduced in renal impairment) in order to prevent this. Allopurinol should be started the day before chemotherapy and continued for as long as a significant bulk of chemotherapy-sensitive tumour tissue remains.

NOTES FOR PRESCRIBERS

Before each course

- Check FBC prior to giving the go-ahead for chemotherapy. Seek advice if the neutrophil count is $<1.5 \times 10^9$/L or the platelet count is $<100 \times 10^9$/L at the time of treatment. In a recent European study[1] of 5-day BEP, full-dose treatment was given if the total WBC was $>3.0 \times 10^9$/L and the platelet count was $>100 \times 10^9$/L on day 1 of the treatment cycle. It was withheld if the WBC was $<1.5 \times 10^9$/L or the platelet count was $<50 \times 10^9$/L. For WBCs in the range $1.5–3.0 \times 10^9$/L, treatment was given with the etoposide dose reduced by 25% or 50% if the platelet count was also low (in the range $50–100 \times 10^9$/L).
  Note: This treatment is usually given with curative intent, and dose delays should therefore be avoided if at all possible. In this situation, support with haematopoietic growth factors (G-CSF and GM-CSF) may be appropriate if neutropenia is causing delays in treatment delivery, although this was not found to alter outcome significantly in a recent European study[1] where G-CSF was given on days 6–19 of each cycle. Growth factors should be given according to local policy. Note that although growth factors are normally contraindicated on the days when cytotoxic chemotherapy is given, it is reasonable to administer them on days when bleomycin only is being given. Bleomycin is minimally myelosuppressive, so the risk of exacerbating myelotoxicity by administering a growth factor is very low.
- Renal function should be formally assessed at the start of treatment. Ideally this should be done by EDTA clearance, but estimation using the Cockcroft–Gault equation is acceptable as an interim measure if the patient has stable creatinine levels and no confounding factors (e.g. catabolic states):

CrCl (mL/min)

$$= \frac{1.04 \text{ (females) or } 1.23 \text{ (males)} \times (140 - \text{age in years}) \times \text{weight in kg}}{\text{serum creatinine concentration } (\mu mol/L)}.$$

On subsequent cycles renal function should be reassessed.

[1] Fossa SD, Kaye SB, Mead GM *et al.* (1998) Filgrastim during combination chemotherapy of patients with poor-prognosis metastatic germ-cell malignancy. *J Clin Oncol.* **16**: 716–24.

Doses *must be reduced* if creatinine clearance drops below 60 mL/min. Consideration should be given to reducing bleomycin and etoposide doses in cases of significant renal impairment and etoposide doses in cases of significant hepatic impairment (*see* Appendices 1 and 2).

- Check electrolytes for cisplatin-induced wasting, especially of magnesium, calcium and potassium. Additional supplementation may be required.
- Hydrocortisone 100 mg IV and chlorpheniramine 10–20 mg IV should be prescribed on an 'as-needed' basis to allow bleomycin-induced rigors to be treated promptly, should they occur.
- Ask the patient about symptoms indicative of neurotoxicity (parasthesias, difficulty with motor control) or ototoxicity (tinnitus, deafness), and seek further advice if they report such symptoms.
- Unexplained breathlessness may be indicative of bleomycin-induced lung fibrosis, and should be investigated.

On the day after each cisplatin dose

- Check the fluid balance/body weight. If the patient has gained more than 1.5 L/kg during chemotherapy, extra diuresis should be prescribed.

At each inpatient treatment

- Do not forget to make appropriate arrangements with the patient to ensure that they receive day 8 and 15 bleomycin doses.

NOTES FOR NURSES

- Any patient who is being treated as an inpatient should be on a fluid-balance chart, and daily weights should be recorded. Hydration is intended to produce an average urine output of 100 mL/h or more during and for 6–8 h after cisplatin treatment. Contact the prescriber if the urine output is inadequate or the patient's body weight increases by 1.5 kg from baseline during chemotherapy. For outpatients, efforts should be made to ensure that urine output is adequate (e.g. by ensuring that the patient has passed 500 mL of urine between the start of IV hydration and the commencement of cisplatin infusion).
- Patients who are being treated on an outpatient basis should have daily weights recorded and should be encouraged to drink 3 L of fluid in the 24 h following each day's IV hydration, and to contact the hospital if this is proving impossible (e.g. because of nausea and vomiting).

NOTES FOR PHARMACISTS

Day of prescribing

- Make sure that you know which BEP regimen is being followed (i.e. 3 day/5 day) and at what dose levels. Also ascertain the number of cycles and whether they are all BEP or whether a BEP/EP hybrid is being given.

Endorse any pharmacy records (*see* Appendix 3 for an example) with these details, and include a copy of any trial flowchart to ensure that the patient follows the intended treatment course.

- Check that the FBC has been determined and is acceptable before issuing chemotherapy. As this regimen is usually being given with curative intent, treatment may proceed with a lower blood count than would be acceptable for palliative chemotherapy (especially day 8 and 15 bleomycin doses, which are minimally myelosuppressive). If clinically significant myelotoxicity (defined as symptomatic neutropenia or a neutrophil count that is too low to treat at the start of the next cycle, but not asymptomatic low nadir counts) is preventing treatment being given, haematopoietic growth factor (G-CSF or GM-CSF) support may be justified. See your local policy on growth factors for further details. Note that although growth factors are normally contraindicated on the days when cytotoxic chemotherapy is given, it is reasonable to administer them on days when bleomycin only is being given. Bleomycin is minimally myelosuppressive, so the risk of exacerbating myelotoxicity by administering with a growth factor is very low
- Check that creatinine clearance has been measured/calculated at the start of treatment. Record CrCl and the corresponding creatinine concentration on any pharmacy record sheet (*see* Appendix 3 for an example). Recalculate CrCl if the creatinine concentration changes. Dose reduction of cisplatin is required if CrCl drops below 60 mL/min. Consideration should also be given to reducing the bleomycin dose and etoposide dose in renal impairment and the etoposide dose in hepatic impairment (*see* Appendices 1 and 2 for further guidance).
- Check that anti-emetics appropriate to highly emetogenic chemotherapy have been prescribed according to local policy.

Day after each cisplatin dose

- When visiting the treatment area, check that the patient has not gained more than 1.5 L/kg since the start of IV hydration. If they have, discuss the need for additional diuresis with the prescriber (if this measure has not already been instituted).

SOURCE MATERIAL

5-day regimen

- Fossa SD, Kaye SB, Mead GM *et al.* (1998) Filgrastim during combination chemotherapy of patients with poor-prognosis metastatic germ-cell malignancy. *J Clin Oncol.* **16**: 716–24.
- Williams SD, Birch R, Einhorn LH *et al.* (1987) Treatment of disseminated germ-cell tumors with cisplatin, bleomycin, and either vinblastine or etoposide. *NEJM.* **316**: 1435–40.

3-day regimen

- De Wit R, Roberts JT, Wilkinson PM *et al.* (2001) Equivalence of 3BEP versus 4 cycles and of the 5-day schedule versus 3 days per cycle in good-prognosis germ-cell cancer: a randomised study of the European Organisation for Research and Treatment of Cancer Genitourinary Tract Cancer Cooperative Group and the Medical Research Council. *J Clin Oncol.* **19**: 1629–40.

BIP (bleomycin, ifosfamide, cisplatin)

USUAL INDICATION

Cervical cancer.

DOSES

>   Bleomycin 30 000 units (equivalent to 30 old units or 30 mg) IV on day 1
>   Ifosfamide 5000 mg/m^2 plus mesna 4500 mg/m^2 as an IV continuous infusion
>   over days 2–3
>   Mesna 1000 mg IV bolus prior to starting ifosfamide infusion
>   Mesna 1000 mg/m^2 IV over 8 h after ifosfamide infusion is complete
>   Cisplatin 50 mg/m^2 IV on day 2

ADMINISTRATION

Ifosfamide and mesna

Mesna administration is mandatory with ifosfamide, to prevent the urothelial toxicity (haemorrhagic cystitis) which can be caused by acrolein metabolites of the drug.

A loading dose of mesna is given first as an IV bolus followed by an 18-h infusion of ifosfamide plus mesna, which is in turn followed by an 8-h infusion of mesna alone. The scheduling is designed to ensure that there is adequate mesna in the bladder throughout the period when ifosfamide metabolites are appearing in the urine. Therefore the final infusion of mesna should not be speeded up to make the treatment quicker.

Bleomycin

This is given over a period of 24 h in 2 L of saline. Prolonged infusion enhances the efficacy of this drug. Reducing the volume of fluid in which it is given is not appropriate, as it also acts as pre-hydration for the cisplatin that follows.

Cisplatin

This is given as an infusion in 1 L of saline over a period of 2 h, after pre-hydration with 2 L of saline (i.e. the bleomycin doses), and is followed with intensive post-hydration. Cisplatin is nephrotoxic, and hydration is mandatory to dilute the drug as it is excreted via the kidneys to minimise toxicity. The aim of hydration is to maintain a urine output of 100 mL/h during and for 6–8 h after cisplatin administration. Mannitol is given to ensure that urine output is brisk. Electrolytes are added to compensate for cisplatin-induced electrolyte wasting.

ANTI-EMETICS

High emetogenic potential (see local policy).

CYCLE LENGTH

21 days.

NUMBER OF CYCLES

Usually 6.

SIDE-EFFECTS

Bone-marrow suppression (all blood components affected), total alopecia, haemorrhagic cystitis leading to bladder fibrosis, encephalopathy during the administration period, nephrotoxicity, lung fibrosis, vomiting (may be very severe), sensory, motor and occasionally autonomic neuropathy (sometimes irreversible) including significant potential for ototoxicity, mucositis, rigors.

BLOOD NADIR

Around day 12.

TTOS REQUIRED

• Anti-emetics appropriate to highly emetogenic chemotherapy (according to local protocol).

NOTES FOR PRESCRIBERS

At the time of prescribing each course

• Check the full blood count prior to giving the go-ahead for chemotherapy. Seek advice if the neutrophil count is $<1.5 \times 10^9$/L or the platelet count is

$<100 \times 10^9/L$ at the time of treatment. In the original report of this regimen,[1] treatment was delayed if the WBC was $<2.8 \times 10^9/L$ or the platelet count was $<150 \times 10^9/L$.

- Cisplatin is highly nephrotoxic, and renal function should be formally assessed at the start of treatment. Ideally this should be done by EDTA clearance, but estimation from the serum creatinine concentration using the Cockcroft–Gault equation is acceptable if the patient has stable creatinine levels and no confounding factors (e.g. catabolic states):

CrCl (mL/min)

$$= \frac{1.04 \text{ (females) or } 1.23 \text{ (males)} \times (140 - \text{age in years}) \times \text{weight in kg}}{\text{serum creatinine concentration } (\mu\text{mol/L})}.$$

On subsequent cycles the renal function should be reassessed.

Doses of cisplatin *must be reduced* if creatinine clearance drops below 60 mL/min. Adjustment of bleomycin doses should also be considered if CrCl falls below 50 mL/min (*see* Appendix 2). Poor renal function is not only a contraindication to cisplatin and bleomycin therapy, but is also – together with low serum albumin levels and a large pelvic tumour mass – a risk factor for ifosfamide encephalopathy.

This is an insidious condition which can develop on any treatment course and presents in a variety of ways, although somnolence and confusion feature strongly in the early stages. It can be fatal. Therefore, as well as keeping an eye on renal function, serum albumin levels should be checked on each course. If a patient has two or more risk factors, particularly if these have developed since the last treatment, discuss the appropriateness of treatment with a senior member of the medical team.

- Ifosfamide is also contraindicated in patients with severe hepatic dysfunction (*see* Appendix 1 for further guidance).
- Check electrolytes for cisplatin-induced wasting, especially of magnesium, calcium and potassium. Additional supplementation may be required.
- Prescribe anti-emetics appropriate to highly emetogenic chemotherapy according to local policy.
- Hydrocortisone 100 mg IV and chlorpheniramine 10–20 mg IV should be prescribed 'as required' to allow bleomycin-induced rigors to be treated promptly, should they occur.
- Liaise with the nurses who are looking after the patient, who should be on a fluid-balance chart. Urine should be tested for blood (to detect haemorrhagic cystitis), and the nurses should understand the significance of any changes in mental state which may be indicative of encephalopathy.
- If blood is reported in the urine either during or in the 12 h after ifosfamide administration, then increasing the mesna dose may help. However, urine test sticks are very sensitive, and the lowest levels of blood detected by them may not be an indication to intervene. Consult a senior member of the medical team for advice in this situation.
- If the patient displays changes in mental state which suggest encephalopathy, liaise with an experienced prescriber immediately. In this situation, treatment

---

[1] Buxton EJ, Meanwell CA, Hilton C *et al.* (1989) Combination bleomycin, ifosfamide and cisplatin chemotherapy in cervical cancer. *J Natl Cancer Inst.* **81**: 359–61.

suspension is strongly advised. Administration of methylene blue may also be helpful (50 mg IV three times a day).[2,3] This has been reported to reverse ifosfamide-induced encephalopathy. Note that mesna has no ability to ameliorate CNS toxicity.

- Unexplained breathlessness may be indicative of bleomycin-induced lung fibrosis, and should be investigated.
- Ask the patient about symptoms indicative of neurotoxicity (parasthesias, difficulty with motor control) or ototoxicity (tinnitus, deafness), and seek further advice if they report such symptoms.

On the day after each cisplatin dose

- Check the fluid balance/body weight. If the patient gains 1.5 L/kg or more from the start of hydration, extra diuresis will be required (e.g. furosemide 20–40 mg by mouth).

NOTES FOR NURSES

- Patients should be on fluid-balance charts and have daily weights recorded during treatment. Intensive hydration is given with the aim of maintaining a urine output of 100 mL/h during and for 6–8 h after cisplatin therapy. If urine output is inadequate or the patient gains more than 1.5 L/kg above baseline at any point, the medical team should be contacted with a view to prescribing diuretics.
- Once ifosfamide infusion has commenced, all urine should be tested for blood because of the possibility of ifosfamide-induced haemorrhagic cystitis. If this is detected, it should be reported to the prescriber, as extra mesna may be needed. However, urine test sticks are very sensitive, and the lowest levels of blood detected by them may not be an indication to intervene.
- Because of the possibility of ifosfamide-induced CNS toxicity, any excessive drowsiness or confusion should be reported promptly to the medical team.

NOTES FOR PHARMACISTS

- Check that a full blood count has been done and is within acceptable limits before issuing chemotherapy.
- Check that renal function is acceptable at the start of treatment. Calculate CrCl from serum creatinine levels using the Cockroft–Gault equation, and mark this value on any pharmacy patient record sheet (*see* Appendix 3 for an example), together with the corresponding creatinine concentration. On subsequent courses, recalculate the CrCl if the serum creatinine concentration increases significantly. Poor renal function is a risk factor for ifosfamide encephalopathy, and both cisplatin and to a lesser extent ifosfamide are nephrotoxic.

[2] Kupfer A, Aeschlimann C, Wermuth B *et al.* (1994) Prophylaxis and reversal of ifosfamide encephalopathy with methylene blue. *Lancet.* **343**: 763–4.
[3] Zulian GB, Tullan E and Maton B (1995) Methylene blue for ifosfamide-associated encephalopathy. *NEJM.* **332**: 1239–40.

A reduction in the cisplatin dose is required if the CrCl is <60 mL/min. In addition, bleomycin is renally excreted, and a dose reduction should be considered if
the CrCl drops below 50 mL/min (*see* Appendix 2).

- Ifosfamide is also contraindicated in patients with severe hepatic dysfunction (*see* Appendix 1 for further guidance).
- Check serum albumin levels at the start of each cycle, as low albumin is another risk factor for ifosfamide encephalopathy. The risk is increased if the patient has other risk factors for encephalopathy (poor renal function or a large pelvic tumour mass). If the patient has multiple risk factors, especially if these include low albumin (which is often overlooked, as it is not usually particularly important during chemotherapy), point these out to the prescriber. Multiple risk factors are not an absolute contraindication to ifosfamide therapy, but where there is a choice of therapy, they may point towards an alternative treatment.
- Check that anti-emetics appropriate to highly emetogenic chemotherapy have been prescribed according to local protocol.
- Check that mesna has been prescribed and that the dose is appropriate (i e, if the dose of ifosfamide on the fluid chart has been altered, that the mesna dose has been altered proportionally).
  Note: Mesna is essentially non-toxic, and considerable rounding up of doses is acceptable to make preparation simpler.
- When visiting the treatment area during chemotherapy, check that the patient is not in excessive positive fluid balance — that is, that they have not gained more than 1.5 L/kg from the start of hydration, and that urine output is maintained at a level above 100 mL/h during and for 6–8 h after cisplatin infusion. If excessive fluid retention is occurring, consult with the medical team about the possibility of extra diuretics being prescribed (if this has not already been done).

  In addition, if any urine sample is described as containing blood, discuss with the prescriber the possibility of increasing the mesna dosage. However, urine test sticks are very sensitive, and the lowest levels of blood detected by them may not be an indication to intervene. Guidance on a suitable increase in the mesna dose is difficult to give, but it is not unreasonable to double the dose.

- Any reports of patients being excessively drowsy or confused should be regarded as indicators of ifosfamide encephalopathy. As this is a progressive condition, liaise with the prescriber urgently with a view to halting treatment immediately, and possibly instituting treatment with methylene blue (50 mg IV, three times a day; *see* Source material below). This treatment has been reported to be beneficial, but has not been rigorously assessed. In patients who develop encephalopathy, it should not be relied upon to control the problem — ifosfamide infusion should be halted immediately. In patients with a history of encephalopathy, the risks and benefits of further ifosfamide treatment should be evaluated carefully, rather than relying upon methylene blue as a prophylactic/therapeutic measure.

SOURCE MATERIAL

Cervical cancer

- Buxton EJ, Meanwell CA, Hilton C *et al.* (1989) Combination bleomycin, ifosfamide and cisplatin chemotherapy in cervical cancer. *J Natl Cancer Inst.* **81**: 359–61.

Methylene blue in ifosfamide encephalopathy

- Kupfer A, Aeschlimann C, Wermuth B *et al.* (1994) Prophylaxis and reversal of ifosfamide encephalopathy with methylene blue. *Lancet.* **343**: 763–4.
- Zulian GB, Tullen E and Maton B (1995) Methylene blue for ifosfamide-associated encephalopathy. *NEJM.* **332**: 1239–40.

BOP (bleomycin, vincristine [Oncovin®], cisplatin)

Note: *This has also been combined with VIP to form a hybrid BOP/VIP regimen.*

USUAL INDICATION

Largely experimental in the treatment of germ-cell tumours. Has been used in combination with VIP (etoposide, ifosfamide, cisplatin) or VIP-B (etoposide, ifosfamide, cisplatin-bleomycin) as a hybrid BOP/VIP or VIP-B regimen in the salvage treatment of relapsed germ-cell tumours.

DOSES

Bleomycin 30 000 units (equivalent to 30 old units or 30 mg) IV on day 2
Vincristine 2 mg IV on day 1
Cisplatin 50 mg/m^2 IV on days 1 and 2

ADMINISTRATION

Bleomycin

Bleomycin is given in 1 L of saline as part of the post-hydration necessary after cisplatin administration.

Cisplatin

Cisplatin is nephrotoxic, and hydration is mandatory to dilute the drug as it is excreted via the kidneys to minimise toxicity. The aim of hydration is to maintain a urine output of 100 mL/h during and for 6–8 h after cisplatin administration. Mannitol is sometimes given as an osmotic diuretic to ensure that urine output is brisk. Typically 1 L of saline is administered as pre-hydration, followed by 1 L of saline containing cisplatin and a further 2 L as post-hydration. In order to facilitate outpatient treatment, post-hydration may be reduced to 1 L and the patient instructed to drink at least 3 L of fluid in the 24 h after IV hydration has finished. Electrolytes are added to the hydration fluids to compensate for cisplatin-induced electrolyte wasting.

Vincristine

Vincristine is given by slow IV injection into the side-arm of a free-running saline drip.

Vincristine is a powerful vesicant and should be administered with appropriate precautions to prevent extravasation. If there is any possibility that extravasation has occurred, contact a senior member of the medical team immediately and follow local guidance on dealing with cytotoxic extravasation.

ANTI-EMETICS

High emetogenic potential (apply local policy).

CYCLE LENGTH

10 days (unless it is being used as part of a hybrid regimen with VIP; please check).

NUMBER OF CYCLES

Variable. Often used as part of a hybrid regimen with VIP. Two cycles only have been used as adjuvant treatment for seminomas after orchidectomy. If you are in any doubt, check with a senior member of the medical team.

SIDE-EFFECTS

Nephrotoxicity (dose limiting, due to cisplatin), bone-marrow suppression (all blood components affected, but not particularly myelotoxic), alopecia, nausea and vomiting (may be severe), sensory, motor and occasionally autonomic neuropathy (sometimes irreversible, due to cisplatin and vincristine) including some risk of ototoxicity, mucositis (not usually serious), lung fibrosis (bleomycin induced), rigors (bleomycin induced).

TTOS REQUIRED

- Anti-emetics appropriate to highly emetogenic chemotherapy (according to local policy).
- Consideration should be given to prescribing allopurinol (300 mg once daily by mouth, reduced in renal impairment) to prevent tumour lysis syndrome.

NOTES FOR PRESCRIBERS

Before each course

- Make sure that you know which regimen is being followed (BOP alone? BOP/VIP? How many courses?). This is not a 'typical' regimen in which six identical cycles of chemotherapy are usually given.
- Check the FBC prior to giving the go-ahead for chemotherapy, and seek advice if the neutrophil count is $<1.5 \times 10^9$/L or the platelet count is $<100 \times 10^9$/L at the

time of treatment. In a trial of BOP-VIP chemotherapy,[1] treatment was delayed by 1 week if the neutrophil count was $<1.5 \times 10^9$/L or the platelet count was $<50 \times 10^9$/L.

Note: This treatment is usually being given with curative intent, so dose delays or reductions should be avoided if at all possible. Therefore support of neutrophil numbers with haematopoietic growth factors (G-CSF or GM-CSF) may be appropriate if neutropenia is causing delays in treatment delivery (see your local policy on haematopoietic growth factors for further guidance).

- Renal function should be formally assessed at the start of treatment. Ideally this should be done by measuring EDTA clearance, but estimation of CrCl from the serum creatinine concentration using the Cockcroft–Gault equation is acceptable if the patient has stable creatinine levels and no confounding factors (e.g. catabolic states):

CrCl (mL/min)

$$\frac{1.04 \text{ (females) or } 1.23 \text{ (males)} \times (140 - \text{age in years}) \times \text{weight in kg}}{\text{serum creatinine concentration (μmol/L)}}.$$

On subsequent cycles the renal function should be reassessed.

Cisplatin doses *must be reduced* if creatinine clearance drops below 60 mL/min, and consideration should be given to reducing the bleomycin and cyclophosphamide doses if CrCl drops below 50 mL/min (*see* Appendix 2 for further guidance).

- Check LFTs. If these show serious impairment, a reduction in the vincristine dose may be required (*see* Appendix 1 for further guidance).
- Check electrolytes for cisplatin-induced wasting, especially of magnesium, calcium and potassium. Additional supplementation may be required.
- Make sure that anti-emetics appropriate to highly emetogenic chemotherapy have been prescribed according to local policy on both the inpatient chart and any discharge prescription.
- Germ-cell tumours are often highly sensitive to chemotherapy. Massive tumour lysis is possible at the start of treatment. This can lead to the release of large quantities of uric acid which may precipitate in the renal tubules, leading to renal failure. Consideration should be given to the administration of allopurinol (300 mg by mouth once daily, reduced in renal impairment) to prevent this. This should be started the day before the first cycle of chemotherapy and continued for as long as a significant bulk of chemotherapy-sensitive tumour remains.
- Ask the patient about symptoms indicative of neurotoxicity (parasthesias, difficulty with motor control) or ototoxicity (tinnitus, deafness), and seek further advice if they report such symptoms.
- Unexplained breathlessness may be indicative of bleomycin-induced lung fibrosis, and should be investigated.
- If administering vincristine, *see* Administration section above for notes about its vesicant properties.

---

[1] Kaye SB, Mead GM, Fossa S *et al.* (1998) Intensive induction-sequential chemotherapy with BOP/VIP-B compared with BEP/EP for poor-prognosis metastatic non-seminomatous germ-cell tumours: a randomised Medical Research Council/European Organisation for Research and Treatment of Cancer study. *J Clin Oncol.* **16**: 692–701.

On the day after each cisplatin dose

- For inpatients, check the fluid balance/body weight. If the patient has gained 1.5 L/kg or more since the start of chemotherapy, extra diuresis will be required.

NOTES FOR NURSES

- Patients receive very substantial IV hydration as part of this regimen, with the aim of maintaining an average urine output of 100 mL/h or more during and for 6–8 h after cisplatin administration. For inpatients, fluid balance and body weight should be recorded. Contact the prescriber if the patient's urine output is inadequate or their body weight increases by 1.5 kg from the start of IV hydration, with a view to prescribing additional diuresis. Patients who are being treated as outpatients should have daily weights recorded and be instructed to drink a further 3 L of fluid in the 24 h following the completion of IV hydration.
- If administering vincristine, *see* Administration section above for notes about its vesicant properties.

NOTES FOR PHARMACISTS

On the day of prescribing

- Make sure that you know which regimen is being followed (BOP alone? BOP/ VIP? How many cycles?). Once you have ascertained this, endorse any pharmacy patient record (*see* Appendix 3 for an example) accordingly and, if in a trial, include a photocopy of the treatment flowchart from the protocol and file with this record.
- Check that an FBC has been determined and is within acceptable limits before issuing chemotherapy.
- Check that renal function has been measured/calculated at the start of treatment. Record the CrCl and corresponding creatinine concentration in any pharmacy patient record (*see* Appendix 3 for an example). Recalculate the CrCl if the creatinine concentration changes.
  Note: Cisplatin doses *must be reduced* if the creatinine clearance drops below 60 mL/min, and consideration should be given to reducing the bleomycin and cyclophosphamide doses if the CrCl drops below 50 mL/min (*see* Appendix 2 for further guidance).
- Check LFTs. If these show serious impairment, a reduction in vincristine dose may be required (*see* Appendix 1 for further guidance).
- Check that anti-emetics appropriate to highly emetogenic chemotherapy have been prescribed according to local policy.
- As this regimen is usually being given with curative intent, treatment may proceed on quite a low blood count. Moreover, if significant myelotoxicity (i.e. symptomatic neutropenia or neutrophils counts too low to treat at the start of the next cycle, not asymptomatic low nadir counts) prevents treatment being given as planned, the use of haematopoietic growth factors (G-CSF, GM-CSF) may be justified. See your local policy on haematopoietic growth factors for further details.

On the day after each cisplatin dose

- When visiting the ward (for patients treated as inpatients), check that the patient has not gained more than 1.5 L/kg since the start of the chemotherapy cycle. If they have, discuss the need for additional diuresis with the prescriber (if this has not already been instituted).

SOURCE MATERIAL

BOP

- Dearnaley DP, Fossa SD, Kaye SB *et al.* (1998) Adjuvant bleomycin, vincristine and cis-platin (BOP) for high-risk clinical stage 1 (HRCS1) non-seminomatous germ-cell tumours (NSGCT) – an MRC pilot study. *Proceedings of the American Society of Clinical Oncology* (abstract).

BOP/VIP-B

- Kaye SB, Mead GM, Fossa S *et al.* (1998) Intensive induction-sequential chemotherapy with BOP/VIP-B compared with BEP/EP for poor-prognosis metastatic non-seminomatous germ-cell tumours: a randomised Medical Research Council/European Organisation for Research and Treatment of Cancer study. *J Clin Oncol.* **16**: 692–701.

CAP (cyclophosphamide, doxorubicin ['Adriamycin'], cisplatin)

USUAL INDICATION

Ovarian cancer.

DOSES

Doxorubicin 50 mg/m^2 IV on day 1
Cisplatin 50 mg/m^2 IV on day 1
Cyclophosphamide 500 mg/m^2 IV on day 1

Note: This is the version of CAP used in the ICON III* trial. However, there are variations on this.

ADMINISTRATION

Doxorubicin

By slow IV injection into the side-arm of a free-running saline drip.

Doxorubicin is a powerful vesicant and should be administered with appropriate precautions to prevent extravasation. If there is any possibility that extravasation has occurred, contact a senior member of the medical team immediately and follow local guidance on dealing with extravasation incidents.

Cyclophosphamide

By slow IV injection. It may also be given as a short infusion in 100 mL of saline.

Cisplatin

As an infusion in 1 L of saline over a period of 4 h, after pre-hydration with 1 L of saline, and followed by intensive post-hydration with a further 2 L of saline. Patients who are being treated on a day-case basis may be discharged after only 1 L of post-hydration, but must be encouraged to drink 3 L of fluid in the 24 h following IV hydration. Cisplatin is nephrotoxic, and hydration is mandatory to dilute the drug as it is excreted via the kidneys to minimise toxicity. The aim of hydration is to maintain a urine output of 100 mL/h during and for 6–8 h after cisplatin administration.

---

* Third International Collaborative Study in Ovarian Neoplasms.

Mannitol is also often given to ensure that urine output is brisk. Electrolytes are added to compensate for cisplatin-induced electrolyte wasting.

ANTI-EMETICS

High emetogenic potential (see local policy).

CYCLE LENGTH

21 days.

NUMBER OF CYCLES

Usually 6.

SIDE-EFFECTS

Nephrotoxicity (dose limiting due to cisplatin), bone-marrow suppression (all blood components are affected), alopecia (extensive), nausea and vomiting (may be very severe), sensory and motor neuropathy (sometimes irreversible, due to cisplatin) including significant potential for ototoxicity, mucositis, dilated cardiomyopathy (due to doxorubicin, especially if the cumulative dose exceeds $450\,mg/m^2$). Cyclophosphamide *can* cause haemorrhagic cystitis at high doses. However, the doses used in CAP are not likely to lead to this problem, so prophylactic mesna and urine testing are not required.

BLOOD NADIR

10 days.

TTOS REQUIRED

- Anti-emetics appropriate to highly emetogenic regimen (according to local protocol).

NOTES FOR PRESCRIBERS

At the time of prescribing the first cycle

- Patients over 60 years of age or with a history of heart disease must have had an echocardiogram or MUGA scan prior to treatment to ensure that there is adequate left ventricular function.

- Prior to treatment, hair loss should be discussed with the patient. Scalp cooling is unlikely to be effective, as it provides little protection against cisplatin- or cyclophosphamide-induced hair loss. If appropriate, liaise with nurses with regard to referral to a wig-fitter at the start of treatment and before alopecia is evident.

At the time of prescribing each cycle

- Creatinine clearance should be formally assessed at the start of treatment. Ideally this should be done by EDTA clearance, but estimation from the serum creatine concentration using the Cockcroft–Gault equation is acceptable if the patient has stable serum creatinine levels and no confounding factors (e.g. catabolic states):

CrCl (mL/min)

$$= \frac{1.04 \text{ (females) or } 1.23 \text{ (males)} \times (140 - \text{age in years}) \times \text{weight in kg}}{\text{serum creatinine concentration (}\mu\text{mol/L)}},$$

On subsequent cycles the renal function should be reassessed.

Cisplatin doses *must be reduced* if creatinine clearance drops below 60 mL/min, and consideration should also be given to reducing the cyclophosphamide dose if the CrCl drops below 50 mL/min (*see* Appendix 2 for further guidance).
- Check electrolytes for cisplatin-induced wasting, especially of magnesium, calcium and potassium. Additional supplementation may be required.
- Prescribe anti-emetics appropriate to highly emetogenic chemotherapy on any inpatient drug chart and any discharge prescription as appropriate.
- Seek further advice if the patient reports symptoms indicative of neurotoxicity (parasthesias, difficulty with motor control) or ototoxicity (tinnitus, deafness).
- Check the FBC before giving the go-ahead for chemotherapy. Seek advice if the neutrophil count is $<1.5 \times 10^9$/L or the platelet count is $<100 \times 10^9$/L.
- Check LFTs. If these show serious impairment, a reduction in doxorubicin may be required (*see* Appendix 1 for further guidance).
- If administering doxorubicin, *see* Administration section above for notes on the vesicant nature of doxorubicin.
- The dose of cyclophosphamide is below that which is likely to produce urothelial toxicity. Therefore prophylactic mesna and urine testing are not required.

On the day after each cisplatin dose (for patients treated as inpatients)

- Check the fluid balance/body weight. If the patient gains 1.5 L/kg or more from the start of hydration, extra diuresis will be required (e.g. furosemide 20–40 mg immediately).

NOTES FOR NURSES

- Discuss probable hair loss with the patient and, if appropriate, refer them to a wig-fitter at the start of treatment before alopecia is a problem.

- If administering doxorubicin, *see* Administration section above for notes on its vesicant properties.
- The aim of hydration is to ensure an average urine output of 100 mL/h or more during and for 6–8 h after cisplatin administration. Inpatients should be on a fluid balance chart and daily weights should be recorded. Contact the prescriber if the patient's urine output is inadequate or their body weight increases by 1.5 kg from baseline.

  For outpatients, efforts should be made to ensure that urine output is adequate (e.g. by making sure that the patient has passed 500 mL of urine between the start of IV hydration and the beginning of cisplatin infusion).

  Outpatients should also be encouraged to drink 3 L of fluid in the 24 h following each period of IV hydration, and to contact the hospital if this is impossible because of nausea/vomiting or other problems.
- The dose of cyclophosphamide is lower than that which is likely to produce urothelial toxicity (haemorrhagic cystitis). Therefore prophylactic mesna and urine testing are not required. Any symptoms of mild dysuria may be treated by encouraging oral fluid intake and regular voiding of urine.

NOTES FOR PHARMACISTS

- Check that the FBC has been determined and is within acceptable limits (usually neutrophil count $>1.5 \times 10^9$/L and platelet count $>100 \times 10^9$/L) before issuing chemotherapy.
- Check that the creatinine clearance has been measured/calculated at the start of treatment. Record the CrCl and corresponding serum creatinine concentration on any pharmacy patient record (*see* Appendix 3 for an example).

  Cisplatin doses *must be reduced* if creatinine clearance drops below 60 mL/min, and consideration should also be given to reducing the cyclophosphamide dose if the CrCl drops below 50 mL/min (*see* Appendix 2 for further guidance).
- At the start of treatment, make sure that the patient's LFTs have been checked. The doxorubicin dose may require alteration if there is severe hepatic impairment (*see* Appendix 1 for further guidance).
- Check that anti-emetics appropriate to highly emetogenic chemotherapy have been prescribed according to local policy.
- The dose of cyclophosphamide is below that which is likely to produce urothelial toxicity. Therefore prophylactic mesna and urine testing are not required.
- Keep track of the patient's cumulative dose of doxorubicin, and alert the prescriber if this exceeds 450 mg/m². It is especially important when a patient starts a course of treatment to check any pharmacy records and the patient's medical notes to see whether they have received previous anthracycline therapy in your hospital or elsewhere.
- When visiting the ward the day after chemotherapy, check that any patient who is receiving CAP as an inpatient has not gained more than 1.5 L/kg since the start of hydration. If they have, discuss the need for additional diuresis (e.g. furosemide 20 mg by mouth) with the prescriber (if this measure has not already been instituted).

SOURCE MATERIAL

● Ovarian Cancer Meta-Analysis Project (1991). Cyclophosphamide plus cisplatin versus cyclophosphamide, doxorubicin and cisplatin chemotherapy of ovarian carcinoma: a meta-analysis. *J Clin Oncol.* **9**: 1668–74.

Capecitabine (single-agent)

USUAL INDICATION

First-line treatment of advanced colorectal cancer; salvage treatment of metastatic breast cancer after anthracyclines and taxanes.

DOSES

2500 mg/m^2/day by mouth on days 1–14.

ADMINISTRATION

By mouth as two divided doses each day, taken with food.

ANTI-EMETICS

Low emetogenic potential (see local policy).

CYCLE LENGTH

21 days.

NUMBER OF CYCLES

Until there is disease progression or unacceptable toxicity.

SIDE-EFFECTS

Palmar-plantar erythrodysasthesia (hand-and-foot syndrome), diarrhoea, mucositis, abdominal pain, bone-marrow suppression (severe myelotoxicity is uncommon), alopecia (usually restricted to moderate hair thinning), nausea and vomiting, mucositis, asymptomatic increases in bilirubin and liver enzymes.

BLOOD NADIR

No discrete nadir.

TTOS REQUIRED

- Anti-emetics appropriate to weakly emetogenic chemotherapy.
- Antidiarrhoeals to be taken on an 'as required' basis may be appropriate, especially in patients who have experienced problems on previous courses.

NOTES FOR PRESCRIBERS

- Check the FBC prior to giving the go-ahead for chemotherapy. Seek advice if the neutrophil count is $<1.5 \times 10^9$/L or the platelet count is $<100 \times 10^9$/L.
- The creatinine clearance should be checked before prescribing. Estimation from the serum creatinine concentration using the Cockcroft–Gault equation is appropriate if the patient has stable creatinine levels and no confounding factors (e.g catabolic states):

CrCl (mL/min)

$$= \frac{1.04 \text{ (females) or } 1.23 \text{ (males)} \times (140 - \text{age in years}) \times \text{weight in kg}}{\text{serum creatinine concentration } (\mu\text{mol/L})}.$$

On subsequent cycles the renal function should be reassessed.

Capecitabine should be *AVOIDED* in patients with CrCl < 30 mL/min, and the starting dose should be reduced by 25% in patients with moderate renal impairment (CrCl in the range 51–80 mL/min).

- Check the LFTs prior to prescribing. Administration of capecitabine should be interrupted if there is treatment-related elevation of bilirubin $>3.0 \times$ ULN or treatment-related elevation of hepatic aminotransferases (ALT, AST) $>2.5 \times$ ULN. Treatment can be resumed when the elevations resolve or decrease to grade 1. These dose adjustments are appropriate in patients with and without liver metastases (i.e. dose adjustments should be made on the basis of hepatic function, not the presence or absence of metastases).
- The manufacturer of capecitabine gives recommendations for appropriate dosage adjustments to be made in the case of clinically significant toxicity (*see* table below). These should be followed.

Toxicity (NCIC grades)	During a course of treatment	Dose adjustment for next cycle (% of starting dose)
Grade 1	Maintain dose level	Maintain dose level
Grade 2		
First appearance	Interrupt until resolved to grade 0–1	100%
Second appearance	Interrupt until resolved to grade 0–1	75%
Third appearance	Interrupt until resolved to grade 0–1	50%
Fourth appearance	Discontinue treatment permanently	
Grade 3		
First appearance	Interrupt until resolved to grade 0–1	75%
Second appearance	Interrupt until resolved to grade 0–1	50%
Third appearance	Discontinue treatment permanently	

Grade 4
    First appearance   Discontinue permanently
                                  or
                                If physician deems it to be in the   50%
                                patient's best interest to continue,
                                interrupt until resolved to grade 0–1

The grading of toxicity in the above table is that of the National Cancer Institute of Canada (NCIC) common toxicity criteria (version 1), except for hand-and-foot syndrome, where the following scale was used:

Grade 1	Numbness, dysasthesia/parasthesia, tingling, painless swelling or erythema causing discomfort but no disruption of normal activity
Grade 2	Painful erythema and swelling of hands and/or feet and/or discomfort affecting the patient's activities of daily living
Grade 3	Moist desquamation, ulceration, blistering and severe pain of the hands and/or feet, and/or severe discomfort that causes the patient to be unable to work or perform activities of daily living

Since the application of these dose modification schedules requires a knowledge of toxicity on previous courses as well as the most recent course, accurate documentation of toxicity on each course is required, even when that toxicity is only moderate in intensity. Once doses have been reduced for toxicity, they should not be re-elevated.

• Prescriptions should be for an entire 14-day cycle of treatment. When prescribing, take care that the total daily dose is divided into two to give the individual doses. Serious toxicity has occurred when the total daily dose was given twice a day. It should be explained clearly to the patient that the tablets should be taken for 14 days only and then stopped. No attempt should be made to 'catch up' on any missed tablets. Any prescription should make the duration of treatment clear, as should any communication with the patient's GP. *Fatalities have resulted from the inadvertent continuation of short courses of oral chemotherapy.*

• The patient should be encouraged to contact an appropriate person at the treatment centre if they experience any of the following: more than four bowel movements each day, or night-time diarrhoea; more than one vomit in any 24 h; nausea that is interfering with eating; hand-and-foot syndrome or mucositis that causes more than mild discomfort. When patients report these problems, it is important to take the action described in the tables above. Timely treatment interruption and appropriate dose reduction are the key to preventing rare incidents of serious toxicity.

• Prescribed doses should be multiples of 500 and 150 mg. These are the tablet strengths available, and increments smaller than 150 mg are neither practicable nor necessary.

• Capecitabine tablets should not be crushed, and there is no liquid formulation available. Therefore treatment with this drug is unsuitable for patients who cannot swallow tablets.

- Capecitabine may modify the action of warfarin and other coumarin anticoagulants and increase phenytoin levels in patients who are taking it. In patients who are taking these drugs concomitantly with capecitabine, arrangements should be made to monitor PT or INR/phenytoin levels more closely than usual.

NOTES FOR NURSES

- If counselling the patient about their treatment, check that they understand that each cycle of treatment should last for 14 days only, and that 14 days after starting treatment they should stop taking their tablets, *even if they have some left over.* It is important that they do not seek continuation supplies from their GP, except as part of a formal 'shared-care' arrangement. *Fatalities have resulted from the inadvertent continuation of short courses of oral chemotherapy.*
- The likely side-effects of treatment should be explained to the patient. They should be encouraged to contact an appropriate person at the hospital if they experience any of the following: more than four bowel movements each day, or night-time diarrhoea; more than one vomit in any 24 h; nausea that is interfering with eating; hand-and-foot syndrome or mucositis that causes more than mild discomfort. Early identification of toxicity, and dosage adjustment using the scheme described above, are both crucial to the prevention of severe toxicity during capecitabine treatment.

NOTES FOR PHARMACISTS

- When checking prescriptions, ensure that the total daily dose has been divided into two doses. Serious toxicity has occurred when the total daily dose was administered twice a day.
- Check the FBC prior to dispensing tablets. Seek advice if the neutrophil count is $< 1.5 \times 10^9$/L or the platelet count is $< 100 \times 10^9$/L.
- The creatinine clearance should be checked before prescribing. In patients with no confounding characteristics, estimation from the serum creatinine concentration using the Cockcroft–Gault equation is appropriate. Record the calculated CrCl and the corresponding creatinine concentration in any pharmacy patient record (*see* Appendix 3 for an example), and recalculate the CrCl on future courses if the creatinine concentration changes significantly. Capecitabine should be *AVOIDED* in patients with CrCl < 30 mL/min, and the starting dose should be reduced by 25% in patients with moderate renal impairment (CrCl in the range 51–80 mL/min).
- If patients experience treatment toxicity, then the manufacturer's recommendations for dosage adjustment should be followed (*see* Notes for prescribers above).
- Check the LFTs prior to prescribing. Administration of capecitabine should be interrupted if there is treatment-related elevation of bilirubin $< 3.0 \times$ ULN or treatment-related elevation of hepatic aminotransferases (ALT, AST) $> 2.5 \times$ ULN. Treatment can be resumed when the elevations resolve or decrease to grade 1. These dose adjustments are appropriate in patients with and without liver metastases (i.e. dose adjustments should be made on the basis of hepatic function, not the presence or absence of metastases).

- The rounding off of doses to the nearest 150 mg (i.e. smallest whole tablet) is appropriate. The breaking or cutting of tablets is inappropriate.
- Capecitabine tablets should not be crushed, and there is no commercial liquid formulation available. Extemporaneous preparation of such a liquid product has not been reported, and in any case it would be expected to be unpalatable because of the bitter taste of capecitabine. Therefore capecitabine treatment is unsuitable for patients who cannot swallow tablets.
- If counselling the patient about their treatment, check that they understand that each cycle of treatment should last for 14 days only, and that 14 days after starting treatment they should stop taking their tablets, *even if they have some left over.* It is important that they do not seek continuation supplies from their GP, unless a formal 'shared-care' arrangement is in place. *Fatalities have resulted from the inadvertent continuation of short courses of oral chemotherapy.*
- The likely side-effects of treatment should be explained to the patient. They should be encouraged to contact an appropriate person at the hospital if they experience any of the following: more than four bowel movements each day, or night-time diarrhoea; more than one vomit in any 24 h; nausea that is interfering with eating; hand-and-foot syndrome or mucositis that causes more than mild discomfort. Early identification of toxicity, and dosage adjustment using the scheme described above, are both crucial to the prevention of severe toxicity during capecitabine treatment.
- Capecitabine may modify the action of warfarin and other coumarin anticoagulants and increase phenytoin levels in patients who are taking it. In patients who are taking these drugs concomitantly with capecitabine, arrangements should be made to monitor PT or INR/phenytoin levels more closely than usual. Alert the prescriber to this requirement if you are uncertain whether suitable arrangements have been made.

SOURCE MATERIAL

Colorectal cancer

- Hoff PM, Ansari R, Batist G et al. (2001) Comparison of oral capecitabine versus intravenous fluorouracil plus leucovorin as first-line treatment in 605 patients with metastatic colorectal cancer: results of a randomized phase III study. J Clin Oncol. **19**: 2282–92.

Breast cancer

- Blum JL, Jones SE, Buzdar AU et al. (1999) Multicenter phase II study of capecitabine in paclitaxel-refractory metastatic breast cancer. J Clin Oncol. **17**: 485–93.

CAPOMEt (cyclophosphamide, doxorubicin ['Adriamycin'], prednisolone, vincristine [Oncovin®], methotrexate, etoposide)

USUAL INDICATION

High-grade non-Hodgkin's lymphoma.

DOSES

This is a complex regimen consisting of three 4-week phases that are repeated three times.

Weeks 0, 4, 8 and 12 (i.e. days 1, 29, 57 and 85)

Doxorubicin 50 mg/m^2 IV
Cyclophosphamide 400 mg/m^2 IV
Allopurinol 300 mg by mouth, once daily for 28 days starting on day 1

Weeks 1, 3, 5, 7, 9 and 11 (i.e. days 8, 22, 36, 50, 64 and 78)

Vincristine 2 mg (total dose) IV
Prednisolone 60 mg/m^2 by mouth for 5 days
Sodium bicarbonate 2.4 g four times a day by mouth on days 14–17, 42–45, 70–73 (dispense now for use prior to next attendance for chemotherapy)

Weeks 2, 6 and 10 (i.e. days 15, 43 and 71)

Sodium bicarbonate 2.4 g four times a day by mouth for 4 days starting 24 h *before* the following:
Methotrexate 250 mg/m^2 IV
Etoposide 100 mg/m^2 IV followed by 50 mg three times a day by mouth for 3 days (4 days of etoposide treatment in total)
Folinic acid 15 mg four times a day by mouth (for 3 days) starting 24 h *after* methotrexate

ADMINISTRATION

Doxorubicin and vincristine

By slow IV injection into the side-arm of a free-running saline drip.

Doxorubicin and vincristine are powerful vesicants and should be administered with appropriate precautions to prevent extravasation. If there is any possibility that extravasation has occurred, contact a senior member of the medical team immediately and follow local guidance for dealing with extravasation incidents.

Cyclophosphamide

May be given as a slow IV bolus injection or short IV infusion (i.e. in 100 mL of saline over a period of 10–20 min).

Methotrexate

Administered as a 1-h infusion in 0.9% sodium chloride over a period of 30 min.

Treatment should only be commenced after 24 h of treatment with sodium bicarbonate to alkalinise the urine.

Etoposide IV is given in an infusion over 1 h in 0.9% sodium chloride. Rapid infusion may lead to hypotension.

Note: On days when multiple IV drugs are administered, the order of administration is not critical.

ANTI-EMETICS

Weeks 0, 4, 8 and 12 (i.e. days 1, 29, 57 and 85)

High emetogenic potential (see local policy).

Weeks 1, 2, 3, 5, 6, 7, 9, 10 and 11 (i.e. days 8, 15, 22, 36, 43, 50, 64, 71 and 78)

Low emetogenic potential (see local policy). Note that high-dose prednisolone is given as part of this regimen, and therefore extra steroids are not appropriate on odd-numbered weeks.

CYCLE LENGTH

A sequence of four 1-week phases, given sequentially and without gaps. This 1-month treatment cycle is repeated three times, giving a total of 12 weeks of continuous treatment.

NUMBER OF CYCLES

12 weeks of continuous treatment.

SIDE-EFFECTS

Bone-marrow suppression, alopecia, nausea and vomiting, mucositis. Cardiac arrhythmias and dilated cardiomyopathy from doxorubicin (especially at cumulative doxorubicin doses in excess of 450 mg/m^2). Peripheral neuropathy from vincristine. Renal impairment from methotrexate if the patient is inadequately alkalinised prior to treatment. Cyclophosphamide *can* cause haemorrhagic cystitis at high doses. However, the doses used in CAPOMEt are not likely to cause this problem, so prophylactic mesna and urine testing are not required.

The high doses of prednisolone used in this regimen can produce a variety of steroid side-effects, including euphoria/depression, epigastric discomfort, insomnia, psychosis, fluid and sodium retention, proximal myopathy and potassium loss, but the courses are short, and 'tailing-off' is not usually required.

BLOOD NADIR

No discrete nadir is seen, because further chemotherapy is given before the nadir from the previous dose has been reached. The aim is to keep myelosuppression to a chronic, manageable level during treatment.

TTOS REQUIRED

Weeks 0, 4, 8 and 12 (i.e. days 1, 29, 57 and 85)

- Anti-emetics appropriate to highly emetogenic chemotherapy (according to local policy).
- On *day 1*: allopurinol 300 mg each morning (reduced in renal impairment) to prevent tumour lysis syndrome. It is suggested that a 28-day course is prescribed to cover the likely period of tumour lysis early in the treatment course.

Weeks 1, 3, 5, 7, 9 and 11 (i.e. days 8, 22, 36, 50, 64 and 78)

- Anti-emetics appropriate to chemotherapy with a low emetogenic potential (see local policy). Note that patients will already be receiving high-dose steroids at this point, and therefore additional oral steroids as anti-emetics are not appropriate.
- Prednisolone 60 mg/m^2 for 5 days. Doses should be rounded off at least to the nearest 5 mg. Although tablets are available in 5 mg and 25 mg strengths, only the 5 mg strength is available in an enteric-coated format. However, there is probably little point in prescribing enteric-coated tablets, as the evidence for protective effects on the stomach is scarce, and any concomitantly prescribed gastroprotective agent will almost certainly cause the enteric coating to fail.
- Consideration should be given to prescribing an H$_2$-antagonist or other gastro-protective agent to reduce gastric irritation by prednisolone.
- On *weeks 1, 5 and 9 (i.e. days 8, 36 and 64)*, sodium bicarbonate 2.4 g four times daily by mouth for 4 days, starting 24 h before the next planned chemotherapy (methotrexate).
- On *weeks 1 and 3 (i.e days 8 and 22)*, make sure that the patient still has a supply of allopurinol and is still taking this medication (see above). Represcribe if necessary.

Weeks 2, 6 and 10 (i.e. days 15, 43 and 78)

- Anti-emetics appropriate to weakly emetogenic chemotherapy (see local protocol).
- Folinic acid (calcium folinate, calcium leucovorin), 15 mg four times a day by mouth for 3 days, starting 24 h after the methotrexate infusion.
- On *day 15*, make sure that the patient still has a supply of allopurinol and is still taking this medication. Represcribe if necessary.
- Oral etoposide.

NOTES FOR PRESCRIBERS

General

- This is a complex regimen. It includes several short courses of oral treatment. All drug charts, prescriptions and communications with other professionals (e.g. GPs) must specify clearly exactly when drugs should be given and, equally import-antly, when they should be stopped. *Inadvertent chronic administration of steroids or cytotoxic drugs can have tragic consequences.*
- Patients over 60 years of age or with a history of heart disease must have an echocardiogram or MUGA scan prior to treatment to ensure that there is ade-quate left ventricular function before they receive doxorubicin.
- Check the FBC prior to giving the go-ahead for chemotherapy. Seek advice if the neutrophil count is $<1.5 \times 10^9$/L or the platelet count is $<100 \times 10^9$/L. Note that if treatment is being given with curative intent, it may proceed with a lower count than would be acceptable for palliative regimens. The following dose reductions were employed in a large clinical trial of this regimen:[1]

Blood count	Dose modification
Neutrophils $>1.0 \times 10^9$/L Platelets $>50 \times 10^9$/L	Give 100% of all drugs
Neutrophils $0.5-1.0 \times 10^9$/L Platelets $<50 \times 10^9$/L	Give 50% of dose, except full-dose vincristine and prednisolone
Neutrophils $<0.5 \times 10^9$/L Platelets $<50 \times 10^9$/L	Omit all drugs except full-dose vincristine and prednisolone

- If the treatment is being given with curative intent, it is important to maintain dose intensity. Dose delays should be avoided if at all possible. Therefore the use of haematopoietic growth factors (G-CSF or GM-CSF) to support neutrophil numbers may be justified if neutropenia is causing delays in dose delivery. How-ever, note that because G-CSF may worsen neutropenia if given within 24 h of chemotherapy, it may be very difficult to combine it usefully with the CAPOMEt

---

[1] Bailey NP, Stuart NSA, Bessell EM *et al.* (1998) Five-year follow-up of a prospective ran-domised multicentre trial of weekly chemotherapy (CAPOMEt) *versus* cyclical chemo-therapy (CHOP-Mtx) in the treatment of aggressive non-Hodgkin's lymphoma. *Ann Oncol.* **9**: 633–8.

regimen, where the intervals between chemotherapy doses are short. Because vincristine is minimally myelosuppressive, it may be possible to ignore the usual restriction on combining growth factors with chemotherapy on days 8, 22, 36, 50, 67 and 78 (see your local policy on haematopoietic growth factors for further guidance).

- Vincristine can cause peripheral neuropathy. The patient should be questioned about abnormal sensations, jaw pain or constipation that may be indicative of neuropathy. If such symptoms are reported, they should be discussed with a senior member of the medical team with a view to dose modification or switching to vinblastine (another vinca alkaloid which appears to be more myelosuppressive but less neurotoxic than vincristine).

- Lymphomas are very sensitive to chemotherapy, and massive tumour lysis is likely to occur at the start of chemotherapy. This can result in the generation of large amounts of insoluble uric acid which are capable of precipitating in the kidneys, causing renal damage. To prevent this, allopurinol 300 mg once daily should be commenced the day before starting cytotoxic therapy and continued for as long as significant chemotherapy sensitive tumour bulk remains and cytotoxic therapy continues. In general, administering allopurinol for the first month of treatment should be sufficient.

- Check the LFTs. If these show serious impairment, a reduction in doxorubicin, vincristine and etoposide doses may be required (see Appendix 1 for further guidance).

- Renal function should be formally assessed at the start of treatment. Ideally this should be done by EDTA clearance, but estimation from serum creatine levels using the Cockcroft–Gault equation is acceptable if the patient has a stable serum creatinine concentration and no confounding factors (e.g. catabolic states):

CrCl (mL/min)

$$= \frac{1.04 \text{ (females) or } 1.23 \text{ (males)} \times (140 - \text{age in years}) \times \text{weight in kg}}{\text{serum creatinine concentration (}\mu\text{mol/L)}}.$$

On subsequent cycles the renal function should be reassessed.

Consideration should be given to reducing the methotrexate and etoposide doses if the CrCl is below 60 mL/min, and to reducing the cyclophosphamide dose if the CrCl drops below 50 mL/min (see Appendix 2 for further guidance). The allopurinol dose should also be reduced in patients with renal impairment.

- Prior to treatment, hair loss should be discussed with the patient. Scalp cooling is of limited benefit in preventing hair loss with CAPOMEt, because of the prolonged half-lives of cyclophosphamide and etoposide. Liaise with the nurses with regard to referral of the patient to a wig-fitter at the start of treatment, before alopecia is evident, if this is appropriate.

Weeks 0, 4, 8 and 12 (i.e. days 1, 29, 57 and 85)

- If administering IV treatment, see Administration section above for notes on the vesicant nature of doxorubicin.

- Check renal and hepatic function in case dose modifications are needed for doxorubicin or cyclophosphamide (see General notes for prescribers above).
- Monitor the cumulative dose of doxorubicin. Above $450\,mg/m^2$ the risk of cardiac toxicity increases sharply. This dose should only be exceeded with great caution and with regular monitoring of cardiac function.
- Prescribe anti-emetics appropriate to highly emetogenic chemotherapy, according to the local protocol.
- In addition, on *day 1 (week 0)*, institute allopurinol treatment to prevent tumour lysis syndrome. It is suggested that a 1-month supply is provided to avoid patients running out of tablets and stopping treatment prematurely.

Weeks 1, 3, 5, 7, 9 and 11 (i.e. days 8, 22, 36, 50, 64 and 78)

- Note that the dose of vincristine is a standard dose, not based on BSA.
- If administering IV treatment, see Administration section above for notes on the vesicant nature of vincristine.
- Prescribe anti-emetics appropriate to weakly emetogenic chemotherapy (refer to local policy). Note that patients already receive high-dose steroids as part of this regimen (which has a very low emetogenic potential), so additional oral steroids are not appropriate. The use of $5HT_3$-antagonists is seldom if ever justified with this weakly emetogenic treatment.
- Prophylactic H_2-antagonists or other gastroprotective agents are recommended during high-dose prednisolone courses, to provide a measure of protection against gastritis.
- Check the LFTs. Dose adjustment of vincristine may be necessary in cases of severe hepatic impairment (see General notes for prescribers above).
- When prescribing prednisolone, make it clear both on the prescription and to the patient that this is a short course which is not to be continued.
- On *days 8, 36 and 64 (weeks 1, 5 and 9)*, prescribe sodium bicarbonate for the patient to start taking prior to their next chemotherapy admission (for methotrexate).
- On *days 8 and 22 (weeks 1 and 3)*, make sure that the patient still has and is using a supply of allopurinol tablets.

Weeks 2, 6 and 10 (i.e. days 15, 43 and 71)

- Prescribe oral etoposide to complete the course started with IV therapy. Make sure the patient understands that this is a discrete course and that no further supply should be sought from their GP. Make this clear on the prescription, too.
- Prescribe folinic acid rescue medication. Make sure the patient knows that they should not start the tablets until 24 h after methotrexate chemotherapy, and should then take them regularly until they are finished, and report any problems (e.g. vomiting) which would interfere with their folinic acid treatment. Taken straight after methotrexate, folinic acid will negate the effect of the chemotherapy.
- On *day 15 (week 2)*, make sure that the patient still has and is using a supply of allopurinol tablets.
- If the patient is hospitalised, instruct the nursing staff not to administer methotrexate until the patient's urinary pH is above 7, and explain that the urinary pH

needs to be maintained above 7 for 72 h after the start of methotrexate administration. Prescribe sodium bicarbonate 50 mmol IV to be given on an 'as-required' basis if the urinary pH falls. If the patient is an outpatient, make sure that they have received and taken at least 24 h of treatment with oral bicarbonate, prior to methotrexate, and that they have enough tablets remaining to continue treatment on the day of methotrexate administration and for 2 days afterwards. Instruct the nursing staff not to administer methotrexate unless the urinary pH is above 7.0.

- Check the LFTs and renal function. If either of these show impairment, dose reductions for methotrexate and etoposide may be required (*see* General notes for prescribers above).

NOTES FOR NURSES

General

- Prior to treatment, hair loss should be discussed with the patient. Scalp cooling is unlikely to be of much benefit because of the prolonged circulation of cyclophosphamide and etoposide. Referral to a wig-fitter, where appropriate, should be made at the start of treatment, before alopecia is evident.
- This regimen contains several oral medications that are given for short courses, plus a prolonged period of continuous allopurinol treatment at the start of treatment. Make sure that the patient knows which medications are only intended as short courses, and instruct them not to seek further supplies of these from their GP. In addition, some patients will need instruction to ensure that they take medications at the correct time (e.g. start bicarbonate before methotrexate treatment).

Weeks 0, 4, 8 and 12 (i.e. days 1, 29, 57 and 85)

- If administering IV treatment, *see* Administration section above for notes on the vesicant nature of doxorubicin.
- The dose of cyclophosphamide in this regimen is below that which is likely to produce haemorrhagic cystitis. Therefore prophylactic mesna, IV hydration and urine testing are not required. Any mild symptoms of dysuria may be treated by encouraging oral fluid intake and regular voiding of urine.
- Make sure that the patient understands that they should continue allopurinol treatment until they are instructed to stop. A further supply of this medication may be needed once they have used up the tablets issued by the hospital.

Weeks 1, 3, 5, 7, 9 and 11 (i.e. days 8, 22, 36, 50, 64 and 78)

- If administering IV treatment, *see* Administration section above for notes on the vesicant nature of vincristine.
- In addition, on *weeks 1, 5 and 9 (days 8, 36 and 64)*, make sure that the patient takes home a supply of sodium bicarbonate to start 24 h before their next (methotrexate) chemotherapy.

- Make sure the patient understands that their prednisolone is a short course and that no further supply should be sought once the 5 days of treatment have been completed.

Weeks 2, 6 and 10 (i.e. days 15, 43 and 71)

- The patient's urine should be alkalinised by administration of sodium bicarbonate prior to methotrexate chemotherapy. Make sure that this has been prescribed to start 24 h prior to methotrexate. For outpatients, check that they have received the tablets and have remembered to take them correctly. For both outpatients and inpatients, check the urinary pH and ensure that it is above 7 before administering methotrexate. It is unsafe to proceed with this dose of methotrexate without first confirming that the urinary pH is alkaline. Check that bicarbonate has also been prescribed both for the day of methotrexate treatment and for the following 2 days.

  In hospitalised patients, where this is possible the urinary pH should be measured. If it rises above 7 during the 3-day period from the start of methotrexate administration, give extra bicarbonate. This should already be prescribed on an 'as-required' basis. If not, contact the prescriber with a view to obtaining a further prescription (50 mmol IV is appropriate if a prompt reduction in pH is required).

  Note: 8.4% sodium bicarbonate can only be given centrally, because it is extremely irritant. If the bicarbonate is to be given peripherally, ensure that a concentration of 1.26% or 1.4% is administered.

NOTES FOR PHARMACISTS

General

- Check that the FBC has been determined, and that it is within acceptable limits, before making up the chemotherapy. Because this is a potentially curative treatment, it is reasonable to treat on a somewhat lower neutrophil/platelet count than would be considered acceptable for a palliative regimen. However, seek confirmation that treatment is to go ahead before issuing if the neutrophil count is $<1.5 \times 10^9$/L or the platelet count is $<100 \times 10^9$/L.
- Make sure that any short courses of oral medication are labelled with a start date and the treatment duration.
- This treatment may be given with curative intent. In this situation, it is important to maintain dose intensity. Dose delays should be avoided if at all possible, and it may be appropriate to support neutrophil numbers with haematopoietic growth factors (G-CSF or GM-CSF). Scheduling doses of this agent may be difficult, given that it should not be administered within 24 h of chemotherapy. Prescriptions should be checked to ensure that they do not conflict with this rule (see your local policy on haematopoietic growth factors for further guidance). However, since vincristine is minimally myelosuppressive, it is probably reasonable to administer haematopoietic growth factors with vincristine on days 8, 22, 36, 50, 64 and 78.

- Check the LFTs. If these show serious impairment, then a reduction in doxorubicin, vincristine and etoposide doses may be required (*see* Appendix 1 for further advice).
- Renal function should be formally assessed at the start of treatment. Ideally this should be done by EDTA clearance, but estimation from the serum creatinine concentration using the Cockcroft–Gault equation is acceptable if the patient has stable serum creatinine levels and no confounding factors (e.g. catabolic states). Note the CrCl and the corresponding serum creatinine concentration on any pharmacy patient record (*see* Appendix 3 for an example). On subsequent cycles, the CrCl should be recalculated if the serum creatinine concentration has changed significantly. Consideration should be given to reducing the methotrexate and etoposide doses if the CrCl is below 60 mL/min, and to reducing the cyclophosphamide dose if the CrCl drops below 50 mL/min (*see* Appendix 2 for further guidance).

Weeks 0, 4, 8 and 12 (i.e. days 1, 29, 57 and 85)

- Check the LFTs (especially on *day 1*). If these show serious impairment, then a reduction in doxorubicin dose may be required (*see* General notes for pharmacists above).
- Check the CrCl. Dose adjustments may be required in cases of renal impairment (*see* General notes for pharmacists above).
- Check that anti-emetics appropriate to highly emetogenic chemotherapy have been prescribed according to local policy.
- In addition, on *day 1 (week 0)* check that allopurinol, 300 mg once daily by mouth (reduced dose in renal impairment), has been prescribed to prevent tumour lysis syndrome. It is probably sensible to supply sufficient medication for a 1-month period of treatment on day 1, to prevent the patient running out of the drug during this critical period.

  Lymphomas are very sensitive to chemotherapy, and massive tumour lysis is likely to occur at the start of chemotherapy. This can result in the generation of large amounts of insoluble uric acid, which are capable of precipitating in the kidneys, causing renal damage. Allopurinol can prevent this.
- Keep a close watch on the patient's cumulative dose of doxorubicin, and alert the prescriber if it exceeds 450 mg/m^2, at which point the risk of cardiac toxicity increases substantially. It is especially important when a patient starts a course of treatment to check any pharmacy records and the patient's notes to see whether they have received previous anthracycline therapy within your hospital or elsewhere.

Weeks 1, 3, 5, 7, 9 and 11 (i.e. days 8, 22, 36, 50, 64 and 78)

- Check the LFTs. A dose reduction of vincristine may be required in cases of severe hepatic impairment (*see* General notes for pharmacists above).
- Check that the correct dose of vincristine has been prescribed (i.e. 2 mg *in total*, unadjusted for BSA).
- Check that anti-emetics appropriate to weakly emetogenic chemotherapy have been prescribed according to local policy. Note that this part of the regimen has

very low emetogenic potential, and $5HT_3$-antagonists are almost never appropriate. Also note that patients receive high-dose steroids on these days. Therefore the prescribing of further steroids as anti-emetics is unnecessary.

- Check that the appropriate 5-day course of steroids has been prescribed, and that it is labelled as a short course. Make sure that it is clear, on any TTO or prescription being sent elsewhere, that the prednisolone treatment is for a short course of 5 days only. It should not be continued by the GP, nor is 'tailing off' of doses necessary. If the patient is an inpatient, block out any administration boxes on the drug chart after the end of the treatment course. *Fatalities have resulted from inappropriate continuation of short courses of oral steroids.*
- Check that consideration has been given to prescribing an H_2-antagonist or other gastroprotective agent during the period of steroid administration, in order to reduce gastritis.
- The dose of cyclophosphamide is below that which is likely to cause urothelial toxicity. Therefore prophylactic mesna, IV hydration and urine testing are not required.
- On *days 8, 36 and 64 (weeks 1, 5 and 9)*, also check that sodium bicarbonate has been supplied to the patient with instructions to start taking it 24 h before their next (methotrexate) chemotherapy.
- On *days 8 and 22 (weeks 1 and 3)*, also check that the patient has a supply of allopurinol medication and, where possible, check that they are taking it.

Weeks 2, 6 and 10 (i.e. days 15, 43 and 71)

- Make sure that sodium bicarbonate was prescribed to start 24 h before chemotherapy. Ask the nurses to check whether it was taken, and to check that the urinary pH is above 7 before proceeding with methotrexate administration. It is unsafe to proceed with methotrexate treatment at this dose unless the patient's urine is known to be alkaline. Make sure that sodium bicarbonate has also been prescribed for the 3 days after methotrexate treatment, and ensure that sodium bicarbonate 50 mmol IV has been prescribed on an 'as-required' basis for inpatients so that rapid alkalinisation is possible in individuals whose urinary pH rises above 7 during treatment.
- Make sure that oral etoposide has been prescribed for the 3 days after IV treatment. Etoposide should be clearly labelled as a short course. Any TTO prescription or prescription being sent elsewhere should be clearly endorsed to make it clear that etoposide treatment is for 3 days only and should not be continued. In addition, if you are counselling an outpatient, explain to them that they should not obtain any more etoposide from their GP. If the patient is an inpatient, block out any administration boxes on the drug chart after the end of the treatment course.

  Fatalities have resulted from inappropriate continuation of short courses of oral cytotoxic drugs.
- Check that folinic acid has been prescribed to start 24 h after methotrexate. If the patient is an inpatient, block out any administration boxes on the drug chart before the beginning and after the end of the treatment course. If you are counselling an outpatient, explain the importance of starting this drug at the correct time, taking doses regularly, and contacting the hospital if they cannot

take the tablets for any reason (e.g. vomiting, although this is not very likely after methotrexate and etoposide).

- On *day 15 (week 2)*, also check that the patient has a supply of allopurinol and, where possible, check that they are taking it.
- Check LFTs and renal function. Dose adjustments for etoposide and methotrexate may be required in cases of impairment (*see* General notes for pharmacists above).

SOURCE MATERIAL

- Bailey NP, Stuart NSA, Bessell EM *et al.* (1998) Five-year follow-up of a prospective randomised multicentre trial of weekly chemotherapy (CAPOMEt) *versus* cyclical chemotherapy (CHOP-Mtx) in the treatment of aggressive non-Hodgkin's lymphoma. *Ann Oncol.* **9**: 633−8.

Carboplatin (single-agent)

USUAL INDICATION

First-line treatment of ovarian cancer where combination treatment with paclitaxel plus carboplatin is considered to be unsuitable (e.g. because of hypersensitivity to paclitaxel or a strong desire to avoid hair loss). Also used for relapsed ovarian cancer in patients who have had a prolonged (usually > 6 months) disease-free interval after previous platinum treatment.

Note: Because of its relatively low potential for nephrotoxicity, carboplatin is often used as a substitute for cisplatin in combination regimens for patients with impaired renal function. However, it should not be assumed that direct substitution of carboplatin for cisplatin is always acceptable, since the toxicity profile of the two drugs is different and this may alter the overall tolerability of the drug combination.

DOSES

Calculated on the basis of renal function according to the following (Calvert) formula:

$$\text{Dose (mg)} = \text{desired AUC} \times (\text{GFR}^* + 25).$$

The desired AUC is usually 6 in untreated and fit patients, and 5 in frail or extensively pretreated patients.

ADMINISTRATION

IV infusion in 500 mL of 5% dextrose over a period of 1 h. No other hydration is required.

---

* The Calvert equation was developed and validated using ^{15}Cr EDTA clearance to measure GFR. In clinical practice, CrCl calculated from serum creatinine levels using the Cockcroft–Gault equation is often substituted for GFR measurement. It has been reported that this results in carboplatin underdosing, and that a correction factor of 1.1 should be applied to doses calculated using Cockcroft–Gault-derived CrCl values. Any local policy on this matter should be followed.

A simpler correction is often applied, namely the addition of 1 to the target AUC when Cockcroft–Gault-derived CrCl is used instead of isotopically measured GFR. Further corrections have been suggested for renal function determined by urinary creatinine measurement and the Jelliffe formula. However, a discussion of these is beyond the scope of this book.

ANTI-EMETICS

High emetogenic potential (see local policy).

CYCLE LENGTH

21–28 days (platelet recovery can be slow, necessitating a 28-day cycle).

NUMBER OF CYCLES

Usually 6.

SIDE-EFFECTS

Bone-marrow suppression (particularly toxic to platelets), alopecia (fairly frequent), nausea and vomiting, sensory neuropathy, hypersensitivity (rare, but more common than with some drugs), nephrotoxicity (modest relative to that with cisplatin), mucositis (not usually serious).

BLOOD NADIR

14–21 days.

TTOS REQUIRED

● Anti-emetics appropriate to highly emetogenic chemotherapy.

NOTES FOR PRESCRIBERS

● Check the FBC before giving the go-ahead for chemotherapy. Seek advice if the neutrophil count is $<1.5 \times 10^9$/L or the platelet count is $<100 \times 10^9$/L at the time of treatment.
● The creatinine clearance should be formally assessed at the start of treatment to allow an accurate dose calculation. Ideally this should be done by EDTA clearance, but estimation from the serum creatinine concentration using the Cockcroft–Gault equation is acceptable if the patient has stable creatinine levels and no confounding factors (e.g. catabolic state) (*see* note in Doses section above on adjustment of doses for different methods of assessment of renal function, and abide by any local policy or trial protocol governing this).

CrCl (mL/min)

$$= \frac{1.04 \text{ (females) or } 1.23 \text{ (males)} \times (140 - \text{age in years}) \times \text{weight in kg}}{\text{serum creatinine concentration } (\mu\text{mol/L})}.$$

On subsequent cycles the renal function should be reassessed if changes in serum creatinine concentration indicate alteration.

It should be noted that the SPC states that carboplatin is contraindicated if the creatinine clearance is <20 mL/min.

Note: Dose adjustment needs to accompany significant *improvements* in renal function (such as may occur following reduction of a large pelvic tumour mass) as well as *deteriorations*. Improved renal function and fixed doses will result in under-dosing.

- Check that anti-emetics appropriate to highly emetogenic chemotherapy have been prescribed according to the local protocol.

NOTES FOR NURSES

- No special precautions are needed.

NOTES FOR PHARMACISTS

- If the patient's renal function has been estimated using the Cockcroft–Gault equation rather than being measured using EDTA clearance, consideration should be given to adjusting the target AUC to avoid inadvertent under-dosing (*see* Doses section above for further discussion of this).
- Check that the FBC has been determined and is within acceptable limits before preparing chemotherapy.
- Record the serum creatinine concentration at each cycle on any pharmacy patient record (*see* Appendix 3 for an example). Check that the carboplatin dose has been recalculated if the serum creatinine concentration has altered significantly since the last cycle. According to the SPC, carboplatin is contraindicated if the creatinine clearance is <20 mL/min. If the CrCl falls below this level, contact the prescriber.
- Check that anti-emetics appropriate to highly emetogenic chemotherapy have been prescribed according to the local protocol.

SOURCE MATERIAL

Dosing based on renal function

- Calvert AH, Newell DR, Gumbrell LA *et al.* (1989) Carboplatin dosage: prospective evaluation of a simple formula based on renal function. *J Clin Oncol.* **7**: 1748–56.

Use of Cockcroft–Gault equation vs. EDTA clearance

- Dooley MJ, Poole SG, Rischin D *et al.* (2000) Sub-optimal dosing of carboplatin with both the Calvert formula using Cockcroft and Gault (CGF) and Jelliffe (JF) estimations of creatinine clearance (CC) and with the Chatelut formula. *Proc Am Soc Clin Oncol.* **19**: 186 (abstract).

CAV (cyclophosphamide, doxorubicin ['Adriamycin'], vincristine)

Note: This regimen is sometimes alternated with PE to form the CAV/PE hybrid protocol.

USUAL INDICATION

Small-cell lung cancer.

DOSES

Doxorubicin 40 mg/m^2 IV on day 1
Cyclophosphamide 1000 mg/m^2 IV on day 1
Vincristine 1 mg/m^2 (maximum 2 mg; some clinicians use a maximum dose of
1.5 mg in patients over 70 years of age because of a perceived higher risk
of peripheral neuropathy, although evidence for this approach is scarce)
IV on day 1

ADMINISTRATION

Doxorubicin and vincristine

By slow IV injection into the side-arm of a free-running saline drip.

Doxorubicin and vincristine are powerful vesicants and should be administered with appropriate precautions to prevent extravasation. If there is any possibility that extravasation has occurred, contact a senior member of the medical team immediately and follow local guidance on dealing with cytotoxic extravasation.

Cyclophosphamide

May be given as a slow IV bolus injection or a short IV infusion (i.e. in 100 mL of saline over a period of 10–20 min).

Note: The order of administration of the three IV drugs in this regimen is not critical.

ANTI-EMETICS

High emetogenic potential (apply local policy).

CYCLE LENGTH

21 days (42 days if alternated with PE).

NUMBER OF CYCLES

Usually 6 (3 if alternated with PE).

SIDE-EFFECTS

Bone-marrow suppression, alopecia, nausea and vomiting, mucositis, cardiac arrhythmias, dilated cardiomyopathy (especially at cumulative doxorubicin doses in excess of 450 mg/m^2), peripheral neuropathy from vincristine. Cyclophosphamide *can* cause haemorrhagic cystitis at high doses. However, the doses used in CAV are not likely to cause this problem, so prophylactic mesna or hydration are not required.

BLOOD NADIR

10 days.

TTOS REQUIRED

- Anti-emetics appropriate to highly emetogenic chemotherapy (*see* local protocol).
- Allopurinol, 300 mg each morning (reduced in renal impairment), should be considered as prophylaxis against tumour lysis syndrome in patients with a large tumour bulk at the start of treatment.

NOTE FOR PRESCRIBERS

- Patients over 60 years of age or with a history of heart disease must have an echocardiogram or a MUGA scan prior to treatment to ensure that there is adequate left ventricular function.
- Check the FBC prior to giving the go-ahead for chemotherapy. Seek advice if the neutrophil count is $<1.5 \times 10^9$/L or the platelet count is $<100 \times 10^9$/L. In a relatively recent study of CAV (alternated with PE), treatment was delayed by 1 week for patients whose WBC was still $<4.0 \times 10^9$/L or whose platelet count was still $<100 \times 10^9$/L after previous chemotherapy. For patients experiencing neutropenia associated with infection, cyclophosphamide and doxorubicin doses were reduced by 25% on subsequent courses. Vincristine doses were not adjusted for haematological toxicity.[1]

---

[1] Roth BJ, Johnson DH, Einhorn LH *et al.* (1992) Randomized study of cyclophosphamide, doxorubicin and vincristine versus etoposide and cisplatin versus alternation of these two regimens in extensive small-cell lung cancer: a phase III trial of the Southeastern Cancer Study Group. *J Clin Oncol.* **10**: 282–91.

- Check the LFTs. If these show serious impairment, a reduction in doxorubicin and vincristine doses may be required (*see* Appendix 1).
- Check the renal function. A cyclophosphamide dose reduction is required in cases of significant renal impairment (*see* Appendix 2).
- Vincristine can cause peripheral and autonomic neuropathy. Patients should be questioned about abnormal sensations, jaw pain or constipation which may be indicative of neuropathy. Discuss such symptoms with an experienced registrar or consultant with a view to dose modification or switching to vinblastine. The latter appears to be more myelosuppressive but less neurotoxic.
- To limit the potential for neurotoxicity, the dose of vincristine is capped at 2 mg.
- Prior to treatment, hair loss should be discussed with the patient. Scalp cooling is of limited benefit in preventing hair loss with CAV because of the prolonged half-life of cyclophosphamide, but it may be tried if the patient is concerned about hair loss. Liaise with the nurses with regard to referral to a wig-fitter at the start of treatment and before alopecia is evident, if this is appropriate.
- If administering drugs, *see* Administration section above for notes on the vesicant nature of doxorubicin and vincristine.
- Small-cell lung cancer can be very sensitive to chemotherapy, and massive tumour lysis may occur at the start of treatment. This can result in the release of large amounts of insoluble uric acid, which may precipitate in the kidneys, causing renal damage. To prevent this, treatment with allopurinol (300 mg each morning, reduced in cases of renal impairment) should be considered. This should be commenced the day before cytotoxic treatment and continued for as long as a significant chemosensitive tumour bulk remains.

NOTES FOR NURSES

- Prior to treatment, hair loss should be discussed with the patient. Scalp cooling is of limited benefit because of the prolonged circulation of cyclophosphamide, but can be attempted if hair loss is of particular concern to the patient. If appropriate, referral to a wig-fitter should be made at the start of treatment and before alopecia is evident.
- If administering drugs, *see* Administration section above for notes on the vesicant nature of doxorubicin and vincristine.
- The dose of cyclophosphamide is lower than that which is likely to cause haemorrhagic cystitis. Therefore prophylactic mesna, IV hydration and urine testing are not required. Any mild symptoms of dysuria may be treated by encouraging oral fluid intake and regular voiding of urine.

NOTES FOR PHARMACISTS

- Check that the FBC has been determined and is within acceptable limits before issuing chemotherapy.
- Check that the maximum dose for vincristine in this regimen (i.e. 2 mg) has not been exceeded.
- Check that anti-emetics appropriate to highly emetogenic chemotherapy have been prescribed according to the local protocol.

- Check the LFTs. If these show serious impairment, a reduction in doxorubicin and vincristine doses may be required (*see* Appendix 1).
- Check the renal function. A cyclophosphamide dose reduction is required in cases of significant renal impairment (*see* Appendix 2).
- Keep a close eye on the cumulative dose of doxorubicin, and alert the prescriber if this exceeds 450 mg/m^2. It is especially important when a patient starts a course of treatment to check the pharmacy records and the patient's notes to see whether they have received previous anthracycline therapy at your hospital or elsewhere.
- The dose of cyclophosphamide is below that which is likely to cause urothelial toxicity. Therefore prophylactic mesna, IV hydration and urine testing are not required.
- Small-cell lung cancer can be very sensitive to chemotherapy, and massive tumour lysis may occur at the start of treatment. This can result in the release of large amounts of insoluble uric acid, which may precipitate in the kidneys, causing renal damage. To prevent this, treatment with allopurinol (300 mg each morning) is often used. This should be commenced the day before cytotoxic treatment and continued for as long as a significant chemosensitive tumour bulk remains. Check that consideration has been given to the use of allopurinol in patients starting treatment for the first time. The allopurinol dose should be reduced in patients with renal impairment.

SOURCE MATERIAL

- Roth BJ, Johnson DH, Einhorn LH *et al.* (1992) Randomized study of cyclophosphamide, doxorubicin and vincristine versus etoposide and cisplatin versus alternation of these two regimens in extensive small-cell lung cancer: a phase III trial of the Southeastern Cancer Study Group. *J Clin Oncol.* **10**: 282–91.

Chlorambucil with or without prednisolone

USUAL INDICATION

Low-grade lymphoma and chronic lymphocytic leukaemia.

DOSES

Chlorambucil 10 mg by mouth once daily for 10 days

In cases complicated by autoimmune reactions such as idiopathic thrombocytopenic purpura (ITP) or autoimmune haemolytic anaemia, the following may be added:

Prednisolone 40 mg by mouth once daily for 10 days.

Note: These doses are total doses and do not need to be multiplied by patient body surface area.

Although these doses are preferred in the author's own hospital, there are many variations on this regimen.

ADMINISTRATION

Both drugs in this regimen are given orally. Although soluble prednisolone tablets are available, chlorambucil is only available in a solid tablet formulation, so this regimen is only suitable for patients who are able to swallow tablets.

ANTI-EMETICS

Low emetogenic potential (see local policy).

CYCLE LENGTH

28 days.

NUMBER OF CYCLES

Remission plus 2; usually 6 in responders.

SIDE-EFFECTS

Bone-marrow suppression, nausea and vomiting, mucositis, interstitial pulmonary fibrosis (rarely, and usually after prolonged administration). Skin rashes (rarely, Stevens–Johnson syndrome), peripheral neuropathy, liver damage, chemical cystitis. Also typical side-effects of systemic steroid treatment, namely proximal myopathy, adrenal insufficiency, fluid and sodium retention, potassium loss, osteoporosis, cataracts, peptic ulceration, mental disturbances and glucose intolerance.

BLOOD NADIR

Because chlorambucil is given as a prolonged course, a discrete nadir may not be seen and the timing of any nadir is difficult to predict, but it may occur up to 10 days after stopping treatment.

TTOS REQUIRED

- Anti-emetics appropriate to weakly emetogenic chemotherapy.
- The drugs themselves.

NOTES FOR PRESCRIBERS

- Ensure that you are clear whether or not it is intended that the patient should receive prednisolone.
- Check the FBC prior to giving the go-ahead for chemotherapy. Seek advice if the neutrophil count is $<1.5 \times 10^9$/L or the platelet count is $<100 \times 10^9$/L at the time of treatment.
- Renal function should be assessed (formal measurement is not required) at the start of treatment. Individuals with impaired renal function may be more prone to myelosuppression, and should be monitored especially carefully during treatment (*see* Appendix 2 for further advice).
- Hepatic function should be assessed at the start of treatment, and consideration should be given to dose reduction in individuals with grossly abnormal hepatic function (*see* Appendix 1 for further advice).
- The possibility of drug-induced peripheral neuropathy should be considered in patients who report abnormal sensation.
- Prescribing the prednisolone dose to be taken in the morning may help to prevent problems with night-time wakefulness.
- All prescriptions for oral cytotoxic agents, including chlorambucil, should be for a finite period. This should be clearly indicated on any prescription or drug chart. It should also be explained to the patient, in order to prevent them seeking further supplies from their GP. In addition, it should be mentioned in communications with GPs. Similar precautions should also be taken with the short course of prednisolone.
Failure to take these precautions has resulted in inadvertent continuation of treatment and patient fatalities.

NOTES FOR NURSES

- When discussing treatment with the patient, it is important to check that they understand that the treatment course is for 10 days only. They should receive a 10-day course of tablets from the hospital and should *not* need to obtain more from their GP, except as part of a *formal* shared-care arrangement.
- Ensure that any diabetic patients are aware of the need to be extra vigilant about monitoring their blood sugar level during treatment with prednisolone, and advise them to contact their doctor if they have problems with regard to control of their blood sugar level.

NOTES FOR PHARMACISTS

- Ensure that you are clear whether or not it is intended that the patient should receive prednisolone.
- Check that the FBC has been determined and is within acceptable limits before dispensing.
- Check that renal and hepatic function are not grossly abnormal before dispensing. Consideration should be given to dose reduction in the case of severe impairment of either system (*see* Appendices 1 and 2 for further advice).
- Check that anti-emetics appropriate to weakly emetogenic chemotherapy have been prescribed according to local protocol.
- Check that chlorambucil and prednisolone packs are labelled with the treatment duration and/or stop dates and that, where possible, the patient has been told not to obtain further supplies from their GP.

SOURCE MATERIAL

The regimen described above is the one preferred locally. A huge variety of different regimens have been used over the years, and it is almost impossible to reference any one of them as standard. For further recommendations on dosing the reader should consult, among other sources, the manufacturer's product literature.

CHOP (cyclophosphamide, doxorubicin [hydroxydaunorubicin], vincristine [Oncovin®], prednisolone)

USUAL INDICATION

High-grade non-Hodgkin's lymphoma.

DOSES

Doxorubicin 50 mg/m^2 IV on day 1
Cyclophosphamide 750 mg/m^2 IV on day 1
Vincristine 1.4 mg/m^2 (maximum 2 mg; some prescribers use a maximum dose of 1.5 mg in patients over 70 years of age because of a perceived increased risk of peripheral neuropathy, although the evidence for this approach is scarce) IV on day 1
Prednisolone 100 mg by mouth on days 1–5

Note: In the original trials with this regimen prednisone was used, but in the UK this is replaced by prednisolone at the same dose.

ADMINISTRATION

Doxorubicin and vincristine

By slow IV injection into the side-arm of a free-running saline drip.

Doxorubicin and vincristine are powerful vesicants and should be administered with appropriate precautions to prevent extravasation. If there is any possibility that extravasation has occurred, contact a senior member of the medical team immediately and follow local guidance on dealing with cytotoxic extravasation.

Cyclophosphamide

May be given as a slow IV bolus injection or a short IV infusion (i.e. in 100 mL of saline over a period of 10–20 min).

Note: The order of administration of the three IV drugs in this regimen is not critical.

ANTI-EMETICS

High emetogenic potential (follow local policy, although it should be noted that because of the high dose of prednisolone on days 1–5, no additional oral steroid is needed for anti-emetic purposes).

CYCLE LENGTH

21 days.

NUMBER OF CYCLES

Depends on the disease stage. Usually for Stage I disease, 4 cycles with or without radiotherapy to local disease, and for Stage II–IV disease, 6–8 cycles.

SIDE-EFFECTS

Bone-marrow suppression, alopecia, nausea and vomiting, mucositis, cardiac arrhythmias, dilated cardiomyopathy (especially at cumulative doxorubicin doses in excess of $450\,mg/m^2$), peripheral neuropathy from vincristine. Cyclophosphamide *can* cause haemorrhagic cystitis at high doses. However, the doses used in CHOP are not likely to give rise to this problem, so prophylactic mesna or hydration are not required.

The high doses of prednisolone used in this regimen can cause a variety of steroid side-effects, including euphoria/depression, epigastric discomfort, glucose intolerance, insomnia, psychosis, proximal myopathy, sodium and water retention and potassium loss.

BLOOD NADIR

10 days.

TTOS REQUIRED

- Anti-emetics appropriate to highly emetogenic chemotherapy (according to local policy), although additional oral steroids are not required, as the prednisolone in the regimen should be sufficient.
- Allopurinol 300 mg each morning (reduced in cases of renal impairment) to prevent tumour lysis syndrome, especially early in treatment when there is a large tumour bulk.

NOTES FOR PRESCRIBERS

- Patients over 60 years of age or with a history of heart disease must have an echocardiogram or MUGA scan prior to treatment to ensure that there is adequate left ventricular function.
- Check the FBC prior to giving the go-ahead for chemotherapy. Seek advice if the neutrophil count is $<1.5 \times 10^9$/L or the platelet count is $<100 \times 10^9$/L. In an early report on the use of CHOP,[1] doses were reduced by 'at least 20%' if the white

---

[1] McKelvey EM, Gottlieb JA, Wilson HE *et al.* (1976) Hydroxydannomycin (Adriamycin) combination chemotherapy in malignant lymphoma. *Cancer.* **38**: 1484–93.

blood cell count was $<1.5 \times 10^9$/L or the platelet count was $<50 \times 10^9$/L, with apparently acceptable results. Note that because treatment is being given with curative intent, it may proceed on a lower count than would be acceptable for palliative regimens.

- Check the LFTs. If these show serious impairment, a reduction in doxorubicin and vincristine doses may be required (*see* Appendix 1).
- Check the renal function. A cyclophosphamide dose reduction is required in cases of significant renal impairment (*see* Appendix 2).
- This is a potentially curative treatment, and it is important to maintain dose intensity. Dose delays should be avoided if at all possible. Therefore the use of haematopoietic growth factors (G-CSF or GM-CSF) to support neutrophil numbers may be justified. Dosage should be in accordance with local policy on haematopoietic growth factor use.
- Vincristine can cause peripheral neuropathy. The patient should be questioned about abnormal sensations, jaw pain or constipation that may be indicative of neuropathy. Discuss any such symptoms with an experienced prescriber with a view to dose modification or switching to vinblastine. The latter appears to be more myelosuppressive but less neurotoxic.
- To limit the potential for neurotoxicity, the dose of vincristine is usually capped at 2 mg. This limit should be exceeded only with caution and after discussion with a senior member of the medical team.
- Lymphomas are very sensitive to chemotherapy, and massive tumour lysis is possible at the start of chemotherapy. This can result in the generation of large amounts of insoluble uric acid that are capable of precipitating in the kidneys, causing renal damage. To prevent this, allopurinol 300 mg once daily should be commenced the day before starting cytotoxic therapy and continued for as long as there is significant tumour bulk remaining and cytotoxic therapy continues. Allopurinol doses should be reduced in patients with impaired renal function.
- Prophylactic H_2-antagonists or other gastroprotective agents may be justified during high-dose prednisolone courses, especially when platelet counts have been reduced as a consequence of chemotherapy.
- Prior to treatment, hair loss should be discussed with the patient. Scalp cooling is of limited benefit in preventing hair loss with CHOP, because of the prolonged half-life of cyclophosphamide. Liaise with the nurses with regard to referral to a wig-fitter at the start of treatment, before alopecia is evident, if this is appropriate.
- If administering drugs, *see* Administration section above for notes on the vesicant nature of doxorubicin and vincristine.
- Make sure that it is stated clearly on any prescription or in any communication with the patient's GP that the prednisolone treatment is a short course of 5 days only. *Fatalities have resulted from the inadvertent continuation of short courses of steroids.*

NOTES FOR NURSES

- Prior to treatment, hair loss should be discussed with the patient. Scalp cooling is of limited value because of the prolonged circulation time of cyclophosphamide. If appropriate, referral to a wig-fitter should be made at the start of treatment, before alopecia is evident.

- If administering drugs, *see* Administration section above for notes on the vesicant nature of doxorubicin and vincristine.
- The dose of cyclophosphamide is lower than that which is likely to cause haemorrhagic cystitis. Therefore prophylactic mesna, IV hydration and urine testing are not required. Any symptoms of mild dysuria may be treated by encouraging oral fluid intake and regular voiding of urine.
- Ensure that any diabetic patients are aware of the need to be extra vigilant about monitoring their blood sugar concentration during treatment with prednisolone, and advise them to contact their doctor if they have problems with the control of their blood sugar levels.
- If you are issuing prednisolone tablets to patients, explain to them that these should be taken for 5 days only, and that they should not attempt to obtain further supplies from their GP. *Fatalities have resulted from the inadvertent continuation of short courses of steroids.*

NOTES FOR PHARMACISTS

- Check that the FBC has been determined and is within acceptable limits before issuing chemotherapy. Because this is a potentially curative treatment, it is reasonable to treat on a somewhat lower neutrophil/platelet count than would be considered acceptable for a palliative regimen.
- This is a potentially curative treatment, and it is important to maintain dose intensity. Dose delays should be avoided if at all possible. Therefore this is one regimen where the use of haematopoietic growth factors (G-CSF, GM-CSF) may be justified. This should be in accordance with your local policy on haematopoietic growth factor use.
- Check the LFTs. If these show serious impairment, a reduction in doxorubicin and vincristine doses may be required (*see* Appendix 1).
- Check the renal function. A cyclophosphamide dose reduction is required in cases of significant renal impairment (*see* Appendix 2).
- Check that the usual maximum dose for vincristine (i.e. 2 mg) has not been exceeded. If it has, confirm with the prescriber that this was intended.
- Check that anti-emetics appropriate to highly emetogenic chemotherapy have been prescribed according to protocol. However, because CHOP incorporates 5 days of high-dose prednisolone, additional oral steroids are not required.
- Lymphomas are very sensitive to chemotherapy, and massive tumour lysis is possible at the start of chemotherapy. This can result in the generation of large amounts of insoluble uric acid, which are capable of precipitating in the kidneys, causing renal damage. To prevent this, allopurinol 300 mg once daily should be commenced the day before starting cytotoxic therapy, and should be continued for as long as there is significant tumour present and cytotoxic treatment continues. Allopurinol doses should be reduced in patients with renal impairment.
- Keep a close eye on the cumulative doxorubicin dose, and alert the prescriber if it exceeds 450 mg/m^2. It is especially important when a patient starts a course of treatment to check their medical notes and any pharmacy records to see whether they have received previous anthracycline therapy within your hospital or elsewhere.

- The dose of cyclophosphamide is lower than that which is likely to cause urothelial toxicity. Therefore prophylactic mesna, IV hydration and urine testing are not required.
- Make sure that it is stated clearly on any discharge prescription or prescription being sent elsewhere for dispensing that the prednisolone treatment is a short course of 5 days only. *Fatalities have resulted from the inadvertent continuation of short courses of steroids.* This drug should not be continued by the GP, nor is routine 'tailing off' of doses necessary.

SOURCE MATERIAL

- McKelvey EM, Gottlieb JA, Wilson HE *et al.* (1976) Hydroxydaunomycin (Adriamycin) combination chemotherapy in malignant lymphoma. *Cancer.* **38**: 1484–93.

Cisplatin (single-agent)

USUAL INDICATION

This regimen is not a standard treatment for any common tumour, but has been used in a variety of situations, especially where combination therapy is contraindicated for any reason. Most solid tumours are sensitive to cisplatin to some degree. Non-small-cell lung and ovarian cancers are among those for which cisplatin monotherapy has been used.

DOSES

There is no standard dose. However, when this regimen is used empirically, doses of 60–100 mg/m^2 (maximum 120 mg/m^2) every 3 weeks are usually employed. Treatment can be delivered as a single infusion or fractionated over several days. Doses exceeding 100 mg/m^2 should not be prescribed without reference to a specific protocol or seeking expert advice.

ADMINISTRATION

As an infusion in saline, typically in 1 L over 2 h, after pre-hydration with 1 L of saline and followed by intensive post-hydration with a further 2 L of saline. To facilitate outpatient treatment, IV post-hydration is sometimes restricted to 1 L, with the patient being instructed to drink a further 3 L over the following 24 h. The degree of hydration should reflect the dose of cisplatin, but that suggested is suitable for the typical dose range of 50–75 mg/m^2. Cisplatin is nephrotoxic, and the hydration is mandatory to dilute the drug as it is excreted via the kidneys, in order to minimise renal toxicity. The aim of hydration is to maintain a urine output of 100 mL/h during and for 6–8 h after cisplatin administration. Mannitol is often given to ensure that fluid output is brisk. Electrolytes are added to compensate for cisplatin-induced electrolyte wasting.

ANTI-EMETICS

High emetogenic potential (follow local policy).

CYCLE LENGTH

21 days.

NUMBER OF CYCLES

Usually 6.

SIDE-EFFECTS

Nephrotoxicity (dose limiting), bone-marrow suppression (all blood components are affected, but seldom dose limiting), alopecia (rarely extensive), nausea and vomiting (may be very severe), sensory motor and occasionally autonomic neuropathy (sometimes irreversible) including significant potential for ototoxicity, mucositis (not usually serious).

TTOS REQUIRED

- Anti-emetics appropriate to highly emetogenic chemotherapy.

NOTES FOR PRESCRIBERS

Before each course

- Check the FBC prior to giving the go-ahead for chemotherapy. Seek advice if the neutrophil count is $<1.5 \times 10^9$/L or the platelet count is $<100 \times 10^9$/L at the time of treatment.
- Renal function should be formally assessed at the start of treatment. Ideally this should be done by EDTA clearance, but estimation of CrCl from the serum creatinine concentration using the Cockcroft–Gault equation is acceptable if the patient has a stable creatinine concentration and no confounding factors (e.g. catabolic states):

CrCl (mL/min)

$$= \frac{1.04 \text{ (females) or } 1.23 \text{ (males)} \times (140 - \text{age in years}) \times \text{weight in kg}}{\text{serum creatinine concentration } (\mu\text{mol/L})}.$$

On subsequent cycles the renal function should be reassessed.

Doses *must be reduced* if the creatinine clearance drops below 60 mL/min (*see* Appendix 2).

- Check the electrolytes for cisplatin-induced wasting, especially of magnesium, calcium and potassium. Additional supplementation may be required.
- Ensure that anti-emetics suitable for highly emetogenic chemotherapy are prescribed according to local policy before chemotherapy begins.
- Seek further advice if the patient reports symptoms indicative of neurotoxicity (parasthesias, difficulty with motor control) or ototoxicity (tinitus, deafness).

On the day after each cisplatin dose

- For patients who are being treated as inpatients, measure the fluid balance/body weight. In general, if the patient has gained 1.5 L/kg since starting hydration, extra diuresis will be required (e.g. furosemide 20–40 mg by mouth).

NOTES FOR NURSES

- The aim of hydration is to ensure an average urine output of 100 mL/h or more during and for 6–8 h after cisplatin administration. Any patient who is being treated as an inpatient should be on a fluid-balance chart, and daily weights should be recorded. Contact the prescriber if the patient's urine output is inadequate or their body weight increases by 1.5 kg from baseline.

  For outpatients, efforts should be made to ensure that urine output is adequate (e.g. by ensuring that the patient has passed 500 mL of urine between the start of IV hydration and the beginning of cisplatin infusion).

  Outpatients should also be encouraged to drink 3 L of fluid in the 24 h following each period of IV hydration, and to contact the hospital if this is impossible because of nausea/vomiting or other problems.

NOTES FOR PHARMACISTS

On the day of cisplatin treatment

- Check that the FBC has been determined and is within acceptable limits before issuing chemotherapy.
- Check that the renal function has been measured/calculated at the start of treatment. Record the CrCl and the corresponding creatinine concentration on any pharmacy patient record (*see* Appendix 3 for an example). Recalculate the CrCl if the creatinine concentration changes. Doses *must be reduced* if the creatinine clearance drops below 60 mL/min (*see* Appendix 2 for further guidance).
- Check that anti-emetics appropriate to highly emetogenic chemotherapy have been prescribed according to local protocol, to start prior to chemotherapy administration.

On the day after cisplatin treatment

- When visiting the ward, check that any patient who is receiving cisplatin on an inpatient basis has not gained more than 1.5 L/kg since the start of treatment. If they have, discuss additional diuresis with the prescriber (if this measure has not already been instituted).

CMF (cyclophosphamide, methotrexate, 5-fluorouracil)

Note: There are many variants of CMF. Two of the most widely used and best supported by evidence are described here. Make sure that you know which is required, especially if the patient is in a trial, in which case something different again may be required.

USUAL INDICATION

Adjuvant treatment of surgically resected breast cancer and palliative treatment of recurrent or inoperable breast cancer, especially in patients who are unsuitable for anthracycline therapy.

DOSES

Cyclophosphamide 100 mg/m^2 by mouth daily for 14 days

or

Cyclophosphamide 600 mg/m^2 IV on days 1 and 8

plus

Methotrexate 40 mg/m^2 IV on days 1 and 8
5-Fluorouracil 600 mg/m^2 IV on days 1 and 8

Cyclophosphamide tablets are only available in 50 mg strength, and are unscored. Therefore the smallest daily dose increment that can be achieved is 50 mg. However, a 25 mg dose increment can effectively be achieved by giving different doses on alternate days (e.g administering 150 mg and 200 mg on alternate days gives a mean daily dose of 175 mg).

ADMINISTRATION

By IV injection or short IV infusions (10–15 min). The administration sequence is not critical.

ANTI-EMETICS

Oral cyclophosphamide

Low emetogenic potential (see local policy). Oral cyclophosphamide can sometimes cause an unpleasant feeling of 'churning' in the stomach, which seems to be a manifestation of gastritis, and may respond better to H$_2$-antagonists than to anti-emetics.

IV cyclophosphamide

Moderate emetogenic potential (see local policy).

CYCLE LENGTH

28 days.

NUMBER OF CYCLES

Usually 6.

SIDE-EFFECTS

Bone-marrow suppression, alopecia (usually moderate hair thinning), amenorrhoea, nausea and vomiting, mucositis, chemical cystitis due to cyclophosphamide (although at the doses used this is likely to present as urinary discomfort rather than haemorrhagic cystitis, so IV hydration, urine testing and concurrent mesna are not required).

BLOOD NADIR

The pattern of treatment in CMF is such that discrete nadirs may not be seen. In addition, the pattern of myelosuppression will depend on precisely which CMF regimen is used.

TTOS REQUIRED

- Anti-emetics appropriate to moderately emetogenic chemotherapy with IV CMF and appropriate to weakly emetogenic chemotherapy with 'oral' CMF should be given according to local protocols (*see* Anti-emetics section for note on use of H_2-antagonists with 'oral' CMF).
- Folinic acid (calcium folinate/calcium leucovorin) 'rescue' is not routinely required with the doses of methotrexate that are used in CMF. If it is used because of unexpected toxicity on previous courses, or because a patient has a 'third-space' fluid collection (e.g. ascites, effusion or extensive oedema) or renal impairment, a reasonable dose is 15 mg by mouth 6-hourly × 6 doses *starting 24 h after methotrexate*. Starting earlier negates the effects of methotrexate.

NOTES FOR PRESCRIBERS

- Make sure that you know whether the IV or 'oral' regimen is intended. Check with a senior member of the medical team if you are in doubt.
- Renal function should be checked before the start of treatment and before each course. In patients who have a stable serum creatinine concentration and no

confounding factors (e.g. catabolic states), it is reasonable to calculate the creatinine clearance from serum creatinine concentration using the Cockcroft–Gault equation as follows:

CrCl (mL/min)

$$= \frac{1.04 \text{ (females) or } 1.23 \text{ (males)} \times (140 - \text{age in years}) \times \text{weight in kg}}{\text{serum creatinine concentration } (\mu mol/L)}.$$

Consideration should be given to reducing the methotrexate dose if the CrCl falls below 80 mL/min, and to reducing the cyclophosphamide dose if the CrCl falls below 50 mL/min (*see* Appendix 2 for further guidance).

- Check the LFTs before the start of treatment or, if hepatic impairment is anticipated, at any point during treatment. Consideration should be given to dose reductions in patients with moderate to severe hepatic impairment (*see* Appendix 1 for further guidance).
- Check the FBC prior to giving the go-ahead for chemotherapy. Seek advice if the neutrophil count is <1.5 × 10⁹/L or the platelet count is <100 × 10⁹/L. In an early study of *oral* CMF,[1] the following dose reductions were used: white cell count 2.5–3.99 × 10⁹/L or platelet count 75–129 × 10⁹/L, reduce dose by 50%; white cell count <2.5 × 10⁹/L or platelet count <75 × 10⁹/L, delay treatment pending recovery. However, it should be noted that there is now greater experience of the administration of cytotoxic chemotherapy, and clinicians are likely to be somewhat less cautious than these reductions imply.
- Discuss alopecia with the patient prior to starting treatment. Hair loss with CMF is usually moderate, resulting in some hair thinning. For this reason, and also because of the prolonged half-life of methotrexate and cyclophosphamide, scalp cooling cannot be recommended with CMF.
- If the patient has a 'third-space' fluid collection (ascites, effusion or extensive oedema), this may prolong the elimination of methotrexate, enhancing its toxicity. Consider folinic acid rescue in such cases (discuss this with an experienced prescriber). If this measure is to be used, make sure that it is charted to start 24 h *after* methotrexate, as folinic acid administered any earlier will negate the effect of methotrexate as well as its toxicity.
- Cyclophosphamide at the doses used should not cause serious urothelial toxicity. Mesna, urine testing and IV hydration are not required. If mild symptoms of dysuria do develop, encourage the patient to increase their oral fluid intake, to void urine regularly and (where appropriate) to take cyclophosphamide tablets early in the day rather than late in order to avoid the accumulation of toxic metabolites in the bladder overnight.
- There is no oral liquid formulation of cyclophosphamide. Patients who are unable to swallow tablets should be treated with the IV regimen.
- For patients who are receiving oral cyclophosphamide, prescriptions should be for an entire 14-day cycle of treatment. Any prescription should state clearly the duration of treatment, as should any communication with GPs. *Fatalities have resulted from the inadvertent continuation of short courses of oral chemotherapy.*

---

[1] Bonadonna G, Brusamoline E, Valagussa P *et al.* (1976) Combination chemotherapy as an adjuvant treatment in operable breast cancer. *NEJM.* **294**: 405–10.

NOTES FOR NURSES

- If you are counselling patients who are receiving oral chemotherapy about their treatment, check that they understand that each cycle of treatment should last for 14 days only, and that 14 days after starting treatment they should stop taking their tablets, *even if they have some left over*. It is important that they do not seek continuation supplies from their GP. *Fatalities have resulted from the inadvertent continuation of short courses of oral chemotherapy.*
- Discuss hair loss with the patient prior to starting treatment. With CMF this is generally restricted to modest hair thinning rather than extensive hair loss. For this reason, and also because of the prolonged circulation of methotrexate and cyclophosphamide, scalp cooling is not appropriate with CMF.
- If the patient is prescribed folinic acid (calcium folinate/calcium leucovorin), it should be prescribed to *start 24 h after methotrexate*. Folinic acid given any earlier will negate the effect of methotrexate as well as its toxicity. If it is charted to start 24 h after methotrexate, do not give it before. If the start time is not specified, check with the prescriber/pharmacist.
- Cyclophosphamide at the doses used should not cause serious urothelial toxicity. Urine testing, mesna administration and IV hydration are not required. If mild symptoms of dysuria do develop, encourage the patient to increase their oral fluid intake, to void urine regularly and (where appropriate) to take cyclophosphamide tablets early in the day rather than late in order to avoid the accumulation of toxic metabolites in the bladder overnight.

NOTES FOR PHARMACISTS

- Check that the FBC has been determined and is within acceptable limits before issuing chemotherapy. Patients receiving day 8 IV therapy are seldom delayed for low blood counts, and treatment can probably be prepared on the assumption that they will be treated. This will speed patient treatment and is unlikely to lead to significant drug wastage.
- Methotrexate and cyclophosphamide are renally excreted and may require dose modification in cases of renal impairment (CrCl of <80 mL/min and <50 mL/min, respectively) (*see* Appendix 2 for further guidance). On the first cycle of treatment the renal function should be measured or estimated using the Cockcroft–Gault equation. The CrCl together with the corresponding serum creatinine concentration should be entered on any pharmacy patient record (*see* Appendix 3 for an example). On subsequent courses the CrCl should be remeasured/recalculated if there is a significant rise in serum creatinine levels.
- Check the LFTs before the start of treatment or, if hepatic impairment is anticipated, at any point during treatment. Consideration should be given to dose reductions in patients with moderate to severe hepatic impairment (*see* Appendix 1 for further guidance).
- Folinic acid (calcium folinate/calcium leucovorin) rescue is not routinely required. However, if it is used (e.g. in patients with unexpected toxicity on a previous course or 'third-space' fluid collection such as ascites, effusion or oedema), it should be prescribed to start 24 h after methotrexate. If it is given any earlier it will negate the effect of methotrexate as well as its toxicity. If it is charted to

start 24 h after methotrexate, block out any earlier spaces on the drug chart/ endorse any discharge prescription clearly and/or add this instruction to the bottle label. If the start time is not specified, check with the prescriber.

If a patient *does* receive folinic acid with their CMF, make a note of this (together with the reason) on any pharmacy patient record to ensure that they do not miss out on future courses.

- 'Third-space' fluid collections (e.g. ascites, effusions, gross oedema) and renal impairment significantly prolong the half-life of methotrexate, increasing its toxicity. If you know that a patient has such a fluid collection, ask the prescriber whether folinic acid rescue is required (*see* TTO section above for further details).

- Cyclophosphamide at the doses used should not cause significant urothelial toxicity. Urine testing, mesna administration and IV hydration are not required. If mild symptoms of dysuria do develop, they may be alleviated by encouraging the patient to increase oral fluid intake, to void urine regularly and (where appropriate) to take cyclophosphamide tablets early in the day rather than late in order to avoid the accumulation of toxic metabolites in the bladder overnight.

- The smallest dose increment that can be achieved with cyclophosphamide tablets is 50 mg. However, by using different doses on alternate days (*see* Dose section above), an effective increment of 25 mg can be achieved. In general, requests for extemporaneous cyclophosphamide mixtures to allow more exact dosing are not justified and should be resisted. Patients who are unable to swallow tablets should be treated with IV CMF.

- If you are counselling a patient who is receiving oral cyclophosphamide about their treatment, check that they understand that each cycle of treatment should last for 14 days only, and that 14 days after starting treatment they should stop taking their tablets, *even if they have some left over*. It is important that they do not seek continuation supplies from their GP, unless a formal 'shared-care' agreement is in place. *Fatalities have resulted from the inadvertent continuation of short courses of oral chemotherapy.*

SOURCE MATERIAL

'Oral' regimen

- Bonadonna G, Brusamoline E, Valagussa P *et al.* (1976) Combination chemotherapy as an adjuvant treatment in operable breast cancer. *NEJM.* **294**: 405–10.

IV regimen

- Bonadonna G, Valagussa P, Moliterni A *et al.* (1990) Milan adjuvant and neo-adjuvant studies in Stage I and II resectable breast cancer. In ES Salmon (ed.) *Adjuvant Therapy of Cancer VI.* WB Saunders, Philadelphia, PA.

COP-X (cyclophosphamide, vincristine [Oncovin®], prednisolone, liposomal daunorubicin [DaunoXome®])

USUAL INDICATION

Relapsed high-grade non-Hodgkin's lymphoma.

Note: This regimen is currently mainly used in clinical trials. Trial protocols must take precedence over these notes for the purposes of prescribing, dose modification, etc.

DOSES

Liposomal daunorubicin (DaunoXome®) 100 mg/m^2 IV on day 1
Cyclophosphamide 750 mg/m^2 IV on day 1
Vincristine 1.4 mg/m^2 (maximum 2 mg) IV on day 1
Prednisolone 100 mg by mouth on days 1–5

ADMINISTRATION

Liposomal daunorubicin

By infusion in 5% dextrose over a period of 2 h. Infusion times can be extended if infusion-related side-effects (e.g. back pain) are a problem.

Vincristine

By slow IV injection into the side-arm of a free-running saline drip.

Vincristine is a powerful vesicant and should be administered with appropriate precautions to prevent extravasation. Although conventional daunorubicin is also a potent vesicant, the liposomal formulation appears to substantially reduce its potential for causing tissue necrosis. However, extravasation of this drug should still be treated seriously. If there is any possibility that extravasation of either agent has occurred, contact a senior member of the medical team and follow local policy for the management of extravasation of cytotoxic drugs.

Cyclophosphamide

May be given as a slow IV bolus injection or short IV infusion in 100 mL of 0.9% sodium chloride over a period of 10–20 min.

Note: The order of administration of the three IV drugs in this regimen is not critical.

ANTI-EMETICS

High emetogenic potential (follow local policy, but note that because of the high dose of prednisolone on days 1–5, no additional oral steroids are needed).

CYCLE LENGTH

21 days.

NUMBER OF CYCLES

Usually 6–8 courses, but care must be taken not to exceed a safe cumulative dose of anthracycline (most recipients will already have received previous anthracycline-based treatment).

SIDE-EFFECTS

Bone-marrow suppression, alopecia, nausea and vomiting, mucositis, cardiac arrhythmias and dilated cardiomyopathy from daunorubicin (see note below on cumulative anthracycline doses), peripheral neuropathy from vincristine. Liposomal formulations such as DaunoXome® are sometimes associated with infusion-related reactions, including back pain, flushing, chest tightness and hypotension. Cyclophosphamide *can* cause haemorrhagic cystitis at high doses. However, the doses used in COP-X are not likely to cause this problem, so prophylactic mesna, hydration or urine testing are not required.

The high doses of prednisolone used in this regimen can produce a variety of steroid side-effects, including euphoria/depression, epigastric discomfort, glucose intolerance, insomnia, psychosis, fluid and sodium retention, proximal myopathy and potassium loss.

BLOOD NADIR

10 days.

TTOS REQUIRED

- Anti-emetics appropriate to highly emetogenic chemotherapy (according to standard protocol), but without oral dexamethasone (the prednisolone in the regimen should be sufficient).
- Allopurinol 300 mg each morning (reduced in renal impairment) to prevent tumour lysis syndrome, especially early in treatment when there is a large tumour bulk.

NOTES FOR PRESCRIBERS

- Patients over 60 years of age, or with a history of heart disease or who have received a cumulative dose of 400 mg/m² daunorubicin or equivalent anthracyclines (e.g. 450 mg/m^2 doxorubicin) must have an echocardiogram or MUGA scan prior to treatment to ensure that there is adequate left ventricular function.

- Because of its cumulative cardiotoxicity, the manufacturer of liposomal daunorubicin recommends that the left ventricular ejection fraction should be measured after a cumulative dose of 320 mg/m^2, and at intervals of 160 mg/m^2 thereafter. Following this recommendation is not particularly onerous at the smaller doses used in its licensed indication (AIDS-related Kaposi's sarcoma). In clinical trials it has been recommended that an echocardiogram should be performed every other cycle for the first six cycles and then after every cycle. Overall, it is probably reasonable to assess left ventricular function formally after the third or fourth cycle, and after every two cycles thereafter, provided that no evidence of declining function is seen, in which case more frequent monitoring may be appropriate. It is important to take into consideration the contribution of anthracycline treatment (e.g. daunorubicin, doxorubicin, idarubicin, DaunoXome®, Caelyx®) that the patient may have received previously.
- Check the FBC prior to giving the go-ahead for chemotherapy. Dose reductions should be considered if the neutrophil count is <2.0 × 10^9/L or the platelet count is <100 × 10^9/L. The following dose reductions have been used in clinical trials:

Neutrophils ($\times 10^9$/L)		Platelets ($\times 10^9$/L)	Cyclophosphamide dose (%)	DaunoXome® dose (%)
>2.0	and	>100	100	100
1.5–1.9	and	>100	75	75
1.0–1.4	or	50–99	50	50
<1.0	or	<50	0	0

- Vincristine can cause peripheral neuropathy. The patient should be questioned about abnormal sensations, jaw pain or constipation, any of which may be indicative of neuropathy. If such symptoms are reported, discuss them with a senior member of the medical team with a view to dose modification or switching to vinblastine, which appears to be more myelosuppressive but less neurotoxic.
- Lymphomas are very sensitive to chemotherapy, and massive tumour lysis is possible at the start of chemotherapy. This can result in the generation of large amounts of insoluble uric acid, which is capable of precipitating in the kidneys, causing renal damage. To prevent this, allopurinol 300 mg once daily (reduced dose in cases of renal impairment) should be commenced the day before starting cytotoxic therapy and continued for as long as there is significant tumour bulk remaining and cytotoxic therapy continues.
- Prophylactic H$_2$-antagonists or other gastroprotective agents may be justified during prednisolone treatment, especially if platelet counts have been reduced as a consequence of previous chemotherapy.
- Check the LFTs. If these show serious impairment, then a reduction in liposomal daunorubicin and vincristine doses may be required (*see* Appendix 1 for further guidance).

- Check the renal function. Provided that the patient has a stable serum creatinine concentration and no confounding factors (e.g. catabolic state), estimation of the CrCl from serum creatinine levels using the Cockcroft–Gault equation is adequate:

CrCl (mL/min)

$$= \frac{1.04 \text{ (females) or } 1.23 \text{ (males)} \times (140 - \text{age in years}) \times \text{weight in kg}}{\text{serum creatinine concentration } (\mu\text{mol/L})}.$$

A cyclophosphamide dose reduction is required in cases of significant renal impairment (*see* Appendix 2 for further guidance). The dose of allopurinol (when used) should also be reduced in patients with renal impairment.

- Prior to treatment, hair loss should be discussed with the patient. Scalp cooling is likely to be of limited benefit in preventing hair loss with COP-X, because of the prolonged half-life of cyclophosphamide and liposomal daunorubicin. Liaise with the nurses with regard to referral to a wig-fitter at the start of treatment and before alopecia is evident, if this is appropriate.
- If administering the drugs, *see* Administration section above for notes on the vesicant nature of vincristine and, possibly, liposomal daunorubicin.
- This protocol is currently mainly used within clinical trials. For such patients, mark all prescriptions clearly with the trial protocol number and any patient number. For these patients the relevant trial protocol must be consulted and takes precedence over any guidance that is given here.
- State clearly on any prescription or in any communication with the patient's GP, or any prescription being sent elsewhere for dispensing, that the prednisolone is a short course of 5 days only. *Fatalities have resulted from the inadvertant continuation of short courses of steroids.*

NOTES FOR NURSES

- Prior to treatment, hair loss should be discussed with the patient. Scalp cooling is unlikely to be of much benefit because of the prolonged circulation of cyclophosphamide and liposomal daunorubicin. Where appropriate, referral to a wig-fitter should be made at the start of treatment and before alopecia is evident.
- If administering the drugs, *see* Administration section above for notes on the vesicant nature of vincristine and possibly liposomal daunorubicin.
- The dose of cyclophosphamide is below that which is likely to cause haemorrhagic cystitis. Therefore prophylactic mesna, IV hydration and urine testing are not required. Any mild symptoms of dysuria may be treated by encouraging oral fluid intake and regular voiding of urine.
- Liposomal daunorubicin is incompatible with saline. IV lines should be flushed with 5% dextrose before and after the infusion.
- Infusion-related reactions such as backache, flushing and shortness of breath can be controlled by slowing the infusion rate or temporarily interrupting the drug administration.
- Ensure that any diabetic patients are aware of the need to be extra vigilant about monitoring their blood sugar levels during treatment with prednisolone, and advise them to contact their doctor if they have problems with the control of their blood sugar levels.

- If issuing prednisolone tablets to the patient, explain to them that these should be taken for 5 days only, and that they should not attempt to obtain further supplies from their GP. *Fatalities have resulted from the inadvertent continuation of short courses of steroids.*

NOTES FOR PHARMACISTS

- Check that the FBC has been determined and is within acceptable limits before issuing chemotherapy. Because COP-X is usually used as a salvage regimen without curative intent, treatment in the case of low blood counts is likely to be more cautious than is the case with first-line lymphoma regimens such as CHOP. Similarly, supporting treatment with haematopoietic growth factors to maintain dose intensity is probably less justifiable and should not be considered automatically.
- Check the LFTs. If these show serious impairment, then a reduction in liposomal daunorubicin and vincristine doses may be required (*see* Appendix 1 for further guidance).
- Check the renal function. Provided that the patient has a stable serum creatinine concentration and no confounding factors (e.g. catabolic state), estimation of the CrCl from serum creatinine levels using the Cockcroft–Gault equation is adequate.

  Record the calculated CrCl on any pharmacy patient record (*see* Appendix 3 for an example), together with the serum creatinine concentration. On subsequent courses, the CrCl should be recalculated if the serum creatinine level changes significantly.

  A cyclophosphamide dose reduction is required in cases of significant renal impairment (*see* Appendix 2 for further guidance). The dose of allopurinol (when used) should also be reduced in patients with renal impairment.
- Check that the maximum dose for vincristine (i.e. 2 mg) has not been exceeded.
- Check that anti-emetics appropriate to highly emetogenic chemotherapy have been prescribed according to local protocol. However, because COP-X incorporates 5 days of high-dose prednisolone, additional oral steroids are not required.
- Lymphomas are very sensitive to chemotherapy, and massive tumour lysis is possible at the start of chemotherapy. This can result in the generation of large amounts of insoluble uric acid, which is capable of precipitating in the kidneys, causing renal damage. To prevent this, allopurinol 300 mg once daily (reduce dose in cases of renal impairment) should be commenced the day before starting cytotoxic therapy and continued for as long as there is significant tumour load.
- Monitor the total dose of liposomal daunorubicin administered. Alert the prescriber if this exceeds 320 mg/m^2 (unless there is evidence that cardiac function has been checked at this point and is acceptable). Thereafter, it is important that the left ventricular ejection fraction is checked regularly – after every alternate cycle of treatment is probably reasonable (*see* Notes for prescribers above). If you are unclear whether monitoring is being carried out or what the schedule is, discuss this with the appropriate member of the medical team. It is especially important when a patient starts a course of treatment to check the pharmacy records and patient notes to ascertain whether they have received previous therapy. The contribution of other anthracyclines should be considered (e.g. doxorubicin) (normal cumulative maximum dose 450 mg/m^2).

- The dose of cyclophosphamide is below that which is likely to cause urothelial toxicity. Therefore prophylactic mesna, IV hydration and urine testing are not required.
- Make sure that it is stated clearly on any discharge prescription or prescription being sent elsewhere for dispensing that the prednisolone is a short course of 5 days only. *Fatalities have resulted from the inadvertent continuation of short courses of steroids.* Prednisolone should not be continued by the GP, nor is routine 'tailing-off' of doses necessary.

SOURCE MATERIAL

- Nikitin EA, Iahnina EI, Pivik AV *et al.* (1997) *Treatment of primary aggressive lymphoma with liposomal daunorubicin (DaunoXome®) substitution in the CHOP regimen.* Abstract presented at the 39th Annual Meeting and Exposition of the American Society of Haematology, 5–9 December 1997, San Diego, CA.

CT (carboplatin plus paclitaxel [Taxol®])

USUAL INDICATION

First-line treatment of advanced ovarian cancer and inoperable non-small-cell lung cancer.

Note: The manufacturer of paclitaxel recommends its use in combination with cisplatin rather than carboplatin in the product SPC. However, in the UK it is much more frequently combined with carboplatin.

DOSES

Paclitaxel 175 mg/m² IV on day 1
Carboplatin IV on day 1 with dose based on renal function according to the
    following (Calvert) formula:

$$\text{dose (mg)} = \text{desired AUC} \times (\text{GFR}^* + 25)$$

The desired AUC is usually 6 in untreated and fit patients, and 5 in frail or extensively pretreated patients.

Both drugs are administered on the same day, with carboplatin given immediately after paclitaxel.

ADMINISTRATION

Paclitaxel is given first as an IV infusion in dextrose or sodium chloride 0.9% over a period of 3 h after the following *mandatory* premedication:

---

* The Calvert equation was developed and validated using ^{51}Cr EDTA clearance to measure GFR. In clinical practice, CrCl calculated from serum creatinine using the Cockcroft–Gault equation is often substituted for GFR measurement. It has been reported that this results in carboplatin under-dosing, and that a correction factor of 1.1 should be applied to doses calculated using the Cockcroft–Gault-derived CrCl value. Any local policy on this matter should be followed. A simpler correction is often applied, namely the addition of 1 to the target AUC when the Cockcroft–Gault-derived CrCl value is used instead of the isotopically measured GFR.

Further corrections have been suggested for renal function determined by urinary creatinine measurement and the Jelliffe formula. However, a discussion of these is beyond the scope of this book.

Dexamethasone 20 mg by slow IV injection/short infusion immediately prior to chemotherapy.*

Ranitidine 50 mg by slow IV injection immediately prior to chemotherapy

Chlorpheniramine 10 mg IV immediately prior to chemotherapy

Paclitaxel is followed immediately by carboplatin infused over 1 h in 500 mL of 5% dextrose (in non-PVC bag/glass bottle with non-PVC tubing)

ANTI-EMETICS

High emetogenic potential (see local policy).

CYCLE LENGTH

21 days.

NUMBER OF CYCLES

Usually 6.

SIDE-EFFECTS

Bone-marrow suppression (neutropenia and significant thrombocytopenia), total alopecia, nausea and vomiting, arthralgia, myalgia, sensory neuropathy, hypersensitivity, mucositis (not usually serious), nephrotoxicity (modest compared with cisplatin-based regimens).

BLOOD NADIR

Days 10–21 (neutrophil nadir is likely to be towards the beginning of this period, and platelet nadir towards the end).

TTOS REQUIRED

- Anti-emetics appropriate to highly emetogenic chemotherapy (see local policy).

NOTES FOR PRESCRIBERS

- Check the FBC prior to giving the go-ahead for chemotherapy. Seek advice if the neutrophil count is $<1.5 \times 10^9$/L or the platelet count is $<75 \times 10^9$/L at the time of treatment.

---

* In the SPC, the manufacturer of Taxol® recommends a dexamethasone dose of 20 mg 12 h and 20 mg 6 h before chemotherapy taken by mouth. However, the IV regimen is simpler, appears to be as effective, involves a lower total steroid dose and avoids the risk of the patient receiving paclitaxel without prior premedication as a result of com-pliance problems.

- The renal function should be formally assessed at the start of the study to allow dose calculation. Ideally this should be done by EDTA clearance, but estimation from serum creatinine levels using the Cockcroft–Gault equation is acceptable if the patient has a stable creatinine concentration and no confounding factors (e.g. catabolic states) (*see* Doses section above for note on adjustment of doses for different methods of assessment of renal function, and abide by any local policy or trial protocol governing this):

CrCl (mL/min)

$$= \frac{1.04 \text{ (females) or } 1.23 \text{ (males)} \times (140 - \text{age in years}) \times \text{weight in kg}}{\text{serum creatinine concentration } (\mu\text{mol/L})}.$$

On subsequent cycles the renal function should be reassessed if changes in serum creatinine concentration indicate alteration.

Note: Dose adjustment needs to accompany significant *improvements* in renal function (such as may occur as a result of reduction of a large pelvic tumour mass), as well as *deteriorations*. Improved renal function and fixed doses will result in under-dosing.

- Question the patient about abnormal sensations, which may indicate neuropathy, requiring dose modification. Seek advice if such symptoms are reported.
- Make sure that the patient has been prescribed the required premedication. Paclitaxel has been known to cause hypersensitivity reactions.
- The patient should be observed reasonably closely, especially during the first two treatments because of the significant risk of anaphylactoid reactions.

NOTES FOR NURSES

- Make sure that the patient has been prescribed the required premedication and that this has been administered before chemotherapy administration begins. Paclitaxel has been known to cause hypersensitivity reactions.
- The patient should be observed reasonably closely, especially during the first two treatments because of the significant risk of anaphylactoid reactions.
- Inform the prescriber if the patient reports any abnormal sensations which may be indicative of drug-induced neuropathy.
- Try not to agitate paclitaxel infusions, as the solution will froth and the bubbles will interfere with infusion pumps. Paclitaxel should be administered via non-PVC tubing and should be made up in a non-PVC bag or a glass bottle.

NOTES FOR PHARMACISTS

- Check that the FBC has been determined and is within acceptable limits before issuing chemotherapy.
- At the time of the first course, record the calculated/measured GFR on any pharmacy patient record (*see* Appendix 3 for an example). On subsequent courses, check that the carboplatin dose has been recalculated if the serum creatinine concentration has altered significantly.

Note: Doses need to be adjusted in the case of improving as well as deteriorating renal function. Failure to do this may result in under-dosing.

- Check that anti-emetics appropriate to highly emetogenic chemotherapy have been prescribed according to the standard protocol.
- Make sure that the patient has been prescribed premedications to prevent hypersensitivity reactions to paclitaxel.
- Try not to agitate paclitaxel infusions, as the solution will froth and the bubbles will interfere with infusion pumps. Ensure that paclitaxel is made up in a glass bottle/non-PVC bag and is administered via non-PVC tubing.

SOURCE MATERIAL

Ovarian cancer

- Colombo N on behalf of the ICON collaborators (2000) Randomised trial of paclitaxel (PTX) and carboplatin (CBDCA) versus a control arm of carboplatin or CAP (cyclophosphamide, doxorubicin and cisplatin): the Third International Collaborative Ovarian Neoplasm Study (ICON3). *Proc Am Soc Clin Oncol.* **20**: 379 (abstract).

Oral steroid premedication

- Gennari A, Salvadori B, Tognoni A *et al.* (1996) Rapid intravenous premedication with dexamethasone prevents hypersensitivity reactions to paclitaxel. *Ann Oncol.* **7**: 978–9.

C-VAMP (cyclophosphamide, vincristine, doxorubicin ['Adriamycin'], methylprednisolone)

USUAL INDICATION

Multiple myeloma.

DOSES

Cyclophosphamide 500 mg IV on days 1, 8 and 15
Note: This dose is the same for all patients, regardless of body surface area
Doxorubicin ('Adriamycin') 9 mg/m^2/day by continuous IV infusion for 4 days
Vincristine 0.4 mg/day by continuous IV infusion for 4 days
Note: This dose is the same for all patients, regardless of body surface area
Methylprednisolone 1 g/m^2 (maximum 1.5 g) once daily on days 1–5 (normally
as a 1-h IV infusion, but the injection may be given orally to facilitate
outpatient treatment – it is unpalatable!)

Note: The vincristine and cyclophosphamide doses are not adjusted for body surface area.

ADMINISTRATION

Cyclophosphamide

As an IV bolus or short (15–30 min) IV infusion in 100 mL of 0.9% sodium chloride.

Doxorubicin and vincristine

These drugs are combined in the reservoir of a suitable infusion device and given by
continuous infusion over a period of 96 h. Some portable pumps are small enough
for the patient to carry around, so that this regimen may be administered on an
outpatient basis.

Doxorubicin and vincristine are powerful vesicants, and the doxorubicin/vincristine
infusion should only be administered via a central venous access where there is
confidence in its positioning within a large vein.

Methylprednisolone

Methylprednisolone is normally given as a 1-h IV infusion in 500 mL of 0.9%
sodium chloride. The highest strength of tablets available in the UK is 100 mg,

which means that they are unsatisfactory for doses as large as those used in C-VAMP. The injection can be administered orally, although it is unpalatable even when mixed with flavourings, such as orange juice.

ANTI-EMETICS

On days 1, 8 and 15, anti-emetics appropriate to a highly emetogenic regimen should be prescribed according to local policy, and on days 2–4 anti-emetics appropriate to moderately emetogenic chemotherapy should be prescribed. No additional steroids are required for anti-emesis on days 1–5.

CYCLE LENGTH

21 days.

NUMBER OF CYCLES

Until the patient enters complete remission or paraprotein levels stabilise.

SIDE-EFFECTS

Bone-marrow suppression, alopecia, nausea and vomiting (not usually a significant problem), mucositis, cardiac arrhythmias due to doxorubicin (acute cardiac problems are rare with the low dose and prolonged infusion schedule of doxorubicin used in this regimen), dilated cardiomyopathy (especially at cumulative doxorubicin doses in excess of 450 mg/m^2), peripheral neuropathy from vincristine. The high doses of methylprednisolone used in this regimen can produce a variety of steroid side-effects, including euphoria/depression, epigastric discomfort, glucose intolerance, insomnia, psychosis, fluid and sodium retention, and potassium loss.

BLOOD NADIR

Because cytotoxic drugs are being given on a weekly basis, a discrete nadir may not be obvious.

TTOS REQUIRED

- Methylprednisolone for oral use, if the patient is not returning to the hospital for IV therapy.
- Anti-emetics as described in the Anti-emetics section above.
- Allopurinol 300 mg each morning (reduce dose in cases of renal impairment) to prevent tumour lysis syndrome, especially early in treatment when there is a large

tumour bulk. A gastroprotective agent (e.g. an H_2-antagonist) may be appropriate to prevent mucosal irritation in patients who are receiving methylprednisolone orally.

NOTES FOR PRESCRIBERS

When considering treatment options

- Consider whether the patient is suitable for domiciliary treatment, if this is planned. Although modern disposable infusion devices do not require much input from the patient, they may be a cause of excessive anxiety to some patients who would prefer all treatment to take place in the hospital ward or clinic.
- Liaise fully with the nursing and pharmacy staff. Before treatment can be started, arrangements will have to be made for the insertion of a central venous catheter or PICC. If outside agencies (e.g. district nurses) are to be used to disconnect infusions on the last day of treatment, arrangements will also have to be made with this group of professionals before treatment begins. In addition, the filling of infusion devices is time-consuming and pharmacy staff need to be able to schedule this work appropriately.
- Do not forget that the vincristine dose is independent of body surface area – it is 0.4 mg/day for all patients. Similarly, the cyclophosphamide dose is fixed at 500 mg.
- If C-VAMP is being used in ambulatory patients for home treatment, patients must be capable of looking after the requisite infusion pump and associated venous access. This should be considered when treatment options are being reviewed.
- Patients over 60 years of age or with a history of heart disease must have an echocardiogram or MUGA scan prior to treatment to ensure that there is adequate left ventricular function.
- Check the FBC prior to giving the go-ahead for chemotherapy. Seek advice from a senior member of the medical team if the neutrophil count is $<1.5 \times 10^9$/L or the platelet count is $<100 \times 10^9$/L. In the MRC Myeloma VII trial,[1] treatment was withheld for neutrophil counts of $<1 \times 10^9$/L or platelet counts of $<50 \times 10^9$/L.
- Vincristine can cause peripheral neuropathy. The patient should be questioned about abnormal sensations, jaw pain, constipation or difficulty with fine movements that may be indicative of neuropathy. If such symptoms are reported, discuss them with a senior member of the medical team with a view to dose modification.
- Myelomas are relatively sensitive to chemotherapy, and substantial tumour lysis is possible at the start of chemotherapy. This can generate large amounts of insoluble uric acid, which is capable of precipitating in the kidneys, causing renal damage. To prevent this, allopurinol (300 mg once daily) should be commenced the day before starting cytotoxic therapy and continued for as long as there is significant tumour bulk remaining and cytotoxic therapy continues.

---

[1] Davies FE, Forsyth PD, Rawstron AC *et al.* (2001) The impact of attaining a minimal disease state after high-dose melphalan and autologous transplantation for multiple myeloma. *Br J Haematol.* **112**: 814–19.

- Prophylactic H_2-antagonists or other gastroprotective agents may be justified during oral methylprednisolone courses, especially if platelet counts have been reduced as a consequence of chemotherapy.
- Check the LFTs. If these show significant impairment, a reduction in doxorubicin, vincristine and cyclophosphamide doses may be required (*see* Appendix 1 for further advice).
- Renal function should be assessed before treatment. Ideally this should be done by EDTA clearance, but estimation by the Cockcroft–Gault equation from serum creatinine levels is acceptable if the patient has a stable creatinine concentration and no confounding factors (e.g. catabolic states):

CrCl (mL/min)

$$= \frac{1.04 \text{ (females) or } 1.23 \text{ (males)} \times (140 - \text{age in years}) \times \text{weight in kg}}{\text{serum creatinine concentration (}\mu\text{mol/L)}}.$$

On subsequent cycles the renal function should be reassessed.

Consideration should be given to a cyclophosphamide dose reduction in patients with a creatinine clearance of less than 50 mL/min (*see* Appendix 2 for further advice). In the MRC Myeloma VII study, cyclophosphamide was withheld in patients with a serum creatinine concentration of >300 µmol/L.

- Prior to treatment, hair loss should be discussed with the patient. Hair thinning is more likely than total alopecia with this regimen. Scalp cooling is not practicable with C-VAMP because of the prolonged administration schedule that is used.
- If prescribing methylprednisolone injection to be given by mouth, state this clearly on any outpatient prescription so that it can be correctly labelled and the patient can be counselled about the correct mode of administration.
- If administering the drugs, *see* Administration section above for notes on the vesicant nature of doxorubicin and vincristine. Only secure central lines should be used for the infusion of vincristine and doxorubicin.

NOTES FOR NURSES

- For patients who are being treated at home, arrangements need to be in place at the end of each cycle of treatment for removing the empty infusion device and flushing the venous access. It may be possible for a practice nurse or district nurse to do this in or close to the patient's home. However, not all non-oncology nurses are happy with this role, and it should not be *assumed* that they will take it on. Therefore it is important to check this before making any promises to the patient. If the patient is being treated with an electromechanical pump device, it is recommended that disconnection is carried out at the hospital in order to minimise the likelihood of pump loss.
- Patients may find home infusion therapy a source of anxiety. As well as attempting to reassure patients who are receiving the infusional portion of their treatment at home, arrangements should be in place that allow the patient or their carer to contact an informed professional at any time if they experience problems.
- Prior to treatment, hair loss should be discussed with the patient. Hair thinning is more likely than total alopecia with this regimen. Therefore scalp cooling is

unnecessary with C-VAMP, as well as being impractical because of the prolonged administration schedule that is used.

- If administering the drugs, *see* Administration section above for notes on the vesicant nature of doxorubicin and vincristine. The doxorubicin/vincristine combination should only be administered via a secure central venous access device.
- If you are involved in issuing methylprednisolone for injection to patients for oral use, make sure that they understand how to prepare it, withdraw it from the vial and administer it.
- Vincristine can cause peripheral neuropathy. If the patient mentions abnormal sensations, jaw pain, constipation or difficulty with fine movements that may be indicative of neuropathy, alert the medical team.
- Ensure that any diabetic patients are aware of the need to be extra vigilant about monitoring their blood sugar levels during treatment with methylprednisolone, and advise them to contact their doctor if they experience problems with the control of their blood sugar levels.

NOTES FOR PHARMACISTS

- Check that the FBC has been determined and is within acceptable limits before issuing the chemotherapy. Seek confirmation from the prescriber if the neutrophil count is $<1.5 \times 10^9$/L or the platelet count is $<100 \times 10^9$/L. In the MRC Myeloma VII trial, treatment was withheld for neutrophil counts of $<1 \times 10^9$/L or platelet counts of $<50 \times 10^9$/L.
- Vincristine can cause peripheral neuropathy. If the patient mentions abnormal sensations, jaw pain, constipation or difficulty with fine movements that may be indicative of neuropathy, alert the medical team.
- Check the LFTs. If these show significant impairment, a reduction in doxorubicin, vincristine and cyclophosphamide doses may be required (*see* Appendix 1 for further advice).
- Renal function should be assessed before treatment. Ideally this should be done by EDTA clearance, but estimation by the Cockcroft–Gault equation from serum creatinine levels is acceptable if the patient has a stable creatinine concentration and no confounding factors (e.g. catabolic states). Note the CrCl and the corresponding serum creatinine concentration in any pharmacy patient record (*see* Appendix 3 for an example). On subsequent cycles the renal function should be reassessed if the creatinine concentration has changed significantly.

   Consideration should be given to cyclophosphamide dose reduction in patients with a creatinine clearance of <50 mL/min (*see* Appendix 2 for further advice). In the MRC Myeloma VII study, cyclophosphamide was withheld in patients with a serum creatinine concentration of $>300\,\mu$mol/L.
- Do not forget that the vincristine dose is independent of body surface area – it is 0.4 mg/day for all patients. Similarly, the cyclophosphamide dose is fixed at 500 mg.
- Check that appropriate anti-emetics have been prescribed (see above). The high doses of methylprednisolone in this regimen mean that additional steroids are not required for anti-emesis, and the infusion of doxorubicin at low daily doses over 4 days means that routine $5HT_3$-antagonists are not required.

- Myelomas are fairly sensitive to chemotherapy, and substantial tumour lysis is possible at the start of chemotherapy. This can result in the generation of large amounts of insoluble uric acid, which is capable of precipitating in the kidneys, causing renal damage. To prevent this, allopurinol 300 mg once daily should be commenced the day before starting cytotoxic therapy and continued for as long as significant tumour bulk remains.
- Keep a close eye on the cumulative dose of doxorubicin and alert the prescriber if it exceeds 450 mg/m^2. It is especially important when a patient starts a course of treatment to check the pharmacy records and the patient's notes to ascertain whether they have received previous anthracycline therapy in your department or elsewhere. The contributions to the total anthracycline dose of previous daunorubicin, epirubicin, idarubicin and aclarubicin, as well as doxorubicin, must also be considered.
- If you are involved in issuing methylprednisolone for injection for oral use, make sure that the patient understands how to reconstitute the product and withdraw and measure doses. 'Tailing off' of doses is not required with the short courses of methylprednisolone used in this regimen.

SOURCE MATERIAL

- Davies FE, Forsyth PD, Rawstron AC *et al.* (2001) The impact of attaining a minimal disease state after high-dose melphalan and autologous transplantation for multiple myeloma. *Br J Haematol.* **112**: 814–19.
- Raje N, Powles R, Kulkarni S *et al.* (1997) A comparison of vincristine and doxorubicin infusional chemotherapy with methylprednisolone (VAMP) with the addition of weekly cyclophosphamide (C-VAMP) as induction treatment followed by autografting in previously untreated myeloma. *Br J Haematol.* **97**: 153–60.

de Gramont regimen and modified de Gramont (5-fluorouracil plus folinic acid, 5-FU/FA, 5-FU/LV)

USUAL INDICATION

First-line palliative treatment of recurrent or inoperable colorectal cancer.

DOSES

de Gramont

Folinic acid (FA)* 200 mg/m^2 (or 100 mg/m^2 L-folinic acid – conventional FA is a mixture of two stereoisomers, one of which is inactive) IV infusion on days 1 and 2

5-Fluorouracil (5-FU) 400 mg/m^2 IV bolus on days 1 and 2

5-FU 600 mg/m^2 IV infusion (over 22 h) on days 1 and 2

Modified de Gramont

Folinic acid 350 mg flat dose (or 175 mg L-folinic acid – conventional FA is a mixture of two stereoisomers, one of which is inactive) IV infusion on day 1

5-FU 400 mg/m^2 IV bolus on day 1

5-FU 2800 mg/m^2 protracted infusion (over 46 h) on days 1 and 2

Note: There are *many* other regimens of 5-FU and FA in use. Some are completely different to those described above (*see* chapter on Mayo regimen), and others are modifications of the de Gramont-type regimen. The modified de Gramont regimen described above is a specific variant that is quite widely used in the UK and which features in the MRC FOCUS study.

ADMINISTRATION

de Gramont

A 2-h IV infusion of FA in 500 mL of 0.9% sodium chloride is followed by an IV bolus loading dose of 5-FU and then by a 22-h IV infusion of 5-FU. This sequence is repeated on day 2. The prolonged infusion of 5-FU can be administered using a conventional technique (i.e. infusion into a peripheral vein of the requisite dose of

---

*Folinic acid is also known as 'folinate', 'calcium folinate', 'leucovorin' (LV) and 'calcium leucovorin'.

5-FU in 0.9% sodium chloride). However, this requires 2 days of hospitalisation. Therefore the infusion is most commonly delivered using a concentrated solution contained in a portable infusion pump (usually a disposable elastomeric device) which enables the patient to return home with the infusion running. In this case a secure central line or PICC must be in place.

Modified de Gramont

A 2-hour IV infusion of FA in 500 mL of 0.9% sodium chloride is followed by a short IV bolus loading dose of 5-FU and then by a 46-h IV infusion of 5-FU. The prolonged infusion of 5-FU can be administered using a conventional technique (i.e. infusion into a peripheral vein of an infusion containing the requisite dose of 5-FU in 0.9% sodium chloride). However, this requires 2 days of hospitalisation. Therefore the infusion is most commonly delivered using a concentrated solution contained in a portable infusion pump (usually a disposable elastomeric device) which enables the patient to return home with the infusion running. In this case a secure central line or PICC must be in place.

ANTI-EMETICS

Low emetogenic potential (see local policy).

CYCLE LENGTH

14 days.

NUMBER OF CYCLES

Until disease progression.

SIDE-EFFECTS

Bone-marrow suppression, alopecia (usually mild), nausea and vomiting (very rare), mucositis (can be dose limiting), diarrhoea (can be dose limiting), palmar-plantar erythrodysasthesia (hand-and-foot syndrome – much less common than with continuously infused 5-FU). A small proportion of patients who are deficient in the 5-FU-metabolising enzyme dihydropyrimidine dehydrogenase (DPD) may experience unexpectedly severe toxicity.

BLOOD NADIR

Because of the 2-weekly treatment schedule and the modest myelotoxicity of this regimen, a discrete nadir may not be seen.

TTOS REQUIRED

- Anti-emetics appropriate to weakly emetogenic chemotherapy.
- Unless it is contraindicated, low-dose warfarin therapy (1 mg/day) should be instituted once any central venous line (but not PICC line) is *in situ*, in order to prevent line thrombosis.

NOTES FOR PRESCRIBERS

When considering treatment options

- Consider whether the patient is suitable for domiciliary treatment. Although modern disposable infusion devices do not require much input from the patient, they may be a cause of excessive anxiety to some patients who would prefer all treatment to take place in the hospital ward or clinic.
- Liaise fully with the nursing and pharmacy staff. Before treatment can be started, arrangements will have to be made for the insertion of a central venous catheter or PICC. If outside agencies (e.g. district nurses) are to be used to disconnect infusions on the last day of treatment, arrangements will also have to be made with this group of professionals before treatment begins. In addition, filling infusion devices is time-consuming, and pharmacy staff need to be able to schedule this work appropriately.

When prescribing

- Make sure that you are clear which regimen of 5-FU and FA the patient is to receive. Is it de Gramont, modified de Gramont or one of the many others that are in use? Be particularly careful if patients are in clinical trials.
- Check the FBC prior to giving the go-ahead for chemotherapy. Seek advice from a senior member of the medical team if the neutrophil count is $<1.5 \times 10^9$/L or the platelet count is $<100 \times 10^9$/L (the lower limits for treatment in the pivotal trial of the original de Gramont regimen).
- Prior to prescribing, check the LFTs and renal function for evidence of moderate or severe dysfunction. Consideration should be given to 5-FU dose reductions in the case of severe renal dysfunction or moderate hepatic dysfunction (*see* Appendices 1 and 2 for further advice).
- If prescribing low-dose warfarin (*see* TTO section above), ensure that arrangements are made for either the GP or the hospital to check the INR about 1 week after starting therapy to ensure that the patient is not hypersensitive to its effects. Communicate to the GP that this dose of warfarin is not intended to alter the INR significantly and should not be increased without consultation.
- Pyridoxine (50 mg three times a day by mouth) is sometimes used to treat 'hand-and-foot' syndrome and mucositis, but its value is dubious and it should not be relied upon as the sole measure for dealing with significant toxicity.
- Infusion devices are time-consuming to prepare, and are likely to be prepared by pharmacy ahead of time in order to keep patient waiting times down to an acceptable level. However, once they have been filled, it is impossible to alter their infusion rate. Therefore, for patients on established treatment, it is unhelpful to make dose alterations without good reason and adequate notice, so try to

avoid this if possible. For example, dosage adjustment for small degrees of weight loss or weight gain in patients who are tolerating their treatment well is not urgent — it may be appropriate to request a small dose change for the *next* cycle, but to maintain the dose unchanged on the current cycle.

NOTES FOR NURSES

- Arrangements need to be in place at the end of each cycle of treatment for removing the empty infusion device and flushing the venous access. It may be possible for this to be done by a practice nurse or district nurse in or close to the patient's home. However, not all non-oncology nurses are happy with this role, and it should not be *assumed* that they will take it on. This should be checked before any promises are made to the patient.
- If the patient is taking low-dose warfarin to prevent thrombosis of the venous access, take any appropriate opportunity to check they understand that they should take a fixed dose of 1 mg daily. This may help to prevent problems if anyone (e.g. the patient's GP) tries to increase the dose inappropriately.
- Some patients may find home infusion therapy a source of anxiety. As well as attempting to reassure them, arrangements should be in place that allow the patient or their carer to contact an informed professional at any time if they experience problems.
- Because disposable infusion devices have fixed flow rates, care should be taken that the timing of day 2 and day 3 clinic appointments coincides with the projected end of 5-FU infusions. If they have not finished when the patient arrives, it is impossible (and would in any case be undesirable) to speed them up in order to finish them. Similarly, for patients receiving de Gramont, a gap between day 1 and day 2 treatment is undesirable. Therefore the day 2 appointment should be as close as possible to 24 h after the start of treatment on day 1.

NOTES FOR PHARMACISTS

- Check that the FBC has been determined and is within acceptable limits before issuing treatment. However, many patients tolerate this regimen extremely well, and it may be reasonable to prepare treatments ahead of confirmation. This will reduce the waiting time.
- Make sure that you are clear which regimen of 5-FU and FA the patient is to receive. Is it de Gramont, modified de Gramont or one of the many others that are in use? Be particularly careful if patients are in clinical trials.
- Check the LFTs and renal function at the time of prescribing for evidence of moderate or severe dysfunction. Consideration should be given to dose reductions in the case of severe renal dysfunction or moderate hepatic dysfunction (*see* Appendices 1 and 2 for further guidance).
- This protocol is only weakly emetogenic, so any use of $5HT_3$-antagonists should be questioned. Patients with severe gastrointestinal symptoms may have a psychogenic component to their symptoms which may respond to haloperidol and/or lorazepam.

- If the patient is not prescribed low-dose warfarin at the start of treatment, check whether this is needed (*see* TTO section above). If it is contraindicated, mark this on any pharmacy patient record (*see* Appendix 3 for an example) to prevent future prescribing.
- Pyridoxine 50 mg three times a day is sometimes used to treat 'hand-and-foot' syndrome and mucositis, but its value is dubious and it should not be relied upon as the sole measure for managing significant toxicity.

SOURCE MATERIAL

de Gramont

- de Gramont A, Bosset J-F, Milan C *et al.* (1997) Randomized trial comparing monthly low-dose leucovorin and fluorouracil bolus with bimonthly high-dose leucovorin and fluorouracil bolus plus continuous infusion for advanced colorectal cancer: a French Intergroup study. *J Clin Oncol.* **15**: 808–15.

Modified de Gramont

- Seymour MT, Wilson G, Dent JT *et al.* (1998) Dose escalation study of a modified 'de Gramont' regimen, better suited to the chemotherapy day unit. *Ann Oncol.* **9 (Supplement 4):** 47.

de Gramont regimen plus irinotecan (IrdG) and modified de Gramont plus irinotecan (IrMdG) (5-fluorouracil, folinic acid, irinotecan)

USUAL INDICATION

First-line palliative treatment of recurrent or inoperable colorectal cancer.

DOSES

Irinotecan plus de Gramont (IrdG)

Irinotecan 180 mg/m^2 IV infusion on day 1
Folinic acid (FA)* 200 mg/m^2 (or 100 mg/m^2 L-folinic acid — conventional FA is a mixture of two stereoisomers, one of which is inactive) IV infusion on days 1 and 2
5-Fluorouracil (5-FU) 400 mg/m^2 IV bolus on days 1 and 2
5-FU 600mg/m^2 IV infusion (over 22 h) on days 1 and 2

Irinotecan plus modified de Gramont (IrMdG)

Irinotecan 180 mg/m^2 IV infusion on day 1
Folinic acid (FA)* 350 mg flat dose (or 175 mg of L-folinic acid — conventional FA is a mixture of two stereoisomers, one of which is inactive) IV infusion on day 1
5-FU 400 mg/m^2 IV bolus on day 1
5-FU 2400 mg/m^2 (note that this is lower than the dose used in MdG without irinotecan) protracted infusion (over 46 h) on days 1 and 2

Note: There are other regimens of 5-FU plus FA plus irinotecan in use, often as part of a clinical trial. These include the so-called Saltz regimen, which is similar to the Mayo regimen of 5-FU plus FA with irinotecan added. However, in Europe, variations on de Gramont plus irinotecan are more often used. IrMdG has not been the subject of extensive published clinical trials, but is included here because it features in the large MRC FOCUS study.

ADMINISTRATION

de Gramont plus irinotecan

Treatment starts with a 30-min infusion of irinotecan in 250 mL of 0.9% sodium chloride. This is followed by a 2-h IV infusion of FA in 500 mL of 0.9% sodium chloride

---

*Folinic acid is also known as 'folinate', 'calcium folinate', 'leucovorin' (LV) and 'calcium leucovorin'.

followed immediately by the IV bolus loading dose of 5-FU and then by a 22-h IV infusion of 5-FU. On day 2 the sequence of FA and 5-FU is repeated, without any further irinotecan. The prolonged infusion of 5-FU can be administered using a conventional technique (i.e. infusion into a peripheral vein of an infusion containing the requisite dose of 5-FU in 0.9% sodium chloride). However, this requires 2 days of hospitalisation. Therefore the infusion is most commonly delivered using a concentrated solution contained in a portable infusion pump (usually a disposable elastomeric device) which enables the patient to return home with the infusion running. In this case a secure central line or PICC must be in place.

Modified de Gramont plus irinotecan

Treatment starts with a 30-min infusion of irinotecan in 250 mL of 0.9% sodium chloride. This is followed by a 2-h infusion of FA in 500 mL of 0.9% sodium chloride followed immediately by the bolus loading dose of 5-FU and then by a 46-h IV infusion of 5-FU. The prolonged infusion of 5-FU can be administered using a conventional technique (i.e. infusion into a peripheral vein of infusions containing the requisite dose of 5-FU in 0.9% sodium chloride). However, this requires 2 days of hospitalisation. Therefore the infusion is most commonly delivered using a concentrated solution contained in a portable infusion pump (usually a disposable elastomeric device) which enables the patient to return home with the infusion running. In this case a secure central line or PICC must be in place.

ANTI-EMETICS

High (day 1) and low (day 2) emetogenic potential (according to local policy).

CYCLE LENGTH

14 days.

NUMBER OF CYCLES

Until disease progression.

SIDE-EFFECTS

Acute cholinergic syndrome (early diarrhoea, sweating, abdominal cramping, lachrymation, myosis, salivation) at the time of irinotecan infusion, bone-marrow suppression, alopecia (usually mild), nausea, vomiting, mucositis, diarrhoea — including very severe diarrhoea starting around 72 h after irinotecan infusion (can be dose limiting), palmar-plantar erythrodysasthesia ('hand-and-foot' syndrome, as a result of prolonged exposure to 5-FU, but much less common than with continuously infused 5-FU).

BLOOD NADIR

Around day 10. However, the nadir may be less predictable after the second and subsequent courses, because the 14-day cycle can result in further chemotherapy being given before the blood count has fully recovered from the previous cycle.

TTOS REQUIRED

- Anti-emetics appropriate to highly emetogenic chemotherapy (day 1) and weakly emetogenic chemotherapy (day 2) according to local policy.
- Loperamide to start if late-onset diarrhoea occurs. The recommended dose is 2 capsules (4 mg) with the first loose stool, then 1 capsule (2 mg) every 2 h for at least 12 h after the last loose stool and for a maximum of 48 h. This is higher than the standard loperamide dose.
- A course of a broad-spectrum antibiotic (e.g. ciprofloxacin 250 mg twice a day) to take if diarrhoea continues for more than 48 h.
  Note: Loperamide and ciprofloxacin need not be issued at every course provided that the patient still has an unused supply of this medication *and knows where it is*.
- Unless it is contraindicated, low-dose warfarin therapy (1 mg/day) should be instituted once any central venous line (but not PICC line) is *in situ*, in order to prevent line thrombosis.

NOTES FOR PRESCRIBERS

When considering treatment options

- Consider whether the patient is suitable for domiciliary treatment. Although modern disposable infusion devices do not require much input from the patient, they may be a cause of excessive anxiety to some patients who would prefer all treatment to take place in the hospital ward or clinic.
- Consider the general performance status of the patient. Irinotecan is a toxic treatment and the manufacturer cautions that it should only be used with great circumspection in patients with an Eastern Cooperative Oncology Group (ECOG) performance status of <2.
- Liaise fully with the nursing and pharmacy staff. Before treatment is started, arrangements will have to be made for the insertion of a central venous catheter or PICC. If outside agencies (e.g. district nurses) are to be used to disconnect infusions on the last day of treatment, arrangements will also have to be made with this group of professionals before treatment begins. In addition, filling infusion devices is time-consuming, and pharmacy staff need to be able to schedule this work appropriately.

When prescribing

- Make sure that you are clear which chemotherapy regimen the patient is to receive. Is it de Gramont plus irinotecan, modified de Gramont plus irinotecan or another combination of irinotecan, 5-FU and FA? Be particularly careful if patients are in clinical trials.

- Check the FBC prior to giving the go-ahead for chemotherapy. Irinotecan is contraindicated if the neutrophil count is $<1.5 \times 10^9$/L or the platelet count is $<75 \times 10^9$/L. Patients who experienced febrile neutropenia after a previous cycle or whose neutrophil nadir was $<0.5 \times 10^9$/L (even if they remained well) should have a dose reduction of 15–20% on subsequent cycles.

- Because irinotecan can be quite toxic, the next cycle should not be given until all toxicities have resolved to grade 0 or 1 on the National Cancer Institute common toxicity criteria (NCI-CTC) grading system and treatment-related diarrhoea has resolved completely. Any patients who experienced grade 3–4 non-haematological toxicity on a previous course should have their dose reduced by 15–20%.

- Check hepatic function. Irinotecan is contraindicated if the bilirubin level is $>1.5 \times$ ULN. If the bilirubin is $1–1.5 \times$ ULN, the patient should be treated with particular caution. Consideration should also be given to reducing 5-FU doses in patients with moderate hepatic dysfunction (see Appendix 1).

- Check the renal function prior to prescribing. Consideration should be given to a 5-FU dose reduction in the case of severe renal dysfunction (see Appendix 2).

- On the first course of treatment, a 300 µg subcutaneous dose of atropine should be charted 'as required' in case the patient develops an acute cholinergic syndrome. On subsequent courses, atropine should be charted either as a regular premedication or 'as required', depending on whether it was needed with the first course.

- Prescribe anti-emetics appropriate to highly emetogenic chemotherapy for day 1 and weakly emetogenic chemotherapy for day 2 according to local policy.

- Advise the patient on what to do if late diarrhoea develops (i.e. how to take the prescribed medication), and emphasise the importance of contacting the hospital if diarrhoea persists for more than 48 h, is not controlled by loperamide, or is accompanied by vomiting/fever. In such cases the patient should be admitted for IV hydration. This is a potentially life-threatening condition and it needs to be treated vigorously.

- If the patient is prescribed low-dose warfarin (see TTO section above), ensure that arrangements are made for either the patient's GP or the hospital to check the patient's INR about 1 week after starting the drug to ensure that they are not hypersensitive to it. Communicate clearly to the patient's GP that this dose of warfarin is not intended to alter the INR significantly, and that the dose should not be increased without consultation.

- Pyridoxine 50 mg three times a day is sometimes used to treat 'hand-and-foot' syndrome and mucositis arising from 5-FU treatment, but its value is dubious and it should not be relied upon as the sole measure for dealing with significant toxicity.

- Infusion devices containing 5-FU are time-consuming to prepare, and are likely to be prepared by pharmacy ahead of time in order to keep patient waiting times down to an acceptable level. However, once these devices have been filled, it is impossible to alter the infusion rate. Therefore for patients on established treatment it is unhelpful to make dose alterations without good reason and adequate notice, so try to avoid this if possible. For example, dosage adjustments for small degrees of weight loss or weight gain in patients who are tolerating their treatment well are not urgent − it may be appropriate to request a small dose change for the next cycle, but to maintain the dose unchanged on the current cycle.

NOTES FOR NURSES

- If the patient develops an acute cholinergic syndrome (stomach cramps, salivation, sweating, pupillary constriction) during the irinotecan infusion, this may be treated with 300 μg of atropine SC. This should have been prescribed on an 'as-required' basis, or as part of the routine premedication for patients who developed the syndrome on an earlier course.

- Advise the patient on what to do if late diarrhoea develops (i.e. how to take their prescribed medication), and emphasise the importance of contacting the hospital if diarrhoea persists for more than 48 h, is not controlled by loperamide, or is accompanied by vomiting/fever. In such cases the patient should be admitted for IV hydration. This is a potentially life-threatening problem and it needs to be treated vigorously.

- Arrangements need to be in place at the end of each cycle of treatment for removing the empty infusion device and flushing the venous access. It may be possible for this to be done by a practice nurse or district nurse in or close to the patient's home. However, not all non-oncology nurses are happy with this role, and it should not be assumed that they will take it on. This should be checked before any promises are made to the patient.

- If the patient is taking low-dose warfarin to prevent thrombosis of the venous access, take any appropriate opportunity to make sure they understand that they should take a fixed dose of 1 mg daily. This may help to prevent problems if anyone (e.g. the patient's GP) tries to increase the dose inappropriately.

- Some patients may find home infusion therapy a source of anxiety. As well as attempting to reassure them, arrangements should be in place that allow the patient or their carer to contact an informed professional at any time if they experience problems.

- Because disposable infusion devices have fixed flow rates, care should be taken that the timing of day 2 and day 3 clinic appointments coincides with the projected end of 5-FU infusions. If the device still contains 5-FU when the patient arrives, it is impossible (and would in any case be undesirable) to speed it up in order to complete the infusion. Similarly, for patients receiving de Gramont plus irinotecan, a gap between day 1 and day 2 treatment is undesirable. Therefore the day 2 appointment should be as close as possible to 24 h after the start of treatment on day 1.

NOTES FOR PHARMACISTS

- Make sure that the FBC has been checked and is within satisfactory limits before issuing the chemotherapy. Irinotecan is contraindicated if the neutrophil count is $<1.5 \times 10^9$/L or the platelet count is $<75 \times 10^9$/L. Check the nadir count where possible. This is one of the few regimens where asymptomatic low nadir neutrophil counts are an indication for treatment modification. Patients with a nadir neutrophil count of $<0.5 \times 10^9$/L should have their next irinotecan dose reduced by 15–20%, as should patients who experienced febrile neutropenia after the last course.

- Because irinotecan can be quite toxic, the next course should not be given until all toxicities have resolved to grade 0 or 1 on the NCI-CTC grading system and treatment-related diarrhoea has resolved completely. Any patients who experienced grade 3–4 non-haematological toxicity on a previous course should have their dosage reduced by 15–20%. If you have any reason to believe that the patient experienced severe toxicity after a previous cycle or has inadequately resolved treatment toxicity, discuss this with the prescriber if dose reductions have not already been made.

- Make sure that you are clear which chemotherapy regimen the patient is to receive. Is it de Gramont plus irinotecan, modified de Gramont plus irinotecan or one of the other combinations of irinotecan, 5-FU and FA that are in use? Be particularly careful if patients are in clinical trials.
- Check hepatic function. Irinotecan is contraindicated if the bilirubin level is >1.5 × ULN. If the bilirubin level is 1–1.5 × ULN, the patient should be treated with particular caution. Consideration should also be given to reducing 5-FU doses in patients with moderate hepatic dysfunction (see Appendix 1).
- Check the renal function prior to prescribing. Consideration should be given to a 5-FU dose reduction in the case of severe renal dysfunction (see Appendix 2).
- Make sure that on the first course of treatment a 300 µg SC dose of atropine is prescribed 'as required' in case the patient develops acute cholinergic syndrome. On subsequent courses, atropine should be charted either as a regular premedication or 'as required', depending on whether it was needed with the first course.
- Make sure that anti-emetics suitable for highly emetogenic chemotherapy (day 1) and weakly emetogenic chemotherapy (day 2) have been prescribed according to local policy, and that loperamide and a broad-spectrum antibiotic have been included on the TTO at the appropriate doses (unless you are sure that the patient still has a supply of these unused from a previous course and knows where they are). The TTO will need to be clearly endorsed to ensure that these agents are correctly labelled by non-specialist dispensing staff, especially as the loperamide dosing regimen exceeds the normal maximum dose.
- Check that the patient has been advised (or advise them yourself) on what to do if late diarrhoea develops (i.e. how to take their prescribed medication) and to contact the hospital if diarrhoea persists for more than 48 h, is not reasonably controlled by loperamide, or is accompanied by vomiting/fever. In such cases patients will require admission for IV hydration.
- If the patient is not prescribed low-dose warfarin at the start of treatment, check whether this is needed (see TTO section above). If it is contraindicated, mark this clearly on any pharmacy patient record (see Appendix 3 for an example).
- Pyridoxine 50 mg three times a day is sometimes used to treat 'hand-and-foot' syndrome and mucositis, but its value is dubious and it should not be relied upon as the sole measure for managing significant toxicity.

SOURCE MATERIAL

Irinotecan plus de Gramont

- Douillard JY, Cunningham D, Roth AD et al. (2000) Irinotecan combined with fluorouracil compared with fluorouracil alone as first-line treatment for metastatic colorectal cancer: a multicentre randomised trial. Lancet. 355: 1041–7.

de Gramont regimen plus oxaliplatin (OxdG) and modified de Gramont plus oxaliplatin (OxMdG)

USUAL INDICATION

First-line palliative treatment of recurrent or inoperable colorectal cancer.

DOSES

Oxaliplatin plus de Gramont (OxdG)

Oxaliplatin 85 mg/m^3 IV infusion on day 1
Folinic acid (FA)* 200 mg/m^2 (or 100 mg/m^2 L-folinic acid − conventional FA is a mixture of two stereoisomers, one of which is inactive) IV infusion on days 1 and 2
5-Fluorouracil (5-FU) 400 mg/m^2 IV bolus on days 1 and 2
5-FU 600 mg/m^2 IV infusion on days 1 and 2

Oxaliplatin plus modified de Gramont (OxmdG)

Oxaliplatin 85 mg/m^2 IV infusion on day 1
Folinic acid (FA)* 350 mg flat dose (or 175 mg of L-folinic acid − conventional FA is a mixture of two stereoisomers, one of which is inactive) IV infusion on day 1
5-FU 400 mg/m^2 IV bolus on day 1
5-FU 2400 mg/m^2 (note that this is lower than the dose used in MdG without oxaliplatin) protracted infusion on days 1 and 2.

Note: There are other regimens of 5-FU plus FA plus oxaliplatin in use, often as part of a clinical trial. OxMdG has not been the subject of extensive published clinical trials, but is included because it features in the large MRC FOCUS study.

ADMINISTRATION

de Gramont plus oxaliplatin

Before chemotherapy administration is commenced, the venous access should be flushed with 5% dextrose. Treatment starts with a 2-h IV infusion of FA in 250 mL

---

*Folinic acid is also known as 'folinate', 'calcium folinate', 'leucovorin' (LV) and 'calcium leucovorin'.

of 5% dextrose infused concurrently with oxaliplatin, which is also administered as a 2-h infusion in 250 mL of 5% dextrose. The venous access is then flushed with 5% dextrose prior to administration of the IV bolus loading dose of 5-FU, which is followed by a 22-h IV infusion of 5-FU. On day 2 the sequence of FA and 5-FU is repeated, without any further oxaliplatin. The prolonged infusion of 5-FU can be administered using a conventional technique (i.e. infusion into a peripheral vein of an infusion containing the requisite dose of 5-FU in 0.9% sodium chloride).

However, this requires 2 days of hospitalisation. Therefore the infusion is most commonly delivered using a concentrated solution contained in a portable infusion pump (usually a disposable elastomeric device) which enables the patient to return home with the infusion running. In this case a secure central line or PICC must be in place.

Modified de Gramont plus oxaliplatin

Before chemotherapy administration is commenced, the venous access should be flushed with 5% dextrose. Treatment starts with a 2-h IV infusion of FA in 250 mL of 5% dextrose infused concurrently with oxaliplatin, which is also administered as a 2-h infusion in 250 mL of 5% dextrose. The venous access is then flushed with 5% dextrose prior to administration of the IV bolus loading dose of 5-FU, which is followed by a 46-h IV infusion of 5-FU. The prolonged infusion of 5-FU can be administered using a conventional technique (i.e. infusion into a peripheral vein of an infusion containing the requisite dose of 5-FU in 0.9% sodium chloride). However, this requires 2 days of hospitalisation. Therefore the infusion is most commonly delivered using a concentrated solution contained in a portable infusion pump (usually a disposable elastomeric device) which enables the patient to return home with the infusion running. In this case a secure central line or PICC must be in place.

ANTI-EMETICS

High (day 1) and low (day 2) emetogenic potential (see local policy).

CYCLE LENGTH

14 days.

NUMBER OF CYCLES

Until disease progression.

SIDE-EFFECTS

Bone-marrow suppression (usually mild, predominantly neutropenia), alopecia (usually mild), nausea, vomiting, diarrhoea (sometimes severe), mucositis, palmar-plantar erythrodysasthesia ('hand-and-foot' syndrome, as a result of prolonged exposure to 5-FU, but much less common than with continuously infused 5-FU), peripheral sensory neuropathy characterised by dysasthesia and/or parasthesia of the extremities with or without cramps and often triggered by cold (induced by oxaliplatin). Acute pharyngolaryngeal dysasthesia (subjective sensations of dysphagia and dyspnoea, jaw spasm and abnormal tongue sensations) during or shortly after oxaliplatin infusion, renal impairment and ototoxicity induced by oxaliplatin have been reported, but are rare and are seldom severe.

BLOOD NADIR

Around day 10. However, the nadir may be rather unpredictable after the first course because the 14-day cycle can result in further chemotherapy being given before the blood count has fully recovered from the previous cycle.

TTOS REQUIRED

- Anti-emetics appropriate to highly emetogenic chemotherapy (day 1) and weakly emetogenic chemotherapy (day 2) (see local policy).
- Unless it is contraindicated, low-dose warfarin therapy (1 mg/day) should be instituted once any central venous line (but not PICC line) is *in situ*, in order to prevent line thrombosis.

NOTES FOR PRESCRIBERS

When considering treatment options

- Consider whether the patient is suitable for domiciliary treatment. Although modern disposable infusion devices do not require much input from the patient, they may be a cause of excessive anxiety to some patients who would prefer all treatment to take place in the hospital ward or clinic.
- Liaise fully with the nursing and pharmacy staff. Before treatment can be started, arrangements will have to be made for the insertion of a central venous catheter or PICC. If outside agencies (e.g. district nurses) are to be used to disconnect infusions on the last day of treatment, arrangements will also have to be made with this group of professionals before treatment begins. In addition, the filling of infusion devices is time-consuming, and pharmacy staff must be able to schedule this work appropriately.

When prescribing

- Make sure that you are clear which chemotherapy regimen the patient is to receive. Is it de Gramont plus oxaliplatin, modified de Gramont plus oxaliplatin or another combination of oxaliplatin, 5-FU and FA? Be particularly careful if patients are in clinical trials.

- Check the FBC prior to giving the go-ahead for chemotherapy. Oxaliplatin is contraindicated if the neutrophil count is $<1.5 \times 10^9$/L or if the platelet count is $<50 \times 10^9$/L. The manufacturer of oxaliplatin recommends that patients who experience febrile neutropenia after oxaliplatin or whose neutrophil count falls to $<1.0 \times 10^9$/L or whose platelet count falls to $<50 \times 10^9$/L (even if they remain well) should have an oxaliplatin dose reduction to 65 mg/m^2 on subsequent cycles. In such circumstances, consideration should be given to making similar reductions in the 5-FU dose. Consult an experienced prescriber if you are in any doubt.
- Neurological toxicity after oxaliplatin treatment is common. Patients who have already received any previous doses of oxaliplatin should be specifically questioned about neurological symptoms, and doses should be adjusted as follows.

  If symptoms last longer than 7 days and are troublesome, the subsequent oxaliplatin dose should be reduced from 85 to 65 mg/m^2.

  If parasthesia without functional impairment persists until the next course of treatment, the subsequent oxaliplatin dose should be reduced from 85 to 65 mg/m^2.

  If parasthesia with functional impairment persists until the next cycle, oxaliplatin should be discontinued.

  If these symptoms improve following discontinuation of therapy, consideration can be given to reintroducing oxaliplatin.

  5-FU and FA are not expected to contribute to peripheral neurotoxicity, and their doses do not need modification for this reason.
- Any patient who has experienced acute pharyngolaryngeal dysasthesia during or shortly after oxaliplatin infusion *may* be retreated with caution. Any subsequent drug infusions should be over 6 h.
- Oxaliplatin doses should also be reduced from 85 to 65 mg/m^2 in patients who have experienced grade 4 diarrhoea after previous cycles. Similar dose reductions in 5-FU should also be considered. Seek advice from a senior member of the medical team if you are unsure about this.
- Check hepatic function. Consideration should be given to reducing 5-FU doses in patients with moderate hepatic dysfunction (*see* Appendix 1). Similar caution is advised with regard to the use of oxaliplatin in patients with severe hepatic impairment, since there is little experience of its use in this situation.
- Check renal function prior to prescribing. Estimation from serum creatinine levels by the Cockcroft–Gault equation is acceptable if the patient has a stable creatinine concentration and no confounding factors (e.g. catabolic states):

CrCl (mL/min)

$$= \frac{1.04 \text{ (females) or } 1.23 \text{ (males)} \times (140 - \text{age in years}) \times \text{weight in kg}}{\text{serum creatinine concentration (}\mu\text{mol/L)}}.$$

Oxaliplatin is contraindicated in patients with severe renal impairment (CrCl < 30 mL/min). Consideration should also be given to 5-FU dose reduction in the case of severe renal dysfunction (*see* Appendix 2).
- Prescribe anti-emetics appropriate to highly emetogenic chemotherapy for day 1 and weakly emetogenic chemotherapy for day 2, according to local protocol.
- Since peripheral neuropathy is common, the patient should be warned of the possibility and reassured that any symptoms which they do experience are likely to be transient. They should be encouraged to keep any affected body part warm,

as exposure to cold is likely to precipitate or aggravate symptoms. Keeping warm also reduces the risk of acute pharyngolaryngeal dysasthesia. The patient should be warned about this possible side-effect which, although rare, can be distressing, especially if it is unexpected.

- If the patient is prescribed low-dose warfarin (*see* TTO section above), ensure that arrangements are made for either the patient's GP or the hospital to check the patient's INR about 1 week after starting the drug, to ensure that they are not hypersensitive to it. Communicate clearly to the patient's GP that this dose of warfarin is not intended to alter the INR significantly, and that the dose should not be increased without consultation.
- Pyridoxine 50 mg three times a day is sometimes used to treat 'hand-and-foot' syndrome and mucositis arising from 5-FU treatment, but its value is dubious and it should not be relied upon as the sole measure for dealing with significant toxicity.
- Disposable 5-FU infusion devices are time-consuming to fill, and are likely to be prepared by pharmacy ahead of time in order to keep patient waiting times down to an acceptable level. However, once these devices have been filled, it is impossible to alter the infusion rate. Therefore for patients on established treatment it is unhelpful to make dose alterations without good reason and adequate notice, so try to avoid this if possible. For example, dosage adjustment for small degrees of weight loss or weight gain in patients who are tolerating their treatment well are not urgent — it may be appropriate to request a small dose change for the *next* cycle, but to maintain the dose unchanged on the current cycle.

NURSES NOTE

- It is important to flush the venous access with 5% dextrose before and after oxaliplatin, as this drug is incompatible with saline and with other drugs.
- Since peripheral neuropathy is common, the patient should be warned of the possibility and reassured that any symptoms which they do experience are likely to be transient. They should be encouraged to keep any affected body part warm, as exposure to cold is likely to precipitate or aggravate symptoms. Keeping warm also reduces the risk of pharyngolaryngeal dysasthesia. The patient should be warned about this possible side-effect of oxaliplatin which, although rare, can be distressing, especially if it is unexpected.
- Laryngopharyngeal symptoms during and shortly after oxaliplatin infusion are fairly rare, but are likely to be alarming to the patient. If any patient does experience abnormal sensations in the mouth or tongue, or subjective feelings of dyspnoea or dysphagia, the infusion should be stopped and the patient reassured that their symptoms, although unpleasant, are likely to resolve rapidly without treatment. Of course, dyspnoea *with evidence of bronchospasm* may represent an allergic response, in which case prompt intervention is required, as for any anaphylactic episode. If the decision is made to retreat any patient who has experienced pharyngolaryngeal dyasthesia with oxaliplatin, it should be infused over 6 h rather than 2 h.
- Arrangements must be in place at the end of each cycle of treatment for removing the empty infusion device and flushing the venous access. It may be possible for this to be done by a practice nurse or district nurse in or close to the

patient's home. However, not all non-oncology nurses are happy with this role, and it should not be *assumed* that they will take it on. This should be checked before any promises are made to the patient.

- If the patient is taking low-dose warfarin to prevent thrombosis of the venous access, take any appropriate opportunity to make sure they understand that they should take a fixed dose of 1 mg daily. This may help to prevent problems if anyone (e.g. the patient's GP) tries to increase the dose inappropriately.

- Some patients may find home infusion therapy a source of anxiety. As well as attempting to reassure them, arrangements should be in place that allow the patient or their carer to contact an informed professional at any time if they experience problems.

- Because disposable infusion devices have fixed flow rates, care should be taken that the timing of day 2 and day 3 clinic appointments coincides with the projected end of 5-FU infusions. If the latter have not finished when the patient arrives, it is impossible (and would in any case be undesirable) to speed them up in order to finish them. Similarly, for patients who are receiving de Gramont plus oxaliplatin, a gap between day 1 and day 2 treatment is undesirable. Therefore the day 2 appointment should be as close as possible to 24 h after the start of treatment on day 1.

NOTES FOR PHARMACISTS

- Do not forget that in this regimen the FA must be infused in 5% dextrose, as it has to be administered concomitantly with oxaliplatin, which is incompatible with saline and 5-FU.

- Make sure that you are clear which chemotherapy regimen the patient is to receive. Is it de Gramont plus oxaliplatin, modified de Gramont plus oxaliplatin or another combination of oxaliplatin, 5-FU and FA? Be particularly careful if patients are in clinical trials.

- Make sure that the FBC has been checked and is within an acceptable range prior to issuing the chemotherapy. Oxaliplatin is contraindicated if the neutrophil count is $<1.5 \times 10^9$/L or the platelet count is $<50 \times 10^9$/L. The manufacturer of oxaliplatin recommends that patients who experience febrile neutropenia after oxaliplatin, or whose neutrophil count falls to $<1.0 \times 10^9$/L or whose platelet count falls to $<50 \times 10^9$/L (even if they remain well) should have an oxaliplatin dose reduction to 65 mg/m^2 on subsequent cycles, so the nadir count should also be checked if one is available. In such circumstances, consideration should be given to making similar reductions in the 5-FU dose.

- Specific dose reductions are recommended for oxaliplatin in patients who experience neuropathy or grade 4 diarrhoea as a result of oxaliplatin treatment. If you are aware that the patient has experienced such toxicity, check that the appropriate dose reductions have been made (for further details of suggested reductions, *see* Notes for prescribers above). Note the reasons for and the degree of dose reduction in any pharmacy patient record (*see* Appendix 3 for an example).

- Check hepatic function. Consideration should also be given to reducing 5-FU and oxaliplatin doses in patients with moderate hepatic dysfunction (*see* Appendix 1).

- Check the renal function prior to prescribing. Oxaliplatin is contraindicated in patients with severe renal impairment (CrCl < 30 mL/min). Consideration should be given to 5-FU dose reduction patients with severe renal dysfunction (*see* Appendix 2).

- Make sure that anti-emetics suitable for highly emetogenic chemotherapy (day 1) and weakly emetogenic chemotherapy (day 2) have been prescribed according to local policy.
- If you are counselling the patient, suggest that they try to keep their extremities warm, as this will minimise their risk of experiencing neuropathic symptoms. In addition, keeping warm reduces the risk of pharyngolaryngeal dysasthesia. The patient should also be warned about this possible side-effect of oxaliplatin which, although rare, can be distressing, especially if it is unexpected.
- If the patient is not prescribed low-dose warfarin at the start of treatment, check whether this is needed (*see* TTO section above). If it is contraindicated, record this on any pharmacy patient record to prevent future prescribing.
- If it is proposed to retreat a patient who you know has experienced pharyngolaryngeal symptoms on a previous cycle, make sure that the oxaliplatin infusion time is extended to 6 h.
- Pyridoxine 50 mg three times a day is sometimes used to treat 'hand-and-foot' syndrome and mucositis, but its value is dubious and it should not be relied upon as the sole measure for managing significant toxicity.

SOURCE MATERIAL

Oxaliplatin plus de Gramont

- de Gramont A, Figer M, Seymour M *et al.* (1998) A randomized trial of leucovorin (LV) and 5-fluorouracil (5-FU) with or without oxaliplatin in advanced colorectal cancer (CRC). *Proc Am Soc Clin Oncol.* **17**: 257 (abstract).

DHAP (dexamethasone, cytarabine, cisplatin)

USUAL INDICATION

Relapsed lymphoma and myeloma.

DOSES

Dexamethasone 40 mg PO/IV once daily for 4 days
Cisplatin 100 mg/m^2 IV over 24 h on day 1
Cytarabine (cytosine arabinoside, Ara-C) 2000 mg/m^2 IV every 12 h for two doses only on day 2

ADMINISTRATION

Cisplatin is administered as a continuous infusion over a period of 24 h. It is nephrotoxic, especially at the high dose used in this regimen, and extensive hydration is mandatory to dilute the drug and minimise toxicity as it is excreted via the kidneys. The aim of hydration is to maintain a urine output of 100 mL/h during and for 6–8 h after cisplatin administration. Mannitol is usually given to ensure that urine output is brisk. Electrolytes are added to compensate for cisplatin-induced electrolyte wasting.

Cytarabine is administered as a 4-h infusion in 500 mL of 0.9% sodium chloride. If dexamethasone is being administered intravenously, it should be given as a slow IV bolus or short infusion (over at least 5 min) to prevent perineal discomfort as a result of histamine release.

ANTI-EMETICS

High emetogenic potential (see local policy), although because of the high doses of dexamethasone incorporated into the regimen, extra steroids should not be prescribed routinely.

CYCLE LENGTH

21 days.

NUMBER OF CYCLES

Variable. As a salvage regimen, it may be used to test chemosensitivity/achieve remission prior to high-dose chemotherapy and stem-cell transplantation.

SIDE-EFFECTS

Nephrotoxicity (dose-limiting), ototoxicity, bone-marrow suppression, alopecia (rarely extensive), nausea and vomiting (may be very severe), sensory, motor and occasionally autonomic neuropathy (sometimes irreversible) from cisplatin, plus CNS toxicity (commonly cerebellar, and usually resolves within 4–7 days, although sometimes irreversible/fatal) from cytarabine, mucositis (not usually serious). Chemical conjunctivitis from cytarabine. Erythema, 'flu-like' syndrome and (rarely) respiratory distress from cytarabine. The high doses of dexamethasone used in this regimen can produce a variety of steroid side-effects, including euphoria/depression, epigastric discomfort, glucose intolerance, insomnia and psychosis.

TTOS REQUIRED

- Anti-emetics appropriate to highly emetogenic chemotherapy (according to local policy, although note that because of the high-dose dexamethasone incorporated into the regimen, additional steroids are unlikely to be required).
- Steroid eyedrops (e.g. Predsol®, two drops in each eye four times a day) starting on day 2 and continuing for 7 days after cytarabine administration, to prevent chemical conjunctivitis.
- Allopurinol (300 mg by mouth, once daily, reduced dose in renal impairment) to prevent tumour lysis syndrome.
- Sufficient dexamethasone to complete the treatment course if this is unfinished at the time of hospital discharge.
- Consideration should be given to prescribing a gastroprotective agent (e.g. ranitidine 150 mg twice daily by mouth) for the duration of dexamethasone treatment, in order to prevent gastritis.

NOTES FOR PRESCRIBERS

- Check the FBC prior to giving the go-ahead for chemotherapy. Seek advice if the neutrophil count is $<1.5 \times 10^9$/L or the platelet count is $<100 \times 10^9$/L at the time of treatment. The following dose reductions were used in the trial by Velasquez et al.,[1] with almost 50% of the 90 patients treated requiring hospitalisation for infections (many clinicians will adopt a more conservative approach):

[1] Velasquez WS, Cabanillas F, Salvador P et al. (1988) Effective salvage therapy for lymphoma with cisplatin in combination with high-dose ara-C and dexamethasone (DHAP). *Blood.* **71**: 117–22.

Blood count	Cytarabine dose	Cisplatin dose
Neutrophils $<0.2 \times 10^9$/L	1000 mg/m^2	100 mg/m^2
Platelets $<20 \times 10^9$/L	1000 mg/m^2	100 mg/m^2
Neutropenic sepsis	500 mg/m^2	100 mg/m^2

- The creatinine clearance should be formally assessed at the start of treatment. Ideally this should be done by EDTA clearance, but estimation by the Cockcroft–Gault equation from the serum creatinine concentration is acceptable if the patient has stable creatinine levels and no confounding factors (e.g. catabolic states):

CrCl (mL/min)

$$= \frac{1.04 \text{ (females) or } 1.23 \text{ (males)} \times (140 - \text{age in years}) \times \text{weight in kg}}{\text{serum creatinine concentration } (\mu mol/L)}$$

On subsequent cycles the renal function should be reassessed.

Doses *must be reduced* if the creatinine clearance drops below 60 mL/min (*see* Appendix 2 for further guidance).
- Check electrolytes for cisplatin-induced wasting, especially of magnesium, calcium and potassium. Additional supplementation may be required.
- Check the LFTs. A cytarabine dose adjustment is necessary in patients with severe hepatic dysfunction (*see* Appendix 1 for further guidance).
- Prescribe anti-emetics appropriate to highly emetogenic chemotherapy according to local policy, although note that because of the high doses of dexamethasone included in this regimen, additional steroids are not required.
- If the patient reports symptoms indicative of neurotoxicity (parasthesias, difficulty with motor control) or ototoxicity (tinnitus, deafness), seek further advice on whether to continue or modify treatment.
- Prescribe 4 days only of dexamethasone 40 mg once daily on the inpatient chart (and any days of treatment remaining on the TTO prescription at discharge). Make sure that it is clearly stated on any prescription or in any communication with the patient's GP that the dexamethasone is a short course of 4 days only. *Fatalities have resulted from the inadvertent continuation of short courses of steroids.*
- Consider prescribing a gastroprotective agent (e.g. ranitidine 150 mg twice daily by mouth) for the days on which high-dose dexamethasone is given, in order to reduce gastritis.
- Prescribe allopurinol (300 mg once daily by mouth, reduced dose in cases of renal impairment) continuously from the start of DHAP therapy in order to prevent the formation of large quantities of uric acid from products released during cell lysis. Urate is poorly soluble, and there is a risk of it precipitating in the kidneys and causing renal failure (urate nephropathy or tumour lysis syndrome). Allopurinol should be continued for as long as a significant bulk of chemosensitive tumour remains.
- Prescribe steroid eyedrops (e.g. Predsol®, two drops in each eye four times a day) to start before cytarabine and to continue for 7 days afterwards, in order to minimise the risk of cytarabine-induced conjunctivitis.

- The fluid balance/body weight should be monitored throughout the hydration period. In general, if the patient gains 1.5 L/kg or more from the start of hydration, extra diuresis will be required (e.g. furosemide 20–40 mg by mouth).

NOTES FOR NURSES

- The patient should be on a fluid-balance chart and daily weights should be recorded during IV therapy, which is intended to achieve an average urine output of 100 mL/h or more during and for 6–8 h after cisplatin. Contact the prescriber if the urine output is inadequate or body weight increases by 1.5 kg or more from baseline.
- Unfortunately, dexamethasone tablets *do not* come in larger sizes than 2 mg, so patients *do* have to take 20 tablets per dose. Ideally, all 20 tablets should be taken in the morning with or after food.
- If you are issuing dexamethasone tablets to the patient, explain to them that these should be taken for 4 days only (including any taken in hospital), and that they should not attempt to obtain further supplies from their GP. *Fatalities have resulted from the inadvertent continuation of short courses of steroids.*
- Ensure that any diabetic patients are aware of the need to be extra vigilant about monitoring their blood sugar levels during treatment with dexamethasone, and emphasise that they should contact their doctor if they experience problems with the control of their blood sugar levels.

NOTES FOR PHARMACISTS

- The acronym DHAP is derived from **D**examethasone, **H**igh-dose Ara-C (cytarabine), **P**latinum (cisplatin).

On the day of prescribing

- Ensure that the FBC has been checked and is within acceptable limits before making up the chemotherapy.
- Check that the creatinine clearance has been measured/calculated at the start of treatment. Record the CrCl and the corresponding creatinine concentration on any pharmacy patient record (*see* Appendix 3 for an example). Recalculate the CrCl if the creatinine concentration changes. Doses *must be reduced* if the creatinine clearance drops below 60 mL/min (*see* Appendix 2 for further guidance).
- Check the LFTs. A cytarabine dose adjustment is necessary in patients with severe hepatic dysfunction (*see* Appendix 1 for further guidance).
- Check that anti-emetics appropriate to highly emetogenic chemotherapy have been prescribed according to local protocol, although note that because of the high-dose dexamethasone included in this regimen, additional steroids are not required.
- Check that allopurinol (300 mg once daily by mouth, reduced dose in cases of renal impairment) has been prescribed prior to starting chemotherapy. This should be given continuously during chemotherapy to prevent the formation of

large quantities of uric acid from products released during cell lysis. Urate is poorly soluble, and there is a risk of it precipitating in the kidneys and causing renal failure (urate nephropathy or tumour lysis syndrome). Allopurinol should be continued for as long as a significant bulk of chemosensitive tumour remains.

- Check that dexamethasone is prescribed according to protocol on the inpatient chart and, if necessary, on any discharge prescription to give a total of 4 days of treatment. Ensure that any inpatient dexamethasone prescription has a stop date, and that any discharge dexamethasone is labelled with a duration. A steroid card or 'tailing off' of doses are not routinely required with this 4-day course. If you are issuing tablets, explain to the patient that they should not attempt to obtain a repeat prescription from their GP.
- Unfortunately, dexamethasone tablets do not come in larger sizes than 2 mg, so patients *do* have to take 20 tablets per dose. Ideally, all 20 tablets should be taken in the morning with or after food.
- Check that ranitidine (150 mg twice a day by mouth) or another gastroprotective has been considered to cover the period of dexamethasone administration, in order to reduce gastritis.
- Check that steroid eyedrops (e.g. Predsol®, two drops in each eye four times a day) have been prescribed to start before cytarabine and to continue for 7 days afterwards, in order to minimise the risk of cytarabine-induced conjunctivitis.
- When visiting the ward, check that the patient has not gained more than 1.5 L/kg since the start of IV hydration. If they have, discuss the need for additional diuresis with the prescriber (if this measure has not already been instituted).

SOURCE MATERIAL

- Velasquez WS, Cabanillas F, Salvador P *et al.* (1988) Effective salvage therapy for lymphoma with cisplatin in combination with high-dose ara-C and dexamethasone (DHAP). *Blood.* **71**: 117–22.

Docetaxel (Taxotere®) (single-agent)

USUAL INDICATION

Anthracycline-resistant metastatic breast cancer and non-small-cell lung cancer relapsing after first-line chemotherapy.

DOSES

Breast cancer

100 mg/m^2 IV on day 1

Relapsed non-small-cell lung cancer

75 mg/m^2 IV on day 1

Note:
1 Dose reduction is mandatory in cases of significant hepatic impairment (see below).
2 This is a highly myelosuppressive regimen, and in patients with breast cancer and poor bone-marrow reserve (due to extensive prior treatment/bone metastases/ extensive skeletal irradiation) or poor performance status, an empirical first-course dose reduction to 75 mg/m^2 has been made with a view to increasing to the full dose if it is well tolerated. It should be noted that this practice is not recommended by the manufacturer.
3 Lower doses have been given on a weekly basis in clinical trials in an attempt to improve the therapeutic index of docetaxel. However, these cannot yet be recommended for routine use.

ADMINISTRATION

IV infusion in 5% dextrose over a period of 1 h after the following premedication:

Dexamethasone 8 mg by mouth twice a day for 3 days starting the morning of the day prior to chemotherapy (i.e. day -1).

ANTI-EMETICS

Low emetogenic potential (see local policy), although note that patients will be receiving dexamethasone in any case as part of the regimen.

CYCLE LENGTH

21 days.

NUMBER OF CYCLES

Usually 6.

SIDE-EFFECTS

Bone-marrow suppression (mainly neutropenia), total alopecia, nausea and vomiting, myalgia/arthralgia, fluid retention, allergic skin reactions, sensory neuropathy, hypersensitivity, mucositis.

BLOOD NADIR

Day 7.

TTOS REQUIRED

- Anti-emetics appropriate to weakly emetogenic chemotherapy (according to local policy).
- Dexamethasone 8 mg by mouth twice a day for 3 days (the day before, the day of and the day after docetaxel) to prevent fluid retention and hypersensitivity reactions. The prescription should direct the patient to 'Take 8 mg (4 × 2 mg tablets) twice daily for 2 days, including the day of docetaxel (Taxotere) treatment, and start taking it again on the morning of the day before the next docetaxel (Taxotere) treatment'. The objective is 3 days of continuous dexamethasone treatment (8 mg twice a day) starting the day before each dose of docetaxel.

NOTES FOR PRESCRIBERS

- Check the FBC prior to giving the go-ahead for chemotherapy. Seek advice if the neutrophil count is $<1.5 \times 10^9$/L or the platelet count is $<100 \times 10^9$/L. The doses should be reduced from 100 mg/m^2 to 75 mg/m^2, or from 75 mg/m^2 to 60 mg/m^2, in patients who experienced either febrile neutropenia or prolonged, profound neutropenia (neutrophil count $<0.5 \times 10^9$/L for more than 5 days) on the previous course.
- Because the standard dose of docetaxel is so close to the maximum tolerated dose, strong consideration should be given to treating obese patients according to their ideal rather than their actual body weight in order to minimise the risk of toxicity.
- Check the patient's LFTs. *Dose reduction is mandatory in significant hepatic impairment* (*see* Appendix 1 or the manufacturer's SPC for detailed advice).

- Investigate weight gain on subsequent courses. This may be the result of docetaxel-induced fluid retention, and therefore not an indication to increase the docetaxel dose.
- Ask the patient if they have experienced any abnormal sensations or skin rashes. These may indicate neuropathy/cutaneous reactions that require dose modification. Seek advice if they report such symptoms. Detailed advice on dose reduction in the event of cutaneous or neurological toxicity can be found in the manufacturer's SPC.
- Make sure that the patient has taken oral premedication at home/in hospital, and do not forget to prescribe steroids for them to take home for use after this course and prior to the next one (see above). Steroids are needed to prevent acute hypersensitivity reactions. Correct steroid co-medication may also reduce skin reactions and fluid retention. The steroid regimen used is an unusual one, so make sure that any prescriptions state the dosage regimen clearly. In particular, make it clear in any communication that the dexamethasone courses are of only 3 days' duration and should not be extended by the patient's GP.
- The patient should be observed reasonably closely during treatment, especially during the first two treatment cycles, because acute hypersensitivity reactions have been reported.
- Prior to treatment, hair loss should be discussed with the patient. It is likely to be extensive in most patients, and scalp cooling is unlikely to prevent it. Liaise with nurses with regard to referral to a wig-fitter at the start of treatment and before alopecia is evident if this is appropriate.

NOTES FOR NURSES

- Make sure that the patient has taken oral dexamethasone premedication at home/ on the ward. Docetaxel has been known to produce hypersensitivity reactions, and proper steroid co-medication will also reduce the risk of fluid retention and skin reactions.
- The patient should be observed reasonably closely during the treatment, especially during the first two cycles, because acute hypersensitivity reactions have been reported.
- Inform the prescriber if the patient reports any abnormal sensations that may be indicative of drug-induced neuropathy.
- Make sure that new patients understand how to take their take-home dexamethasone tablets, as the schedule can be a little confusing.
- Mucositis can be a problem with docetaxel, and the patient should be instructed on how to deal with this side-effect if it arises (e.g. use of soft toothbrushes, avoidance of spicy foods, etc.).
- Ensure that any diabetic patients are aware of the need to be extra vigilant about monitoring their blood sugar levels during treatment with dexamethasone, and emphasise that they should contact their doctor if they experience problems with the control of their blood sugar levels.
- Prior to treatment, hair loss should be discussed with the patient. It is likely to be extensive in most patients, and scalp cooling is unlikely to prevent it. Refer the patient to a wig-fitter at the start of treatment and before alopecia is evident if this is appropriate.

NOTES FOR PHARMACIST'S

- Ensure that the FBC has been checked prior to issuing chemotherapy. Seek confirmation of the prescription if the neutrophil count is $<1.5 \times 10^9/L$ or the platelet count is $<100 \times 10^9/L$, as this is a highly myelosuppressive treatment. The doses should be reduced from $100 \, mg/m^2$ to $75 \, mg/m^2$, or from $75 \, mg/m^2$ to $60 \, mg/m^2$, in patients who experienced either febrile neutropenia or prolonged, profound neutropenia (neutrophil count $<0.5 \times 10^9/L$ for more than 5 days) on the previous course.
- Because the standard dose of docetaxel is so close to the maximum tolerated dose, strong consideration should be given to treating obese patients according to their ideal rather than their actual body weight, in order to minimise the risk of toxicity.
- Check the patient's LFTs. *Dose reduction is mandatory in significant hepatic impairment* (*see* Appendix 1 or the manufacturer's SPC for detailed advice).
- If a dosage increase has been requested on the basis of significant weight gain since the previous course, check whether this is true weight gain or the result of docetaxel-induced fluid retention. The latter is not an indication to increase the docetaxel dose.
- If the patient is on their first course of treatment, make sure that they were previously prescribed oral dexamethasone premedication and have taken it prior to treatment.
- Make sure that dexamethasone post-/premedication tablets are included in the patient's discharge medications. If oral steroid premedications are not given as part of the patient's discharge medication for any reason (e.g. because the patient is thought to be on their last treatment cycle), annotate clearly any pharmacy patient record (*see* Appendix 3 for an example) to ensure that if the patient is retreated, care is taken to check that they receive premedication.

  Ensure that any dexamethasone prescription sent for dispensing clearly states the dose schedule and how to label the tablets. This is an unusual regimen and difficult to interpret if one is not used to it.
- Make sure that new patients understand how to take their dexamethasone post-premedication tablets, as the schedule can be rather confusing. Ensure they understand that the dexamethasone treatment is a short course only, and that they should not attempt to obtain a further supply from their GP.

SOURCE MATERIAL

Lung cancer

- Shepherd FA, Dancey J, Ramlau R *et al.* (2000) Prospective randomized trial of docetaxel versus best supportive care in patients with non-small-cell lung cancer previously treated with platinum-based chemotherapy. *J Clin Oncol.* **18**: 2095–103.

Breast cancer

- Nabholtz J-M, Senn HJ, Bezwoda WR *et al.* (1999) Prospective randomized trial of docetaxel versus mitomycin plus vinblastine in patients with metastatic breast cancer progressing despite previous anthracycline-containing chemotherapy. *J Clin Oncol.* **17**: 1413–24.

Doxorubicin (single-agent)

Note: This chapter refers to conventional doxorubicin. The information cannot necessarily be applied to liposomal formulations.

USUAL INDICATION

Anthracycline-naive breast cancer.

DOSES

50–75* mg/m^2 IV on day 1

ADMINISTRATION

By slow IV injection into the side-arm of a free-running saline drip.

Doxorubicin is a powerful vesicant and should be administered with appropriate precautions to prevent extravasation. If there is any possibility that extravasation has occurred, contact a senior member of the medical team immediately and follow the local guidance for dealing with extravasation injuries.

ANTI-EMETICS

High emetogenic potential (see local policy).

CYCLE LENGTH

21 days.

NUMBER OF CYCLES

Usually 6.

---

*In general, lower doses are used for less fit patients and higher doses for fitter patients. Doses should not normally exceed 75 mg/m^2 without further consultation with an experienced prescriber, and usually as part of a research protocol.

SIDE-EFFECTS

Bone-marrow suppression, alopecia, nausea and vomiting, mucositis, cardiac arrhythmias, dilated cardiomyopathy (especially at cumulative doses in excess of $450 \, mg/m^2$).

BLOOD NADIR

10 days.

TTOS REQUIRED

- Anti-emetics appropriate to highly emetogenic chemotherapy (see local policy).

NOTES FOR PRESCRIBERS

- Patients over 60 years of age or with a history of heart disease must have an echocardiogram or MUGA scan prior to treatment to ensure that there is adequate left ventricular function.
- Check the LFTs. If these show serious impairment, a reduction in doxorubicin dose may be required (*see* Appendix 1 for further guidance).
- Check the FBC prior to giving the go-ahead for chemotherapy. Seek advice if the neutrophil count is $<1.5 \times 10^9/L$ or the platelet count is $<100 \times 10^9/L$. Note that the early studies cited in this chapter used nadir blood counts as the basis for dosage adjustment, which does not generally reflect current clinical practice.
- Prior to treatment, hair loss should be discussed with the patient. Scalp cooling can be planned for those who are particularly concerned about this, although it should be made clear to the patient that this is not universally or completely effective. Liaise with the nurses with regard to referral to a wig-fitter at the start of treatment and before alopecia is evident if this is appropriate.
- If administering the drug, *see* Administration section above for notes on the vesicant nature of doxorubicin.
- Prescribe anti-emetics appropriate to highly emetogenic chemotherapy according to local protocol.
- Check the cumulative dose of doxorubicin on this and any previous treatment course at your hospital or elsewhere. Because of the risk of cardiotoxicity, a cumulative dose of $450 \, mg/m^2$ should only be exceeded with extreme caution, after a formal assessment of cardiac function and discussion with the senior member of the medical team. The impact of previous treatment with other anthracyclines (e.g. aclarubicin, epirubicin, daunorubicin, idarubicin) must also be considered.

NOTES FOR NURSES

- Prior to treatment, hair loss should be discussed with the patient. Scalp cooling can be planned for those who are particularly concerned about this, although it should be made clear to the patient that this is not universally or completely effective. If appropriate, refer the patient to a wig-fitter at the start of treatment before alopecia is evident.

- If administering the drug, *see* Administration section above for notes on the vesicant nature of doxorubicin.

NOTES FOR PHARMACISTS

- Check that the FBC has been determined and is within acceptable limits before issuing the chemotherapy.
- Check the LFTs. If these show serious impairment, a reduction in the doxorubicin dose may be required (*see* Appendix 1 for further guidance).
- Check that anti-emetics appropriate to highly emetogenic chemotherapy have been prescribed according to local protocol.
- Keep a close eye on the patient's cumulative dose of doxorubicin, and alert the prescriber if it exceeds $450\,mg/m^2$. It is especially important when a patient starts a course of treatment to check your records and the patient's notes to see whether they have received previous anthracycline therapy at your hospital or elsewhere. The impact of previous treatment with other anthracyclines (e.g. aclarubicin, epirubicin, daunorubicin, idarubicin) must also be considered.

SOURCE MATERIAL

First-line treatment

- Hoogstraten B, George SL and Samal B (1976) Combination chemotherapy and adriamycin in patients with advanced breast cancer. *Cancer.* **38**: 13–20.

Second-line treatment

- Gottlieb JA, Rivkin SE, Spigel SC *et al.* (1974) Superiority of Adriamycin over oral nitrosoureas in patients with advanced breast carcinoma. *Cancer.* **35**: 519–26.

DTIC (dacarbazine) (single-agent)

USUAL INDICATION

Malignant melanoma.

DOSES

Dacarbazine 800* mg/m^2 on day 1

ADMINISTRATION

Dacarbazine is administered by IV infusion, normally in 1000 mL of 0.9% sodium chloride over a period of 1 h. Increasing the infusion time may be helpful in patients who experience venous pain at the infusion site. Extravasation generally results in very severe pain but little tissue damage.

ANTI-EMETICS

High emetogenic potential (apply local policy).

CYCLE LENGTH

28 days.

NUMBER OF CYCLES

Usually 6.

SIDE-EFFECTS

Bone-marrow suppression, alopecia (generally modest), facial flushing during infusion, nausea and vomiting, mucositis (rare).

---

* Doses of 1000 mg/m^2 have been used and are reasonably well tolerated, but there is no evidence that they are more active than 800 mg/m^2, which seems to be more widely used.

BLOOD NADIR

10 days.

TTOS REQUIRED

Anti-emetics appropriate to highly emetogenic chemotherapy (see local protocol).

NOTES FOR PRESCRIBERS

- Check the FBC prior to giving the go-ahead for chemotherapy. Seek advice if the neutrophil count is $<1.5 \times 10^9$/L or the platelet count is $<100 \times 10^9$/L.
- Check the LFTs. If these show serious impairment, a reduction in dacarbazine dose may be required, as the drug is activated in the liver and is also hepatotoxic (see Appendix 1 for further advice).
- The renal function should be formally assessed at the start of treatment. Estimation from serum creatinine levels using the Cockcroft–Gault equation is acceptable if the patient has a stable creatinine concentration and no confounding factors (e.g. catabolic states):

CrCl (mL/min)

$$= \frac{1.04 \text{ (females) or } 1.23 \text{ (males)} \times (140 - \text{age in years}) \times \text{weight in kg}}{\text{serum creatinine concentration } (\mu mol/L)}.$$

Consideration should be given to reducing the dacarbazine dose in patients with a CrCl of <60 mL/min (see Appendix 2 for further advice).

- Prior to treatment, hair loss should be discussed with the patient. Hair loss is generally limited with dacarbazine. Scalp cooling is of limited benefit in preventing alopecia caused by dacarbazine, because of the prolonged half-life of the drug.
- If venous pain is a problem during the dacarbazine administration, try slowing down the infusion to 120 min. If this fails to solve the problem, it is worth trying a GTN patch downstream of the infusion site to counteract any vasospastic component of the pain.

NOTES FOR NURSES

- Prior to treatment, hair loss should be discussed with the patient. With dacarbazine, hair loss is usually modest. Scalp cooling is unlikely to be of much benefit because of the prolonged circulation of the drug.
- The administration time and volume for dacarbazine are not critical. Therefore if venous pain is a problem during infusion, slowing down the infusion to 120 min may help.

NOTES FOR PHARMACISTS

- Check that the FBC has been determined and is within acceptable limits before issuing the chemotherapy.

- Check the LFTs. If these show ser[i] required, as dacarbazine is a[n] hepatotoxic (see Appendix 1
- Check that the renal f[n] treatment. Record the any pharmacy patient the CrCl if the creatinin[e] should be considered if th[e] further guidance).
- Check that anti-emetics appro[p] been prescribed according to the
- The administration time and volum[e] venous pain is a problem during infus[ion] 120 min may help. If this fails to solve patch downstream of the infusion to cou[nteract] the pain.

SOURCE MATERIAL

- Chapman PB, Einhorn LH, Meyers ML et al. (1999) Phase III [trial] of the Dartmouth regimen versus dacarbazine in patients wi[th] J Clin Oncol. 17: 2745–51.

ECF (epirubicin, cisplatin, 5-fluorouracil)

USUAL INDICATION

Adjuvant and palliative treatment of gastric and oesophageal cancer; treatment of advanced breast and ovarian cancers.

DOSES

Epirubicin 50 mg/m^2 IV on day 1
Cisplatin 60 mg/m^2 IV on day 1
5-Fluorouracil (5-FU) 200 mg/m^2/day on days 2–21 by continuous IV infusion

ADMINISTRATION

Epirubicin

By slow IV injection into the side-arm of a free-running saline drip.

Epirubicin is a powerful vesicant and should be administered with appropriate precautions to prevent extravasation. If there is any possibility that extravasation has occurred, contact a senior member of the medical team immediately and follow local guidance on dealing with extravasation incidents.

Cisplatin

As an infusion in 1 L over 2 h, after pre-hydration with 1 L of saline and followed by post-hydration with a further 1 L of saline. Cisplatin is nephrotoxic, and hydration is mandatory to dilute the drug as it is excreted via the kidneys, to minimise toxicity. The patients should be encouraged to drink a further 3 L of fluid during the 24 h after completion of IV hydration. The aim of hydration is to maintain a urine output of 100 mL/h during and for 6–8 h after cisplatin administration. Mannitol is also often given to ensure that urine output is brisk. Electrolytes are added to compensate for cisplatin-induced electrolyte wasting.

5-FU

By continuous IV infusion via a permanently implanted IV access (PICC, Hickman or Groschong line).

ANTI-EMETICS

High emetogenic potential (see local policy) on day 1; minimal emetogenic potential on days 2–21.

CYCLE LENGTH

21 days.

NUMBER OF CYCLES

Usually 6.

SIDE-EFFECTS

Nephrotoxicity (dose limiting due to cisplatin), bone-marrow suppression (all blood components are affected), alopecia (extensive), nausea and vomiting (may be very severe), sensory, motor and autonomic neuropathy (sometimes irreversible due to cisplatin) including significant potential for ototoxicity, mucositis (especially due to 5-FU), diarrhoea (mainly due to 5-FU), palmar-plantar erythrodysasthesia ('hand-and-foot' syndrome, due to 5-FU), dilated cardiomyopathy (due to epirubicin, especially if the cumulative dose exceeds $900 \, mg/m^2$).

BLOOD NADIR

Around 10 days.

TTOS REQUIRED

- Anti-emetic regimen appropriate to highly emetogenic chemotherapy (see local policy).
- Unless it is contraindicated, low-dose warfarin therapy (1 mg/day) should be instituted once a central venous line (Hickman or Groshong, but *not* PICC) is *in situ*, in order to prevent line thrombosis.

NOTES FOR PRESCRIBERS

When considering treatment options

- Ask yourself *whether the patient will really be able to cope with the demands of looking after an infusion pump*. This is important. Home infusion therapy, particularly with an electromechanical pump, requires the patient or their immediate carers to take an active part in their treatment. If they are unwilling or unable to do so, other treatment options should be explored. Normally patients should also have access to a telephone in case problems occur at home.

Note: Not all community nursing and medical staff are familiar with home chemotherapy. It cannot be assumed that they will take on responsibility for looking after the patient's pump at home. If this is intended, contact must be made and consent for such an approach obtained at an early stage.

- If your department has a finite number of infusion pumps available, liaise with whoever looks after them to see whether there is a free infusion pump available at the moment, *before* you promise the patient treatment. These pumps are often in short supply.
- Liaise in advance with those responsible for setting up the pump and educating the patient about their treatment. Both processes can be time-consuming, and in a busy department both need to be scheduled in advance.

At the time of prescribing

- Patients over 60 years of age or with a history of heart disease must have an echocardiogram or MUGA scan prior to their first course of treatment to ensure that there is adequate left ventricular function.
- Prior to treatment, hair loss should be discussed with the patient. Scalp cooling is likely to be only partially effective, as it provides little protection against cisplatin-induced hair loss. Liaise with the nurses with regard to referral to a wig-fitter at the start of treatment and before alopecia is evident, if this is appropriate.
- Unless it is contraindicated, prescribe low-dose warfarin (*see* TTO section above) and ensure that arrangements are made for either the GP or the hospital to check the INR about 1 week after starting the drug to ensure that the patient is not hypersensitive to it. Communicate to the GP that this dose of warfarin is not intended to alter the INR significantly and that it should not be increased without consultation.
- Renal function should be formally assessed at the start of treatment. Ideally this should be done by an EDTA clearance test, but estimation from the serum creatinine level using the Cockcroft–Gault equation is acceptable if the patient has a stable creatinine concentration and no confounding factors (e.g. catabolic states):

CrCl (mL/min)

$$= \frac{1.04 \text{ (females) or } 1.23 \text{ (males)} \times (140 - \text{age in years}) \times \text{weight in kg}}{\text{serum creatinine concentration } (\mu\text{mol/L})}.$$

On subsequent cycles, the renal function should be reassessed.

Cisplatin doses *must be reduced* if the creatinine clearance drops below 60 mL/min (*see* Appendix 2 for further guidance). In the major trial of ECF in breast cancer,[1] carboplatin (AUC 5) was substituted for cisplatin in patients with a GFR of <50 mL/min.

[1] Jones AI, Smith IE, O'Brien ME *et al.* (1994) Phase II study of continuous fluorouracil with epirubicin and cisplatin in patients with metastatic and locally advanced breast cancer: an active new regime. *J Clin Oncol.* **12**: 1259–65.

- Check electrolytes for cisplatin-induced wasting, especially of magnesium, calcium and potassium. Additional supplementation may be required.
- Prescribe anti-emetics appropriate to highly emetogenic chemotherapy according to local policy to cover cisplatin administration.
- Check the FBC prior to giving the go-ahead for chemotherapy. Seek advice if the neutrophil count is $<1.5 \times 10^9/L$ or the platelet count is $<100 \times 10^9/L$. In the major trial of ECF in breast cancer,[1] epirubicin and cisplatin were delayed by 7 days if the total WBC was $<3.0 \times 10^9/L$ or the platelet count was $<100 \times 10^9/L$ (5-FU was continued). If counts had not then recovered, treatment was delayed by a further 7 days and epirubicin and 5-FU doses were reduced by 25%. If doses were delayed further because of haematological toxicity, the doses of both epirubicin and 5-FU were reduced by 50%.
- Check the LFTs before treatment. The epirubicin dose should be reduced in cases of significant hepatic impairment. Consideration should also be given to reducing the 5-FU dose in cases of severe hepatic impairment (*see* Appendix 1 for further guidance).
- Ask the patient about symptoms indicative of neurotoxicity (parasthesias, difficulty with motor control) or ototoxicity (tinnitus, deafness), and seek further advice if they report such symptoms.
- If administering drugs, *see* Administration section above for notes on the vesicant nature of epirubicin.
- This treatment has specific toxicities associated with 5-FU infusion ('hand-and-foot' syndrome, mucositis, diarrhoea). If these symptoms are causing more than mild discomfort, this is an indication for a treatment break. 'Hand-and-foot' syndrome, mucositis and diarrhoea all resolve very rapidly (within 5–7 days) after stopping treatment. Empirical dose reductions should be of the order of 25% if they are to be worthwhile. In the major trial of ECF in breast cancer,[1] severe palmar-plantar erythrodysasthesia and persistent diarrhoea were both managed by a 1-week interuption of 5-FU infusion, followed by a 25% dose reduction.

   Note: Some individuals lack the 5-FU-metabolising enzyme dihydropyrimidine dehydrogenase (DPD), and may be particularly sensitive to the effects of 5-FU.
- Prescribe 5-FU supplies for a suitable period depending on local arrangements. For example, is the patient returning to the hospital periodically for pump reservoir changes, or are they having this done in the community by a visiting nurse or doing it themselves? However long this period is, it is recommended that the patient is seen 10–14 days after starting treatment, to ensure that there are no problems.

On the day after the cisplatin dose (if the patient is an inpatient)

- Monitor the fluid balance/body weight. If the patient has gained 1.5 L/kg or more from the start of hydration, extra diuresis will be required (e.g. furosemide 20 to 40 mg by mouth).

NOTES FOR NURSES

- Discuss probable hair loss with the patient, and refer them to a wig-fitter at the start of treatment and before alopecia is a problem, if this is appropriate. Scalp cooling is of limited value because of the prolonged exposure of the patient to cisplatin in this regimen.

- Patients with home infusion pumps will need support at home, including advice on problems with their treatment, their pump and their venous access. They are also likely to need practical help with dressing venous line insertion sites, changing infusion reservoirs and flushing unused lumens on the venous line in accordance with local policies. Local arrangements for this support must be formalised and robust. District and practice nurses may be unfamiliar with this type of treatment, and it should not be assumed that they will be willing to support patients. It is important to liaise with them first.
- Details of setting up 5-FU pumps, etc., are beyond the scope of this chapter. If this is being undertaken by nursing staff, it should be the subject of robust and formal local procedures.
- If pharmacy staff set up infusion pumps, and if the patient's dose has been adjusted, ensure as far as is possible that the infusion rate on any variable-rate infusion pump (where the dose is governed by the infusion rate) is reset to deliver the correct dose.
- The aim of hydration is to ensure an average urine output of 100 mL/h or more during and for 6–8 h after cisplatin administration. Any patient who is being treated as an inpatient should have a fluid-balance chart, and daily weights should be recorded. If the patient's urine output is inadequate or their body weight increases by 1.5 kg from baseline, contact the prescriber.

  For outpatients, efforts should be made to ensure that urine output is adequate (e.g. by ensuring that the patient has passed 500 mL of urine between the start of IV hydration and the beginning of cisplatin infusion).

  Outpatients should also be encouraged to drink 3 L of fluid in the 24 h following each period of IV hydration, and they should be advised to contact the hospital if this is impossible because of nausea/vomiting or other problems.
- If administering epirubicin, *see* Administration section above for notes on the vesicant nature of this drug.

NOTES FOR PHARMACISTS

- Check that the FBC has been determined and is within acceptable limits before issuing the chemotherapy.
- Check that the creatinine clearance has been measured/calculated at the start of treatment. Record the CrCl and the corresponding creatinine concentration on any pharmacy patient record (*see* Appendix 3 for an example). Recalculate the CrCl if the creatinine concentration changes. A cisplatin dose reduction is needed if the CrCl drops below 60 mL/min (*see* Appendix 2 for further guidance).
- Check that anti-emetics appropriate to highly emetogenic chemotherapy have been prescribed according to local protocol.
- Monitor the cumulative dose of epirubicin and alert the prescriber if it exceeds 900 mg/m^2. It is especially important when a patient starts a course of treatment to check the pharmacy records and patient notes to see whether the patient has received previous therapy. Consider the possible contribution of previous treatment with other anthracyclines (doxorubicin, daunorubicin, idarubicin).

- At the start of treatment, make sure that the patient's LFTs have been checked, and note any abnormalities on the pharmacy patient record. An epirubicin dose adjustment is needed in cases of significant hepatic dysfunction, and consideration should be given to a 5-FU dose reduction in cases of severe hepatic impairment (*see* Appendix 1 for further guidance).
- Details of setting up 5-FU pumps, etc. are beyond the scope of this chapter. If this is being undertaken by pharmacy staff, it should be the subject of robust and formal local procedures.
- If the patient's 5-FU dose has been altered, ensure as far as is possible that the infusion rate on any variable-rate infusion pump (where the dose is governed by the infusion rate) is reset to deliver the correct dose.
- When calculating 5-FU requirements for a given period of time, remember to allow enough overage to ensure that the patient will not run out of the drug before their next supply is due. The overage required will depend on the type of pump that is being used.
- If the patient is an inpatient, when visiting the ward the day after chemotherapy check that they have not gained more than 1.5 L/kg since the start of treatment. If they have, discuss additional diuresis (e.g. furosemide 20–40 mg by mouth) with the prescriber (if this measure has not already been instituted).
- If the patient is not prescribed low-dose warfarin at the start of treatment, check whether this is needed. If it is contraindicated, mark this clearly on the patient's pharmacy record to prevent future prescribing.

SOURCE MATERIAL

Breast cancer

- Jones AI, Smith IE, O'Brien ME *et al.* (1994) Phase II study of continuous fluorouracil with epirubicin and cisplatin in patients with metastatic and locally advanced breast cancer: an active new regime. *J Clin Oncol.* **12**: 1259–65.

Ovarian cancer

- Ahmed FY, King DM, Nicol B *et al.* (1995) Preliminary results of infusional chemotherapy (cisplatin, epirubicin and 5-fluorouracil, ECF) for refractory and relapsed epithelial ovarian cancer. *Proc Am Soc Clin Oncol.* **14**: 280.

Gastro-oesophageal cancer

- Highley MS, Parnis FX, Trotter GA *et al.* (1994) Combination chemotherapy with epirubicin, cisplatin and 5-fluorouracil for the palliation of advanced gastric and oesophageal adenocarcinoma. *Br J Surgery* **81**: 1763–5.

EMI (IME, IMVP-16) (ifosfamide, methotrexate, etoposide)

USUAL INDICATION

Relapsed high-grade lymphoma.

DOSES

Etoposide 100 mg/m^2 IV on days 1, 2 and 3
Ifosfamide 1000 mg/m^2 IV on days 1–5
Mesna 1000 mg/m^2 IV on days 1–5
Methotrexate 30 mg/m^2 IV on days 3 and 10
Folinic acid (calcium folinate/calcium leucovorin) 15 mg PO/IV every 6 h for six
        doses starting 24 h after each methotrexate dose

ADMINISTRATION

Ifosfamide and mesna

Mesna administration is mandatory with ifosfamide, to prevent the urothelial toxicity which can be caused by acrolein metabolites of the drug.

Mesna is administered as an IV bolus loading dose immediately prior to ifosfamide (which is given as a slow infusion in saline over a period of 1 h) and a slow infusion over the 12 h following ifosfamide administration. This scheduling is designed to ensure that there is adequate mesna in the bladder throughout the period when ifosfamide metabolites are appearing in the urine. The mesna infusion that is given after ifosfamide should not be speeded up to make the regimen quicker. Although mesna can be given as repeated IV bolus doses, this is considered to be less satisfactory, since it increases the risk that doses will be either omitted in error or given at the wrong time, resulting in a loss of protection.

If outpatient treatment is a possibility, mesna can be given orally to patients who are able and willing to comply with a strict dosing schedule. Dosing details are available in the SPC for oral mesna tablets.

Etoposide

As an IV infusion in 0.9% sodium chloride over a period of 60 min. Etoposide infusions should not be speeded up, as rapid infusion can cause hypotensive reactions.

Methotrexate

As an IV bolus.

Folinic acid

By mouth, unless the patient is vomiting severely or unable to swallow, in which case IV bolus doses may be given.

ANTI-EMETICS

High emetogenic potential (see local policy).

CYCLE LENGTH

21 days.

NUMBER OF CYCLES

Variable. May be used to induce a remission prior to high-dose chemotherapy with stem-cell transplantation.

SIDE-EFFECTS

Bone-marrow suppression (all blood components are affected), total alopecia, haemorrhagic cystitis leading to bladder fibrosis, encephalopathy during or soon after the ifosfamide administration period, vomiting (may be severe), nephrotoxicity, mucositis.

BLOOD NADIR

Around day 12.

TTOS REQUIRED

- Anti-emetics appropriate to highly emetogenic chemotherapy (see local protocol).
- Folinic acid rescue (15 mg by mouth every 6 h for six doses) to start 24 h after methotrexate administration on days 4 and 11.

NOTES FOR PRESCRIBERS

At the time of prescribing each course

- Check the FBC prior to giving the go-ahead for chemotherapy. Seek advice if the neutrophil count is $<1.5 \times 10^9$/L or the platelet count is $<100 \times 10^9$/L at the time of treatment. In the study by Cabanillas et al.,[1] treatment was delayed if the platelet count was $<100 \times 10^9$/L or the absolute granulocyte count was $<1.0 \times 10^9$/L, although it should be noted that almost 20% of cycles were complicated by infection.

Note: This treatment is usually being given with curative intent, and dose delays should therefore be avoided if at all possible. Haematopoietic growth factor (G-CSF, GM-CSF) support of neutrophil numbers may be appropriate if neutropenia is causing delays in treatment delivery (see your local policy on haematopoietic growth factors for further guidance).

- Ifosfamide is modestly nephrotoxic, and impaired renal function predisposes to ifosfamide encephalopathy. For both of these reasons, renal function should be assessed at the start of treatment. If the patient has a stable serum creatinine concentration and there are no confounding factors (e.g. catabolic states), estimation of the GFR from the serum creatinine level using the Cockcroft–Gault equation is acceptable:

CrCl (mL/min)

$$= \frac{1.04 \text{ (females) or } 1.23 \text{ (males)} \times (140 - \text{age in years}) \times \text{weight in kg}}{\text{serum creatinine concentration (}\mu\text{mol/L)}}.$$

On subsequent cycles the renal function should be reassessed.

Consideration should also be given to reducing the doses of methotrexate and etoposide if the CrCl falls below 60 mL/min (see Appendix 2 for further guidance).

- As well as poor renal function, low serum albumin levels and a large pelvic tumour mass are also risk factors for ifosfamide encephalopathy. This insidious condition can develop on any treatment course and it presents in a variety of ways, although somnolence and confusion feature strongly in the early stages. It can be fatal. Therefore as well as keeping an eye on renal function, serum albumin levels should be checked on each course. If a patient has two or more risk factors, particularly if these have developed since the previous treatment, discuss this situation with an experienced prescriber before proceeding with treatment.
- Prescribe anti-emetics appropriate to a highly emetogenic chemotherapy regimen according to local policy.
- Check the LFTs. If these show severe impairment, dose adjustments may be required for all three drugs (see Appendix 1 for further guidance).
- Liaise with the nurses who are looking after the patient to ensure that all urine voided during chemotherapy administration is tested for blood (in the case of haemorrhagic cystitis). Confirm that the nurses understand the significance of any changes in mental state which may be indicative of encephalopathy.
- If blood is reported in the urine, then increasing the mesna dose may help if ifosfamide is still being administered, or if it has been administered within the last 12 h. However, it is important to be aware that most urine test strips for blood are very sensitive, and the lowest blood levels detected by them probably do not require intervention. Consult an experienced prescriber for advice in this situation.

[1] Cabanillas F, Hagemeister FB, Bodey GP et al. (1982) An effective regimen for patients with lymphoma who have relapsed after initial combination chemotherapy. Blood. **60**: 693–7.

- If the patient displays changes in mental state which suggest encephalopathy, liaise with a senior member of the medical team immediately. Treatment suspension is strongly advised. Treatment with methylene blue (50 mg IV three times a day), which has been reported to reverse encephalopathy in this situation, should be considered. Note that mesna has no ability to ameliorate CNS toxicity.
- Folinic acid (calcium folinate, calcium leucovorin) rescue should be prescribed to reduce methotrexate toxicity. Because folinic acid is a methotrexate antagonist, it should be prescribed to start 24 h after methotrexate administration. This should be stated clearly on any prescription. If it is prescribed on an inpatient chart, the administration spaces for the 24 h after methotrexate administration should be blocked out to prevent folinic acid being given during this period.
- Poor renal function and 'third-space' fluids (pleural effusions and ascites) prolong the elimination of methotrexate, and this may increase its toxicity. If methotrexate must be given under these circumstances, prolonged folinic acid treatment (72 h is suggested) may be advisable.

NOTES FOR NURSES

- All urine should be tested for blood because of the possibility of ifosfamide-induced haemorrhagic cystitis. Extra mesna may be needed if blood is detected during or in the 12 h after mesna administration. However, it is important to be aware that most urine test strips for blood are very sensitive, and the lowest blood levels detected by them probably do not require intervention.
- Because of the importance of providing protection for the bladder throughout the ifosfamide excretion period, the final 12-h mesna infusion should not be speeded up in order to to shorten the treatment period.
- Because of the possibility of ifosfamide-induced CNS toxicity, any excessive drowsiness or confusion should be reported promptly to the medical team.
- Drug administration in this regimen is discontinuous. Each day's treatment should begin approximately 24 h after that of the previous day.
- Folinic acid (calcium folinate, calcium leucovorin) treatment should not be started until 24 h after methotrexate administration. If it is, the desired action of the methotrexate will be counteracted. Check the time of methotrexate treatment before giving any prescribed folinic acid, and explain the importance of good treatment compliance to any self-medicating patient.
- Do not forget that arrangements will need to be made for the patient to receive their mid-cycle methotrexate dose on day 10.

NOTES FOR PHARMACISTS

- Check that the FBC has been determined and is within acceptable limits before issuing chemotherapy. As EMI is often given with curative intent, treatment may proceed with a lower blood count than would be appropriate for palliative chemotherapy. Furthermore, if myelotoxicity (this means symptomatic neutropenia or a neutrophil count too low to treat at the start of the next cycle, *not* asymptomatic low nadir counts) is preventing treatment being given on time, haematopoietic growth factor (G-CSF, GM-CSF) support of neutrophil numbers may be justified (*see* your local policy on haematopoietic growth factors for further guidance).

- Check that renal function is reasonable at the start of treatment. Calculate the creatinine clearance from the serum creatinine level, using the Cockroft–Gault equation, and mark this on any pharmacy patient record sheet (*see* Appendix 3 for an example), together with the corresponding serum creatinine concentration. On subsequent courses, recalculate the CrCl if the serum creatinine concentration increases significantly. Poor renal function is a risk factor for ifosfamide encephalopathy, and ifosfamide is also modestly nephrotoxic. Consideration should also be given to reducing the doses of methotrexate and etoposide if the CrCl falls below 60 mL/min (*see* Appendix 2 for further guidance).
- Check the LFTs. If these show severe impairment, dose adjustments may be required for all three drugs (*see* Appendix 1 for further guidance).
- Check the serum albumin level at the start of treatment. Low albumin levels are another risk factor for ifosfamide encephalopathy. The serum albumin concentration should also be checked on subsequent cycles, especially if the patient has other risk factors for encephalopathy (poor renal function or large pelvic tumour mass). If the patient has multiple risk factors, especially if these include low albumin levels (which are often overlooked, as they are not routinely checked during chemotherapy), point this out to the prescriber. Multiple risk factors are not an absolute contraindication to ifosfamide therapy, but where there is a choice of therapy they may point towards an alternative.
- Check that anti-emetics appropriate to highly emetogenic chemotherapy have been prescribed according to the local protocol.
- Check that mesna has been prescribed and that the dose is appropriate (i.e. if the dose of ifosfamide on the fluid chart has been altered, then the mesna dose should have been altered proportionally).

  Note: Mesna is essentially non-toxic, and considerable rounding up of doses is acceptable to make preparation simpler.
- On visiting the ward, check that the patient's urine is being tested for the presence of blood. If any blood has been detected, discuss with the prescriber the possibility of increasing the mesna dosage. It is difficult to give guidance on a suitable increase in the mesna dose, but it is not unreasonable to double it. Refer to the SPC for further guidance. However, it is important to be aware that most urine test strips for blood are very sensitive, and the lowest blood levels detected by them probably do not require intervention.
- Any reports of patients being excessively drowsy or confused should be regarded as indicators of ifosfamide encephalopathy. As this is a progressive condition, liaise with the prescriber urgently with a view to halting treatment immediately and possibly instituting treatment with methylene blue (50 mg IV three times a day). This treatment has been reported to be beneficial, but it has not been rigorously assessed and should not be relied upon, particularly as a prophylactic measure.
- Folinic acid (calcium folinate, calcium leucovorin) rescue should be prescribed in order to reduce methotrexate toxicity. Because folinic acid is a methotrexate antagonist, it should be prescribed to start 24 h after methotrexate administration. This should be stated clearly on any prescription. If it is prescribed on an inpatient chart, the administration spaces for the 24 h after methotrexate administration should be blocked out to prevent folinic acid being given during this

period. Unless a specific decision has been made to give extended folinic acid (e.g. because of severe mucositis on a previous course of treatment or poor renal function), courses should be limited to six doses only.

- Poor renal function and 'third-space' fluids (pleural effusions and ascites) prolong the elimination of methotrexate, and this may increase its toxicity. If methotrexate must be given under these circumstances, prolonged folinic acid treatment (72 h is suggested) may be advisable.
- Because of the importance of providing protection for the bladder throughout the ifosfamide excretion period, the 12-h mesna infusion should not be speeded up in order to shorten the treatment period.

SOURCE MATERIAL

- Cabanillas F, Hagemeister FB, Bodey GP *et al.* (1982) An effective regimen for patients with lymphoma who have relapsed after initial combination chemotherapy. *Blood.* **60**: 693–7.

Methylene blue in ifosfamide encephalopathy

- Kupfer A, Aeschlimann C, Wermuth B *et al.* (1994) Prophylaxis and reversal of ifosfamide encephalopathy with methylene blue. *Lancet.* **343**: 763–4.
- Zulian GB, Tullen E and Maton B (1995) Methylene blue for ifosfamide-associated encephalopathy. *NEJM.* **332**: 1239–40.

Epirubicin (single-agent)

USUAL INDICATION

Anthracycline-naive breast cancer.

DOSES

Variable: 75–90* mg/m^2 IV on day 1

ADMINISTRATION

By slow IV injection into the side-arm of a free-running saline drip.

Epirubicin is a powerful vesicant and should be administered with appropriate precautions to prevent extravasation. If there is any possibility that extravasation has occurred, contact a senior member of the medical team immediately and follow local guidance on managing extravasation incidents.

ANTI-EMETICS

High emetogenic potential (see local policy).

CYCLE LENGTH

21 days.

NUMBER OF CYCLES

Usually 6.

SIDE-EFFECTS

Bone-marrow suppression, alopecia, nausea and vomiting, mucositis, cardiac arrhythmias, dilated cardiomyopathy (especially at cumulative doses in excess of 900 mg/m^2).

---

* In general, lower doses are used in patients with poor performance status (ECOG level 3) or with extensive bone disease, and a dose of 90 mg/m^2 is used in those with good performance status and limited bone disease. Doses should not exceed 90 mg/m^2 without a senior member of the medical team being consulted.

BLOOD NADIR

10 days.

TTOS REQUIRED

- Anti-emetics appropriate to highly emetogenic chemotherapy.

NOTES TO PRESCRIBERS

- Patients over 60 years of age or with a history of heart disease must have an echocardiogram or MUGA scan prior to treatment to ensure that there is adequate left ventricular function.
- Check the LFTs. If these show serious impairment, a reduction in epirubicin dose may be required (*see* Appendix 1 for further guidance).
- Check the FBC prior to giving the go-ahead for chemotherapy. Seek advice if the neutrophil count is $<1.5 \times 10^9$/L or the platelet count is $<100 \times 10^9$/L.
- Prior to treatment, hair loss should be discussed with the patient. Scalp cooling can be planned for those who are particularly concerned about this, although it should be made clear to the patient that this is neither universally nor completely effective. If appropriate, liaise with the nurses with regard to referral to a wig-fitter at the start of treatment and before alopecia is evident.
- If administering the drug, *see* Administration section above for notes on the vesicant nature of epirubicin.
- Prescribe anti-emetics appropriate to highly emetogenic chemotherapy according to the local protocol.
- Check the cumulative dose of epirubicin received by the patient on this and any previous treatment course at your hospital or elsewhere. Because of the risk of cardiotoxicity, a cumulative dose of 900 mg/m² should only be exceeded with extreme caution, after a formal assessment of cardiac function and discussion with the senior member of the medical team. The impact of previous treatment with other anthracyclines (e.g. daunorubicin, doxorubicin, idarubicin) must also be considered.

NOTES FOR NURSES

- Prior to treatment, hair loss should be discussed with the patient. Scalp cooling can be planned for those who are particularly concerned about this, although it should be made clear to the patient that this is neither universally nor completely effective. If appropriate, refer the patient to a wig-fitter at the start of treatment before alopecia is evident.
- If administering the drug, *see* Administration section above for notes on the vesicant nature of epirubicin.

NOTES FOR PHARMACISTS

- Check that the FBC has been determined and is within acceptable limits before issuing the chemotherapy.

- Check the LFTs. If these show serious impairment, a reduction in epirubicin dose may be required (*see* Appendix 1 for further guidance).
- Check that anti-emetics appropriate to highly emetogenic chemotherapy have been prescribed according to the local protocol.
- Keep a close eye on the cumulative dose of epirubicin and alert the prescriber if it exceeds 900 mg/m^2. It is especially important when a patient starts a course of treatment to check your records and the patient's notes to see whether they have received previous therapy in your hospital or elsewhere. The impact of previous treatment with other anthracyclines (e.g. daunorubicin, doxorubicin, idarubicin) must also be considered.

SOURCE MATERIAL

- van Oosterom A, Andersson M, Wildiers J *et al.* (1987) *Adriamycin (A) versus 4'-epi-adriamycin (E): report of a second-line randomised phase III study in advanced breast cancer.* Proceedings of the Fourth NCI-EORTC Breast Cancer Working Conference, London, 1987.

Etoposide (single-agent) oral

USUAL INDICATION

Ovarian cancer relapsing after platinum and taxane chemotherapy.

DOSES

Cycle 1

Etoposide 50 mg (total dose) PO twice daily on days 1–7

Cycle 2 (dose escalation only to be carried out if there is no grade 3 or 4 toxicity after the first cycle)

Etoposide 50 mg (total dose) PO twice daily on days 1–10

Cycles 3–6 (dose escalation only to be carried out if there is no grade 3 or 4 toxicity after the first or second cycles)

Etoposide 50 mg (total dose) PO twice daily on days 1–14

Note: Other dosing schedules have been used and reported in the medical literature. This protocol using gradual dose escalation is probably safer than the others, given the high inter-individual variation in etoposide absorption after oral treatment.

ADMINISTRATION

By mouth twice daily for 7–14 days (see above).

ANTI-EMETICS

Low emetogenic potential (see local policy).

CYCLE LENGTH

21 days.

NUMBER OF CYCLES

Usually 6.

SIDE-EFFECTS

Bone-marrow suppression, alopecia (usually significant), nausea and vomiting, mucositis, palmar-plantar erythrodysasthesia ('hand-and-foot' syndrome).

BLOOD NADIR

No clear-cut nadir because of the protracted treatment course.

TTOS REQUIRED

- Anti-emetics appropriate to weakly emetogenic chemotherapy (according to standard protocol).

NOTES FOR PRESCRIBERS

- Check the FBC prior to giving the go-ahead for chemotherapy. If the neutrophil count is $<1.5 \times 10^9/L$ or the platelet count is $<100 \times 10^9/L$, treatment should be deferred for 7 days. If the count has not recovered to this level within 1 week, serious consideration should be given to withdrawing treatment. This dosage modification was used in the study by Seymour et al.[1] If you are in any doubt, consult a senior member of the medical team who has experience of this regimen.
- This is a regimen with unpredictable and potentially severe toxicity, partly because of the wide inter-individual variation in absorption of orally administered etoposide. Published data suggest that there is a disproportionately high risk of severe toxicity in elderly patients, those with poor performance status and those with moderate to severe hepatic or renal impairment. It should be noted that in the original trial of this regimen, attempting to compensate for a reduced etoposide clearance by pharmacokinetically guided dose reduction did not prevent fatal toxicity in one patient. This suggests that reduced drug excretion may be indicative of other independent characteristics which predispose to an unacceptable risk of toxicity. Therefore patients with any of the above risk factors should be treated with extreme caution.
- Because toxicity is unpredictable, no attempt should be made to bypass the use of reduced etoposide treatment duration during the first two treatment cycles. In the published trial by Seymour et al.,[1] using 14 days of etoposide treatment for all patients from the first cycle onward led to unacceptable toxicity.
- Renal function should be assessed at the start of treatment. Unless the patient is known to have renal problems which are likely to impair renal function significantly, estimation of the CrCl from serum creatinine levels using the

---

[1] Seymour MT, Mansi JL, Gallagher CJ et al. (1994) Protracted oral etoposide in epithelial ovarian cancer: a phase II study in patients with relapsed or platinum-resistant disease. Br J Cancer. **69**: 191–5.

Cockcroft–Gault equation is acceptable provided that the patient has a stable creatinine concentration and no confounding risk factors (e.g. catabolic states):

CrCl (mL/min)

$$= \frac{1.04 \text{ (females) or } 1.23 \text{ (males)} \times (140 - \text{age in years}) \times \text{weight in kg}}{\text{serum creatinine concentration (}\mu\text{mol/L)}}.$$

On subsequent cycles, renal function should be reassessed if the creatinine concentration rises significantly.

Although etoposide is renally excreted, a dose reduction is unnecessary for mild renal impairment because the treatment starts with a low dose/course which is gradually elevated depending on tolerability. However, treatment in moderate to severe renal impairment (CrCl < 20 mL/min) should only be prescribed with extreme caution (see above).

- Check the LFTs before prescribing. The treatment of patients with moderate to severe hepatic impairment with oral etoposide should be approached with extreme caution.
- Prescribe anti-emetics appropriate to weakly emetogenic chemotherapy according to the local protocol.
- A complete cycle of capsules should always be prescribed. Any prescription should state clearly the total number of days of treatment that are required. The patient should also be made aware of the fact that treatment is for a short, fixed period only, and that they should not attempt to obtain further supplies from their GP. Any communication with the GP or other doctors should make it clear that they are not required to prescribe further supplies of etoposide. *Fatalities have resulted from the inadvertent continuation of short courses of oral cytotoxic drugs.*
- There is no oral liquid formulation of etoposide, and although the injection can be used orally, it is very unpalatable. In addition, it needs to be packed into oral syringes by pharmacy staff, which is very time-consuming. Therefore the oral etoposide regimen should only be used as a last resort in patients who are unable to swallow capsules.
- Prior to treatment, hair loss should be discussed with the patient. It is likely to be extensive in most patients, and the treatment schedule makes any type of scalp cooling impossible. Liaise with the nurses with regard to referral to a wig-fitter at the start of treatment, and before alopecia is evident, if this is appropriate.

NOTES FOR NURSES

- If you are counselling the patient about their treatment, emphasise that treatment is not continuous and that when they have finished the capsules supplied, they should not attempt to obtain repeat prescriptions from their GP. *Fatalities have resulted from the inadvertent continuation of short courses of oral cytotoxic drugs.*
- Prior to treatment, hair loss should be discussed with the patient. It is likely to be extensive in most patients, and the treatment schedule makes any type of scalp cooling impossible. Refer the patient to a wig-fitter at the start of treatment, and before alopecia is evident, if this is appropriate.

NOTES FOR PHARMACISTS

- Check that the FBC has been determined and is within acceptable limits before issuing the chemotherapy. Treatment should normally be deferred for 7 days if the neutrophil count is $<1.5 \times 10^9$/L or the platelet count is $<100 \times 10^9$/L, as in the study by Seymour et al.[1] If recovery has not occurred within 7 days, serious consideration should be given to withdrawing treatment.

- If you are counselling the patient about their treatment, emphasise the length of the treatment cycle and the importance of the fact that once the treatment which has been supplied has been completed, they should not attempt to obtain repeat prescriptions from their GP. *Fatalities have resulted from the inadvertent continuation of short courses of oral cytotoxic drugs.*

- Make sure that renal function has been assessed prior to starting treatment. Estimation of the creatinine clearance by the Cockcroft–Gault equation is acceptable (unless the patient has borderline renal function) if the patient has a stable serum creatinine concentration and no confounding factors (e.g. catabolic states). Although etoposide is renally excreted, a dose reduction is unnecessary for mild renal impairment because the treatment starts with a low dose/cycle which is gradually elevated depending on tolerability. However, treatment in moderate to severe renal impairment (CrCl < 20 mL/min) should only be undertaken with extreme caution, as impaired renal function may be a risk factor for exaggerated toxicity even if the dose is reduced in an attempt to compensate for reduced excretion. Confirm the prescription with the prescriber in cases of moderate to severe renal impairment.

- Check the LFTs before prescribing. The treatment of patients with moderate to severe hepatic impairment with oral etoposide should be approached with extreme caution. Impaired hepatic function may be a risk factor for exaggerated toxicity even if the etoposide dose is reduced in an attempt to compensate for reduced excretion. Confirm the prescription with the prescriber in cases of moderate to severe hepatic impairment.

- Check that anti-emetics appropriate to chemotherapy with low emetogenic potential have been prescribed according to the local protocol.

- If the patient is unable to swallow etoposide capsules, it is *possible* to use the injection orally. However, it is very unpalatable (cola is said to be quite effective for masking the flavour) and needs to be packed into oral syringes within the pharmacy. Therefore this regimen should only be used as a last resort for patients who are unable to swallow capsules. If the injection is to be used orally, it is theoretically necessary to allow for its slightly greater bioavailability compared with capsules. However, since the dosage is started at a relatively low level and titrated upwards according to tolerability, this is not necessary in this case.

SOURCE MATERIAL

- Seymour MT, Mansi JL, Gallagher CJ et al. (1994) Protracted oral etoposide in epithelial ovarian cancer: a phase II study in patients with relapsed or platinum-resistant disease. *Br J Cancer.* **69**: 191–5.

FAC (CAF) (5-fluorouracil, doxorubicin ['Adriamycin'], cyclophosphamide)

USUAL INDICATION

Anthracycline-naive breast cancer.

DOSES

Doxorubicin 50 mg/m^2 IV on day 1
Cyclophosphamide 500 mg/m^2 IV on day 1
5-Fluorouracil (5-FU) 500 mg/m^2 IV on day 1

ADMINISTRATION

Doxorubicin

By slow IV injection into the side-arm of a free-running saline drip.

Doxorubicin is a powerful vesicant and should be administered with appropriate precautions to prevent extravasation. If there is any possibility that extravasation has occurred, contact a senior member of the medical team immediately and follow local guidance on dealing with extravasation incidents.

5-FU and cyclophosphamide

May be given as slow IV bolus injections or short IV infusions (i.e. in 100 mL of 0.9% sodium chloride over a period of 10–20 min).

Note: The order of administration of the three drugs in this regimen is not critical.

ANTI-EMETICS

High emetogenic potential (see local policy).

CYCLE LENGTH

21 days.

NUMBER OF CYCLES

Usually 6.

SIDE-EFFECTS

Bone-marrow suppression, alopecia, nausea and vomiting, mucositis, cardiac arrhythmias, dilated cardiomyopathy (especially at cumulative doxorubicin doses in excess of 450 mg/m^2). Cyclophosphamide *can* cause haemorrhagic cystitis at high doses. However, the doses used in FAC are not likely to cause this problem, so prophylactic mesna and hydration are not required.

BLOOD NADIR

10 days.

TTOS REQUIRED

- Anti-emetics appropriate to highly emetogenic chemotherapy (see local protocol).

NOTES FOR PRESCRIBERS

- Patients over 60 years of age or with a history of heart disease must have an echocardiogram or MUGA scan prior to treatment to ensure that there is adequate left ventricular function.
- Check the LFTs. If these show serious impairment, a reduction in doxorubicin and 5-FU doses may be required (*see* Appendix 1 for further guidance).
- Check the renal function. A cyclophosphamide dose reduction is required in patients with severe renal impairment (*see* Appendix 2 for further guidance).
- Check the FBC prior to giving the go-ahead for chemotherapy. Seek advice if the neutrophil count is $<1.5 \times 10^9$/L, or the platelet count is $<100 \times 10^9$/L.
- Prescribe anti-emetics appropriate to highly emetogenic chemotherapy according to the local protocol.
- Check the cumulative dose of doxorubicin on this and any previous treatment course, at the current hospital or elsewhere. Because of the risk of cardiotoxicity, a cumulative dose of 450 mg/m^2 should only be exceeded with extreme caution, after a formal assessment of cardiac function and discussion with a senior member of the medical team. The impact of previous treatment with other anthracyclines (aclarubicin, epirubicin, daunorubicin, idarubicin) must also be considered.
- Prior to treatment, hair loss should be discussed with the patient. Scalp cooling may be of benefit in reducing hair loss with FAC, but its success is limited by the prolonged half-life of cyclophosphamide. Liaise with the nurses with regard to referral to a wig-fitter at the start of treatment and before alopecia is evident, if this is appropriate.

- If administering the drugs, *see* Administration section above for notes on the vesicant nature of doxorubicin.

NOTES FOR NURSES

- Prior to treatment, hair loss should be discussed with the patient. Scalp cooling may be of benefit in reducing hair loss with FAC, but its success is limited by the prolonged circulation time of cyclophosphamide. If appropriate, refer the patient to a wig-fitter at the start of treatment and before alopecia is evident.
- If administering the drugs, *see* Administration section above for notes on the vesicant nature of doxorubicin.
- The dose of cyclophosphamide is below that which is likely to cause haemorrhagic cystitis. Therefore prophylactic mesna, IV hydration and urine testing are not required. Any mild symptoms of dysuria may be treated by encouraging oral fluid intake and regular voiding of urine.

NOTES FOR PHARMACISTS

- Check that the FBC has been determined and is within acceptable limits before issuing the chemotherapy.
- Check the LFTs. If these show serious impairment a reduction in doxorubicin and 5-fluorouracil doses may be required (*see* Appendix 1 for further guidance).
- Check the renal function. A cyclophosphamide dose reduction is required in patients with significant renal impairment (*see* Appendix 2 for further guidance).
- Keep a close eye on the cumulative dose of doxorubicin, and alert the prescriber if this exceeds 450 mg/m^2. It is especially important when a patient starts a course of treatment to check the pharmacy records and the patient's notes to see whether they have received previous therapy at your hospital or elsewhere. The impact of previous treatment with other anthracyclines (e.g. epirubicin, daunorubicin, idarubicin) must also be considered.
- Check that anti-emetics appropriate to highly emetogenic chemotherapy have been prescribed according to the local policy.
- The dose of cyclophosphamide is below that which is likely to cause urothelial toxicity. Therefore prophylactic mesna, IV hydration and urine testing are not required.

SOURCE MATERIAL

- Hortobagyi GN, Gutterman JU, Blumenschein GR *et al.* (1979) Combination chemoimmunotherapy of breast cancer with 5-fluorouracil, Adriamycin, cyclophosphamide and BCG. *Cancer.* **43**: 1225–33.

FEC (5-fluorouracil, epirubicin, cyclophosphamide)

Note: *This regimen is also sometimes referred to as ECF or EFC, and should not be confused with cisplatin-containing regimens for which the ECF/EFC acronym is also used.*

USUAL INDICATION

Breast cancer: adjuvant and neo-adjuvant treatment as well as treatment of metastatic disease.

DOSES

Epirubicin 60 mg/m^2 IV on day 1
Cyclophosphamide 500 mg/m^2 IV on day 1
5-Fluorouracil (5-FU) 500 mg/m^2 IV on day 1

Note: Other dose levels (up to and including 70:700:700) have been used. In early reports (e.g. Blomqvist *et al.*[1]), lower doses (60:500:500) were administered every 4 weeks, although this would now generally be considered to be very low-intensity treatment.

ADMINISTRATION

Epirubicin

By slow IV injection into the side-arm of a free-running saline drip.

Epirubicin is a powerful vesicant and should be administered with appropriate precautions to prevent extravasation. If there is any possibility that extravasation has occurred, contact a senior member of the medical team immediately and follow local guidance on dealing with extravasation incidents.

5-FU and cyclophosphamide

May be given as slow IV bolus injections or short IV infusions (i.e. in 100 mL of 0.9% sodium chloride over a period of 10–20 min).

Note: The order of administration of the three drugs in this regimen is not critical.

---

[1] Blomqvist C, Elomaa I, Rissanen P *et al.* (1993) Influence of treatment schedule on toxicity and efficacy of cyclophosphamide, epirubicin and fluorouracil in metastatic breast cancer: a randomized trial comparing weekly and every-4-weeks administration. *J Clin Oncol.* **11**: 467–73.

ANTI-EMETICS

High emetogenic potential (see local policy).

CYCLE LENGTH

21 days.

NUMBER OF CYCLES

Usually 6.

SIDE-EFFECTS

Bone-marrow suppression, alopecia, nausea and vomiting, mucositis, cardiac arrhythmias, dilated cardiomyopathy (especially at cumulative epirubicin doses in excess of $900 \, mg/m^2$). Cyclophosphamide *can* cause haemorrhagic cystitis at high doses. However, the doses used in FEC are not likely to cause this problem, so prophylactic mesna and hydration are not required.

BLOOD NADIR

10 days.

TTOS REQUIRED

- Anti-emetics appropriate to highly emetogenic chemotherapy (see local protocol).

NOTES FOR PRESCRIBERS

- Patients over 60 years of age or with a history of heart disease must have an echocardiogram or MUGA scan prior to treatment to ensure that there is adequate left ventricular function.
- Check the LFTs. If these show serious impairment, a reduction in epirubicin and 5-FU doses may be required (*see* Appendix 1 for further guidance).
- Check the renal function. A cyclophosphamide dose reduction is required in significant renal impairment (*see* Appendix 2 for further guidance).
- Check the FBC prior to giving the go-ahead for chemotherapy. Seek advice if the neutrophil count is $<1.5 \times 10^9/L$ or the platelet count is $<100 \times 10^9/L$.
- Prescribe anti-emetics appropriate to highly emetogenic chemotherapy according to the local protocol.
- Check the cumulative dose of epirubicin on this and any previous treatment course at your hospital or elsewhere. Because of the risk of cardiotoxicity,

a cumulative dose of 900 mg/m^2 should only be exceeded with extreme caution, after a formal assessment of cardiac function and discussion with a senior member of the medical team. The impact of previous treatment with other anthracyclines (e.g. daunorubicin, doxorubicin, idarubicin) must also be considered.

- Prior to treatment, hair loss should be discussed with the patient. Scalp cooling may be of some use in reducing hair loss with FEC, but its success is limited by the prolonged half-life of cyclophosphamide. Liaise with the nurses with regard to referral to a wig-fitter at the start of treatment and before alopecia is evident, if this is appropriate.
- If administering the drugs, see Administration section above for notes on the vesicant nature of epirubicin.

NOTES FOR NURSES

- Prior to treatment, hair loss should be discussed with the patient. Scalp cooling may be of some use in reducing hair loss with FEC, but its success is limited by the prolonged circulation time of cyclophosphamide. Liaise with a wig-fitter at the start of treatment and before alopecia is evident, if this is appropriate.
- If administering the drugs, see Administration section above for notes on the vesicant nature of epiribucin.
- The dose of cyclophosphamide is below that which is likely to cause haemorrhagic cystitis. Therefore prophylactic mesna, IV hydration and urine testing are not required. Any mild symptoms of dysuria may be treated by encouraging oral fluid intake and regular voiding of urine.

NOTES FOR PHARMACISTS

- Check that the FBC has been determined and is within acceptable limits before issuing the chemotherapy.
- Check the LFTs. If these show serious impairment, a reduction in epirubicin and 5-fluorouracil doses may be required (see Appendix 1 for further details).
- Check the renal function. A cyclophosphamide dose reduction is required in significant renal impairment (see Appendix 2 for further guidance).
- Keep a close eye on the cumulative dose of epirubicin and alert the prescriber if this exceeds 900 mg/m^2. It is especially important when a patient starts a course of treatment to check the pharmacy records and the patient's notes to see whether they have received previous anthracycline therapy. The impact of other anthracyclines (e.g doxorubicin, daunorubicin, idarubicin, aclarubicin) must be considered as well as that of epirubicin.
- Check that anti-emetics appropriate to highly emetogenic chemotherapy have been prescribed according to the local policy.
- The dose of cyclophosphamide is below that which is likely to cause urothelial toxicity. Therefore prophylactic mesna, IV hydration and urine testing are not required.

SOURCE MATERIAL

- Blomquist C, Elomaa I, Rissanen P *et al.* (1993) Influence of treatment schedule on toxicity and efficacy of cyclophosphamide, epirubicin and fluorouracil in metastatic breast cancer: a randomized trial comparing weekly and every-4-weeks administration. *J Clin Oncol.* **11**: 467–73.

Fludarabine IV (single-agent)

USUAL INDICATION

Licensed for relapsed B-cell chronic lymphocytic leukaemia, but also used for relapsed low-grade lymphomas.

DOSES

Fludarabine 25 mg/m^2 IV on days 1–5

ADMINISTRATION

By IV bolus or short IV infusion.

ANTI-EMETICS

Very low emetogenic potential (see local policy).

CYCLE LENGTH

28 days.

NUMBER OF CYCLES

Usually 6.

SIDE-EFFECTS

Bone-marrow suppression, alopecia, nausea and vomiting, mucositis, neurotoxicity (weakness, agitation, confusion, visual disturbances and peripheral neuropathy; these symptoms are rare at the recommended doses, but increase sharply if the latter are exceeded – take care when dosing obese patients).

BLOOD NADIR

13 days (neutrophils); 16 days (platelets).

TTOS REQUIRED

- Anti-emetics appropriate to chemotherapy with low emetogenic potential (see local protocol).
- Unless it is contraindicated (e.g. in sulphonamide-allergic patients), co-trimoxazole (e.g. 960 mg by mouth three times a week) should be prescribed as *Pneumocystis carinii* pneumonia (PCP) prophylaxis during and for 6–12 months after treatment, because of the profound reduction in lymphocyte numbers caused by fludarabine. It should be remembered that a significant number of patients are allergic to sulphonamides, so all patients should be asked about this before prescribing.

NOTES FOR PRESCRIBERS

- Renal function should be assessed at the start of treatment. Unless the patient is known to have renal problems which are likely to impair renal function significantly, estimation of the CrCl from the serum creatinine concentration using the Cockcroft–Gault equation is acceptable provided that the patient has a stable level and no confounding factors (e.g. catabolic states):

CrCl (mL/min)

$$= \frac{1.04 \text{ (females) or } 1.23 \text{ (males)} \times (140 - \text{age in years}) \times \text{weight in kg}}{\text{serum creatinine concentration } (\mu\text{mol/L})}.$$

On subsequent cycles, the renal function should be reassessed if the creatinine level rises significantly. Fludarabine doses must be reduced once the CrCl falls below 70 mL/min, and the drug is contraindicated in patients with a CrCl of <30 mL/min (*see* Appendix 2 for further guidance).
- Prescribe anti-emetics appropriate to chemotherapy with low emetogenic potential according to local protocol, and also co-trimoxazole prophylaxis against PCP. Fludarabine induces a profound lymphopenia associated with a high risk of opportunistic infections, including PCP.
- Seek further advice if the patient reports symptoms indicative of neurotoxicity (parasthesias, visual disturbances, weakness or agitation).
- Check the FBC prior to giving the go-ahead for chemotherapy. Seek advice if the neutrophil count is $<1.5 \times 10^9$/L or the platelet count is $<100 \times 10^9$/L.

NOTES FOR NURSES

- If presented as a bolus dose, the drug will often be diluted to 10 mL, regardless of dose (in accordance with the manufacturer's directions). If this is local practice, there is therefore no need for concern if two patients with different doses end up with the same *volume* of injection.
- If issuing prophylactic co-trimoxazole to patients, make sure they realise that they need to continue this for as long as they continue fludarabine therapy (and for 6–12 months afterwards).

NOTES FOR PHARMACISTS

- Make sure that the renal function has been assessed prior to starting treatment. Estimation of the CrCl by the Cockcroft–Gault equation is acceptable (unless the patient has borderline renal function) provided that the patient has a stable serum creatinine concentration and no confounding factors (e.g. catabolic states). Dose reductions are necessary in patients with a CrCl of <70 mL/min (see Appendix 2 for further guidance).
- Check that the FBC has been determined and is within acceptable limits before issuing the chemotherapy.
- Check that anti-emetics appropriate to chemotherapy with low emetogenic potential have been prescribed according to local protocol.
- Check that prophylactic co-trimoxazole has been prescribed to prevent PCP infection. Fludarabine is very toxic to lymphocytes and produces prolonged and profound lymphopenia, which predisposes to opportunistic infections, including PCP. If co-trimoxazole is contraindicated, record this on any pharmacy patient record (see Appendix 3 for an example) to prevent inadvertent dispensing in the future.

SOURCE MATERIAL

- Zinzani PL, Lauria F, Rondelli D et al. (1993) Fludarabine in patients with advanced and/or resistant B-chronic lymphocytic leukemia. Eur J Haematol. **51**: 93–7.

Fludarabine oral (single-agent)

USUAL INDICATION

Licensed for relapsed B-cell chronic lymphocytic leukaemia, but also used for relapsed low-grade lymphomas.

DOSES

Fludarabine 40 mg/m^2 by mouth on days 1–5

ADMINISTRATION

By mouth once daily for 5 days.

ANTI-EMETICS

Very low emetogenic potential (see local policy).

CYCLE LENGTH

28 days.

NUMBER OF CYCLES

Usually 6.

SIDE-EFFECTS

Bone-marrow suppression, alopecia, nausea and vomiting, mucositis, chemical cystitis, neurotoxicity (weakness, agitation, confusion, visual disturbances and peripheral neuropathy; these symptoms are rare at the recommended doses, but increase sharply if the latter are exceeded – take care when dosing obese patients).

BLOOD NADIR

13 days (neutrophils); 16 days (platelets).

TTOS REQUIRED

- Anti-emetics appropriate to chemotherapy with low emetogenic potential (see local protocol).
- Unless contraindicated (e.g. in sulphonamide-allergic patients), co-trimoxazole (e.g. 960 mg by mouth, three times a week) should be prescribed as *Pneumocystis carinii* pneumonia (PCP) prophylaxis during and for 6–12 months after treatment, because of the profound reduction in lymphocyte numbers caused by fludarabine. It should be remembered that a significant number of patients are allergic to sulphonamides, so all patients should be asked about this before prescribing.

NOTES FOR PRESCRIBERS

- Oral and IV doses of fludarabine are not interchangeable. If a patient on oral fludarabine requires IV treatment because they are unable to swallow, or for any other reason, the lower IV dose of 25 mg/m^2 must be used.
- Fludarabine tablets come in only one strength − 10 mg. Therefore daily doses need to be given in multiples of 10 mg. More accurate total dosing may be achieved by giving different numbers of tablets on alternate days. In effect, this allows daily dose increments of 5 mg to be achieved.
- Renal function should be assessed at the start of treatment. Unless the patient is known to have renal problems which are likely to impair renal function significantly, estimation of the CrCl from serum creatinine levels using the Cockcroft–Gault equation is acceptable if the patient has a stable creatinine level and no confounding factors (e.g. catabolic states):

CrCl (mL/min)

$$= \frac{1.04 \text{ (females) or } 1.23 \text{ (males)} \times (140 - \text{age in years}) \times \text{weight in kg}}{\text{serum creatinine concentration } (\mu\text{mol/L})}.$$

On subsequent cycles renal function should be reassessed if the creatinine concentration rises significantly. Fludarabine doses must be reduced if the CrCl falls below 70 mL/min, and the drug is contraindicated in patients with a CrCl of <30 mL/min (*see* Appendix 2).
- Prescribe anti-emetics appropriate to chemotherapy with low emetogenic potential according to local protocol, and co-trimoxazole prophylaxis against PCP (2 tablets three times a week). Fludarabine induces a profound lymphopenia associated with a high risk of opportunistic infections, including PCP.
- Seek further advice if the patient reports symptoms indicative of neurotoxicity (parasthesias, visual disturbances, weakness, agitation).
- Check the FBC prior to giving the go-ahead for chemotherapy, and seek advice if the neutrophil count is <1.5 × 10^9/L or the platelet count is <100 × 10^9/L. In the pivotal study of oral fludarabine, doses were delayed (for a maximum of 2 weeks) if the neutrophil count was <0.5 × 10^9/L or the platelet count was <50 × 10^9/L. If after 2 weeks the granulocyte count remained in the range 0.5–1.0 × 10^9/L or the platelet count was in the range 50–100 × 10^9/L, the

dose was reduced to 30 mg/m². If after dose delay the granulocyte counts were $< 0.5 \times 10^9$/L or the platelet counts were $< 50 \times 10^9$/L, the dose was further reduced to 20 mg/m².

- A complete 5-day course of tablets should always be prescribed. Any prescription should make it clear that 5 days of treatment *only* are required. The patient should also be made aware that treatment is for 5 days only, and that they should not attempt to obtain further supplies from their GP. *Fatalities have resulted from the inadvertent continuation of short courses of oral cytotoxic drugs.*

NOTES FOR NURSES

- If you are counselling the patient about their treatment, emphasise that each course of treatment should last for 5 days only, and that they should not attempt to obtain repeat prescriptions from their GP. *Fatalities have resulted from the inadvertent continuation of short courses of oral cytotoxic drugs.*
- If you are issuing prophylactic co-trimoxazole to patients, make sure they realise that they need to continue this for as long as they continue fludarabine therapy (and for 6–12 months afterwards).

NOTES FOR PHARMACISTS

- Oral and IV doses of fludarabine are not interchangeable. If a patient on oral fludarabine requires IV treatment because they are unable to swallow, or for any other reason, the lower IV dose of 25 mg/m² must be used.
- If you are counselling patients about their treatment, emphasise that each course of treatment should last for 5 days only, and that they should not attempt to obtain repeat prescriptions from their GP. *Fatalities have resulted from the inadvertent continuation of short courses of oral cytotoxic drugs.*
- Make sure that renal function has been assessed prior to starting treatment with fludarabine. Estimation of the CrCl using the Cockcroft–Gault equation is acceptable (unless the patient has borderline renal function) provided that the patient has a stable serum creatinine level and no confounding factors (e.g. catabolic states). Dose reductions are necessary in patients with a CrCL of <70 mL/min (*see* Appendix 2).
- Check that the FBC has been determined and is within acceptable limits before issuing chemotherapy.
- Check that anti-emetics appropriate to chemotherapy with low emetogenic potential have been prescribed according to local protocol.
- Check that prophylactic co-trimoxazole has been prescribed (960 mg by mouth three times a week) to prevent PCP infection. Fludarabine is very toxic to lymphocytes and produces prolonged and profound lymphopenia, which predisposes to opportunistic infections, including PCP.
- If you are issuing prophylactic co-trimoxazole to patients, make sure they realise that they need to continue this for as long as they continue fludarabine therapy (and for 6–12 months afterwards).

SOURCE MATERIAL

● Boogaerts MA, Van Hoof A, Catovsky D *et al.* (2001) Activity of oral fludarabine phosphate in previously treated chronic lymphocytic leukemia. *J Clin Oncol.* **19**: 4252–8.

FMD (fludarabine, mitoxantrone, dexamethasone), also known as FND (fludarabine, Novantrone®, dexamethasone) and FMP (fludarabine, mitoxantrone, prednisolone)

USUAL INDICATION

Relapsed low-grade lymphoma.

DOSES

FMD

Fludarabine 25 mg/m^2 IV* on days 1–3
Mitoxantrone 10 mg/m^2 IV on day 1
Dexamethasone 20 mg (total dose) IV or by mouth on days 1–5

FMP

Fludarabine 25 mg/m^2 IV* on days 1–3
Mitoxantrone 10 mg/m^2 IV on day 1
Prednisolone† 40 mg (total dose) by mouth on days 1–5

ADMINISTRATION

Fludarabine is administered by IV bolus or short IV infusion, and mitoxantrone is administered as a slow IV bolus into a free-running saline infusion. The order of administration of IV drugs is not critical. Dexamethasone (FMD) is administered as a slow IV bolus (over a period of 4–5 min – rapid administration leads to histamine release, which causes perineal discomfort) or by mouth (oral administration should be used if possible), and prednisolone (FMP) is administered by mouth.

Mitoxantrone can cause tissue necrosis following extravasation, and should be administered with appropriate precautions to prevent this from occurring. If there is any possibility that extravasation has occurred, contact a senior member of the medical team immediately and follow local procedures for dealing with extravasation incidents.

---

* Published studies were conducted before fludarabine tablets became available. However, it is reasonable to suppose that oral fludarabine at a dose of 40 mg/m^2/day could be substituted for IV fludarabine on days 1–3. Oral fludarabine at this dose has been shown to be equivalent to IV fludarabine 25 mg/m^2 in other situations (*see* chapter on fludarabine monotherapy).

† Published studies have used IV prednisone. This is not available in the UK. Oral prednisolone is often used as a substitute without any requirement for dose adjustment.

ANTI-EMETICS

Low emetogenic potential (see local policy). Note that the steroids included in the regimen will have a substantial anti-emetic effect, so no additional steroids should be prescribed.

CYCLE LENGTH

28 days.

NUMBER OF CYCLES

Usually 6.

SIDE-EFFECTS

Bone-marrow suppression, alopecia (relatively low risk of major hair loss), nausea and vomiting, mucositis, neurotoxicity (weakness, agitation, confusion, visual disturbances and peripheral neuropathy; these neurotoxic effects are rare at the recommended doses of fludarabine). Cardiotoxicity has been reported after mitoxantrone administration, but it is less common than with anthracyclines. It seems to be more likely at cumulative doses in excess of $160\,mg/m^2$, or $100\,mg/m^2$ after previous anthracycline therapy. The high-dose steroids that are used in these regimens can cause a variety of side-effects, including euphoria/depression, epigastric discomfort, glucose intolerance, insomnia and psychosis.

BLOOD NADIR

10–15 days (not well defined – mitoxantrone produces an earlier nadir than fludarabine, resulting in a window of several days where the nadir might occur).

TTOS REQUIRED

- Anti-emetics appropriate to chemotherapy with low emetogenic potential (see local protocol).
- Unless it is contraindicated (e.g. in sulphonamide-allergic patients), co-trimoxazole (e.g 960 mg three times a week) (2 tablets three times a week) should be prescribed as *Pneumocystis carinii* pneumonia (PCP) prophylaxis during and for 6–12 months after treatment. This is because of the profound reduction in lymphocyte numbers that is caused by fludarabine. However, it should be remembered that a significant number of patients are allergic to sulphonamides, so all patients should be asked about this before prescribing.

- Ensure that sufficient dexamethasone (FMD) or prednisolone (FMP) tablets are prescribed to finish the cycle of treatment.
- Allopurinol (300 mg by mouth once a day; reduced in cases of renal impairment) to prevent tumour lysis syndrome should be prescribed while the patient has bulky disease.
- Consideration should be given to prescribing a gastroprotective agent (e.g. ranitidine 150 mg by mouth twice a day) for the duration of steroid treatment, in order to prevent gastritis.

NOTES TO PRESCRIBERS

- Check the FBC prior to giving the go-ahead for chemotherapy. Seek advice if the neutrophil count is $<1.5 \times 10^9$/L or the platelet count is $<100 \times 10^9$/L. In a large trial of FMD,[1] the doses of fludarabine and mitoxantrone were reduced on subsequent cycles if an earlier cycle resulted in any of the following: platelet count $<20 \times 10^9$/L; granulocyte count $<0.1 \times 10^9$/L; mucosal bleeding; sepsis; blood count recovery delayed by >35 days. Therefore nadir blood counts, if available, should also be considered when prescribing chemotherapy. It should be noted that in this study patients who were considered to be particularly at risk of haematological toxicity (poor prior tolerance of chemotherapy, prior extensive radiotherapy, age >65 years) were started on treatment with mitoxantrone and fludarabine doses 20% lower than those described above. Such patients should be treated with particular caution.
- Renal function should be assessed at the start of treatment. Unless the patient is known to have renal problems which are likely to impair renal function significantly, estimation of the CrCl from the serum creatinine levels using the Cockcroft–Gault equation is acceptable provided that the patient has a stable creatinine concentration and no confounding factors (e.g. catabolic states):

CrCl (mL/min)

$$= \frac{1.04 \text{ (females) or } 1.23 \text{ (males)} \times (140 - \text{age in years}) \times \text{weight in kg}}{\text{serum creatinine concentration } (\mu\text{mol/L})}.$$

On subsequent cycles, renal function should be reassessed if the serum creatinine concentration rises significantly. Fludarabine doses must be reduced once the CrCl falls below 70 mL/min, and the drug is contraindicated in patients with a CrCl of <30 mL/min (*see* Appendix 2).
- Mitoxantrone is extensively metabolised in the liver, and a dosage reduction may be necessary in cases of significant hepatic impairment (*see* Appendix 1 for further guidance).
- Prescribe anti-emetics appropriate to chemotherapy with low emetogenic potential according to local protocol.
- Prescribe co-trimoxazole prophylaxis against PCP (e.g. co-trimoxazole 960 mg three times a week). Fludarabine induces a profound lymphopenia associated with

[1] McLaughlin P, Hagemeister FB, Romaguera JE *et al.* (1996) Fludarabine, mitoxantrone and dexamethasone: an effective new regimen for indolent lymphoma. *J Clin Oncol.* **14**: 1262–8.

a high risk of opportunistic infections, including PCP. The prescription and any communication with the patient's GP or other doctors should state clearly that this is long-term prophylaxis that should normally be continued for 6–12 months after fludarabine treatment has been completed.

- Prescribe allopurinol (300 mg once daily by mouth; reduced in cases of renal impairment) continuously from the start of FMD/FMP therapy, and for as long as the patient has a significant bulk of chemosensitive tumour remaining, to prevent the formation of large quantities of uric acid from products released during cell lysis. Urate is poorly soluble, and there is a risk of it precipitating in the kidneys and causing renal failure (urate nephropathy or tumour lysis syndrome).

- Consider prescribing a gastroprotective agent to cover the period of high-dose steroid treatment.

- Sufficient steroids should be prescribed to complete the current treatment cycle. The steroid prescription and any communication with the patient's GP or other doctors should state clearly that the dexamethasone (FMD) or prednisolone (FMP) is being prescribed as a short course only. *This will prevent inappropriate continuation of treatment that can have tragic consequences.*

- Neither dexamethasone (FMD) nor prednisolone (FMP) are available in a liquid formulation for patients who are unable to swallow tablets. Howevever, dexamethasone tablets can be made into a slurry with water immediately before use, and soluble tablets of prednisolone are available.

- Seek further advice if the patient reports symptoms indicative of neurotoxicity (parasthesias, visual disturbances, weakness or agitation).

- If you are administering mitoxantrone, *see* Administration section above for notes on the problems associated with extravasation.

- It is unlikely that, at the doses of mitoxantrone used in FMD/FMP, cumulative cardiac toxicity will be a problem (*see* Side-effects section above). However, great care should be exercised in patients with pre-existing cardiac dysfunction, including that induced by anthracyclines, and in patients who have received large cumulative doses of anthracyclines in the past.

NOTES FOR NURSES

- If fludarabine is presented as a bolus dose, the drug will often be diluted to 10 mL, regardless of dose (in accordance with the manufacturer's directions). There is therefore no need for concern if two patients who are receiving different doses end up with the same *volume* of injection.

- If you are administering mitoxantrone, *see* Administration section above for notes on the problems associated with extravasation.

- If you are issuing prophylactic co-trimoxazole to patients, make sure they realise that they need to continue this for as long as they continue fludarabine therapy (and for 6–12 months afterwards).

- If you are issuing steroids, explain that these are to be taken for 5 days only and then stopped, and that no repeat supply should be sought from the patient's GP. *Inappropriate continuation of high-dose steroids can have tragic consequences.*

- Unfortunately, dexamethasone tablets (for FMD) are not available in larger sizes than 2 mg, so patients *do* have to take 10 tablets per dose. Similarly, prednisolone tablets (for FMP) come in 5 mg and 25 mg strengths, so patients will have to take either eight 5 mg tablets or one 25 mg tablet and three 5 mg tablets. In either case, the patient may need reassurance that it is OK to take so many tablets. Ideally, each day's dose of prednisolone or dexamethasone tablets should be taken in the morning with food.

- Ensure that any diabetic patients are aware of the need to be extra vigilant about monitoring their blood sugar levels during treatment with dexamethasone or prednisolone, and advise them to contact their doctor if they experience problems with the control of their blood sugar levels.

NOTES FOR PHARMACISTS

- Check that the FBC has been determined and is within acceptable limits before issuing the chemotherapy. Nadir counts should also be consulted where these are available (see Notes for prescribers above).
- Make sure that the renal function has been assessed prior to starting treatment. Estimation of the CrCl using the Cockcroft–Gault equation is acceptable (unless the patient has borderline renal function) provided that the patient has a stable serum creatinine concentration and no confounding factors (e.g. catabolic states). Fludarabine dose reductions are necessary in patients with a CrCL of <70 mL/min (see Appendix 2).
- Mitoxantrone is extensively metabolised in the liver, and a dosage reduction may be necessary in cases of significant hepatic impairment (see Appendix 1 for further guidance).
- Check that anti-emetics appropriate to chemotherapy with low emetogenic potential have been prescribed according to protocol.
- Check that prophylactic co-trimoxazole (e.g. 960 mg three times a week) (2 tabs three times a week) has been prescribed to prevent PCP infection. Fludarabine is highly toxic to lymphocytes and produces prolonged and profound lymphopenia, which predisposes to opportunistic infections, including PCP. Co-trimoxazole should normally be continued for 6–12 months after fludarabine treatment has been completed. If the patient is not started on co-trimoxazole, query this with the prescriber. If co-trimoxazole is contraindicated (e.g. because of hypersensitivity), endorse any pharmacy patient record (see Appendix 3 for an example) in order to prevent inadvertent prescribing in the future.
- If a gastroprotective agent and allopurinol have not been prescribed, check with the prescriber whether these medications are needed. Any decision not to prescribe should be recorded in the pharmacy patient record for future reference.
- It is unlikely that, at the doses of mitoxantrone used in FMD/FMP, cumulative cardiac toxicity will be a problem (see Side-effects section above). However, great care should be exercised in patients with pre-existing cardiac dysfunction, including that induced by anthracyclines.
- If you are checking a steroid prescription for dispensing by another member of staff, make sure that it clearly states that the steroid treatment is for 5 days only. The pack of tablets should also be labelled in a way that makes this clear. If you are issuing steroids, explain that these are to be taken for 5 days only and then stopped, and that no repeat supply should be sought from the patient's GP. *Inappropriate continuation of high-dose steroids can have tragic consequences.*

SOURCE MATERIAL

FMD

- McLaughlin P, Hagemeister FB, Romaguera JE *et al.* (1996) Fludarabine, mitoxantrone and dexamethasone: an effective new regimen for indolent lymphoma. *J Clin Oncol.* **14**: 1262–8.

FMP

- Zinzani PL, Bendandi M and Tura S (1995) FMP regimen (fludarabine, mitoxantrone, prednisone) as therapy in recurrent low-grade non-Hodgkin's lymphoma. *Eur J Haematol.* **55**: 262–6.

Gemcitabine (single-agent)

USUAL INDICATION

Pancreatic cancer; non-small-cell lung cancer (NSCLC) in patients who are unfit for cisplatin-based chemotherapy.

DOSES

Gemcitabine 1000 mg/m^2 IV on day 1 weekly for 3 weeks in 4

In patients with pancreatic cancer, initial treatment may be given weekly for up to 7 weeks without a break to induce a response. This is followed by a 1-week break, before continuing with treatment on 3 weeks in every 4.

ADMINISTRATION

As an IV infusion in 500 mL of 0.9% sodium chloride over a period of 30 min. Prolonged infusion increases the treatment toxicity and should be avoided.

ANTI-EMETICS

Weakly emetogenic (see local policy).

CYCLE LENGTH

28 days, but note that in pancreatic cancer induction treatment can be given weekly for up to 7 weeks without a break (*see* Doses section above).

NUMBER OF CYCLES

Until treatment progression or unacceptable toxicity.

SIDE-EFFECTS

Bone-marrow suppression (generally mild), thrombocythaemia, alopecia (usually moderate thinning rather than complete hair loss), nausea and vomiting, mucositis, radiosensitisation (use of radiotherapy within 7 days of gemcitabine should only be undertaken as part of a clinical trial), radiation recall, haemolytic uraemic syndrome. Transient and usually clinically insignificant proteinuria and haematuria are common (50% of patients). Rash is common (25% of patients) and often pruritic, but can usually be managed conservatively. Bronchospasm (an indication for stopping treatment) and dyspnoea (usually mild and self-limiting) and, rarely, other respiratory problems (adult respiratory distress syndrome). Influenza-like symptoms are common (20% of patients), but usually mild and self-limiting. Oedema is common, but usually mild and self-limiting. Pulmonary oedema (rare), somnolence, diarrhoea/constipation and transient increases in serum transaminases.

BLOOD NADIR

Because of the treatment schedule that is used, a clear nadir is not observed.

TTOS REQUIRED

- Anti-emetics appropriate to weakly emetogenic chemotherapy.
- Paracetamol if flu-like symptoms have been a problem on previous courses.
- Emollients/mild steroids if skin rash has been a problem on previous courses.

NOTES FOR PRESCRIBERS

- Make sure that you know which schedule of gemcitabine is being used (weekly for induction in pancreatic cancer, or weekly for 3 weeks in 4) and which treatment week the patient is on (i.e. do not forget the rest week).
- Administration of gemcitabine within 7 days of radiotherapy can lead to serious toxicity because of the drug's radiosensitising action. The combination should normally be avoided outside clinical trials. If radiotherapy has been given or is scheduled within 7 days of gemcitabine, discuss this with a senior member of the medical team before proceeding.
- Check the FBC prior to giving the go-ahead for chemotherapy. The manufacturer has made the following recommendations for dose modifications in the case of haematological toxicity. These should not be deviated from without prior discussion with a senior member of the medical team.

Absolute granulocyte count $(\times 10^9/L)$		Platelet count $(\times 10^9/L)$	Percentage of full dose
>1.0	and	100	100
0.5–1.0	or	50–100	75
<0.5	or	<50	Do not give treatment on this day

In the pivotal study of gemcitabine monotherapy in pancreatic cancer,[1] the initial 7-week period of unbroken weekly treatment was terminated early in the event of ⩾ grade 2 non-haematological toxicity or ⩾ grade 3 haematological toxicity. Similarly, in a study of gemcitabine monotherapy in NSCLC,[2] WHO Grade 3 and 4 non-haematological toxicity was dealt with using the following dose-reduction schedule and the outcomes were satisfactory:

Observed toxicity	Percentage of full dose of gemcitabine
Grade 3 toxicity after first cycle	50 or omit
Grade 3 toxicity after subsequent cycles (except nausea/vomiting or alopecia)	75
Grade 4 toxicity after first cycle	Omit
Grade 4 toxicity after subsequent cycles	50 or omit

- Check the LFTs prior to treatment. No specific guidance is available on dosage modifications, but the manufacturer of gemcitabine recommends caution in patients with severe hepatic impairment.
- Renal function should be assessed at the start of treatment. Estimation by the Cockcroft–Gault equation from serum creatinine levels is acceptable if the patient has a stable creatinine concentration and no confounding factors (e.g. catabolic states):

CrCl (mL/min)

$$= \frac{1.04 \ (\text{females}) \text{ or } 1.23 \ (\text{males}) \times (140 - \text{age in years}) \times \text{weight in kg}}{\text{serum creatinine concentration} \ (\mu\text{mol/L})}.$$

On subsequent cycles the renal function should be reassessed.

Consideration should be given to dose reduction in patients with a CrCl of < 30 mL/min (see Appendix 2 for further guidance).

- Patients should be warned about the possible side-effects of gemcitabine, some of which are not typical of other chemotherapy drugs. In particular, they should be told not to worry if they develop mild dyspnoea a few hours after treatment, as this will quickly wear off, as will flu-like symptoms (which can be treated with paracetamol). Similarly, moderate swelling as a result of fluid retention or an itchy rash are not a major cause for concern.
- Consider prescribing paracetamol and emollients/mild steroids for patients who experienced flu-like symptoms or rash on earlier courses.
- Review treatment with a view to stopping it if the patient develops adverse pulmonary effects (e.g. pulmonary oedema, interstitial pneumonitis, adult respiratory distress syndrome), which may rarely be caused by gemcitabine.

[1] Burris HA III, Moore MJ, Anderson J et al. (1997) Improvements in survival and clinical benefit with gemcitabine as first-line therapy for patients with advanced pancreas cancer: a randomized trial. J Clin Oncol. 15: 2403–13.

[2] Manegold C, Bergman B, Chemaissani A et al. (1997) Single-agent gemcitabine versus cisplatin–etoposide: early results of a randomised phase II study in locally advanced or metastatic non-small-cell lung cancer. Ann Oncol. 8: 525–9.

NOTES FOR NURSES

- Patients should be warned about the possible side-effects of gemcitabine, some of which are not typical of other chemotherapy drugs. In particular, they should be told not to worry if they develop mild dyspnoea a few hours after treatment, as this will quickly wear off, as will flu-like symptoms (which can be treated with paracetamol). Similarly, moderate swelling as a result of fluid retention or an itchy rash are not a major cause for concern.

NOTES FOR PHARMACISTS

- Make sure that you know which schedule of gemcitabine is being used (weekly for induction in pancreatic cancer, or weekly for 3 weeks in 4) and which treatment week the patient is on (i.e. do not forget the rest week).
- Check the FBC prior to issuing chemotherapy. The manufacturer has made recommendations for dose modifications in the case of haematological toxicity (*see* Notes for prescribers above), and any deviation from these should be discussed with the prescriber.
- Check the LFTs prior to treatment. No specific guidance is available on dosage modifications, but the manufacturer of gemcitabine recommends caution in patients with severe hepatic impairment.
- Renal function should be assessed at the start of treatment. Estimation from serum creatinine levels using the Cockcroft–Gault equation is acceptable if the patient has a stable creatinine concentration and no confounding factors (e.g. catabolic states). Record the CrCl and the corresponding creatinine concentration in any pharmacy patient record (*see* Appendix 3 for an example). On subsequent cycles the renal function should be reassessed if the creatinine concentration changes. Consideration should be given to dose reduction in patients with a CrCl of <30 mL/min (*see* Appendix 2 for further guidance).

SOURCE MATERIAL

Pancreatic cancer

- Burris HA III, Moore MJ, Andersen J *et al.* (1997) Improvements in survival and clinical benefit with gemcitabine as first-line therapy for patients with advanced pancreas cancer: a randomized trial. *J Clin Oncol.* **15**: 2403–13.

Non-small-cell lung cancer

- Manegold C, Bergman B, Chemaissani A *et al.* (1997) Single-agent gemcitabine *versus* cisplatin–etoposide: early results of a randomised phase II study in locally advanced or metastatic non-small-cell lung cancer. *Ann Oncol.* **8**: 525–9.

Gemcitabine plus cisplatin

USUAL INDICATION
___

First-line treatment of non-small-cell lung cancer (NSCLC) and bladder cancer.

DOSES
___

Non-small-cell lung cancer

3-weekly schedule

    Gemcitabine 1250 mg/m^2 by IV infusion on days 1 and 8
    Cisplatin 80 mg/m^2 by IV infusion on day 1

4-weekly schedule

    Gemcitabine 1000 mg/m^2 by IV infusion on days 1, 8 and 15
    Cisplatin 80 mg/m^2 by IV infusion on day 1

Note: There are many slight variations on the above used for NSCLC. The above protocols represent common UK practice, with 3-weekly schedules incorporating two (slightly higher) gemcitabine doses only, plus a relatively low dose of cisplatin (the manufacturer of gemcitabine recommends a range of 75–100 mg/m^2 cisplatin every 3–4 weeks). One of the reasons why the regimens used in the UK are popular is because they are suitable for outpatient treatment.

Bladder cancer

    Gemcitabine 1000 mg/m^2 by IV infusion on days 1, 8 and 15
    Cisplatin 70 mg/m^2 by IV infusion on day 1

ADMINISTRATION
___

Cisplatin

Cisplatin is administered after IV pre-hydration, typically with 1 L of 0.9% sodium chloride containing 20 mmol potassium chloride and 1 g of magnesium sulphate, plus an additional 500 mL of 0.9% sodium chloride containing gemcitabine and infused over a period of 30 min.

    Cisplatin is then administered as an IV infusion, typically in 1 L of 0.9% sodium chloride over a period of 2 h, followed by at least 1 L of saline as post-hydration.

If post-hydration is restricted to 1 L, the patient should be instructed to drink a further 3 L of fluid during the 24 h after the end of IV hydration. The aim of hydration is to maintain a urine output of 100 mL/h during and for 6–8 h after cisplatin administration. Electrolytes are usually added to hydration fluids to combat cisplatin-induced electrolyte wasting. Mannitol may also be administered to stimulate diuresis.

Gemcitabine

Gemcitabine is administered as an IV infusion in 500 mL of 0.9% sodium chloride over a period of 30 min. Prolonged infusion of gemcitabine increases treatment toxicity and should be avoided.

ANTI-EMETICS

Day 1

High emetogenic potential (see local policy).

Day 8 (and day 15 in 4-weekly schedules)

Low emetogenic potential (see local policy).

CYCLE LENGTH

21 or 28 days, depending on the schedule used.

NUMBER OF CYCLES

Usually 6.

SIDE-EFFECTS

Nephrotoxicity (potentially dose limiting – due to cisplatin), bone-marrow suppression (all blood components are affected, but seldom dose limiting), alopecia (rarely extensive), nausea and vomiting (may be very severe), sensory motor and autonomic neuropathy (sometimes irreversible) including significant potential for ototoxicity (due to cisplatin), mucositis (not usually serious), radiosensitisation (use of radiotherapy within 7 days of gemcitabine should only be undertaken as part of a clinical trial), radiation recall, haemolytic uraemic syndrome. Transient and usually clinically insignificant proteinuria and haematuria are common (50% of patients). Rash is common (25% of patients) and often pruritic, but can usually be managed conservatively. Bronchospasm (an indication for stopping treatment) and dyspnoea (usually mild and self-limiting) and, rarely, other respiratory problems (adult respiratory distress syndrome) may occur. Influenza-like symptoms are common (20% of patients), but usually mild and self-limiting. Oedema is common, but usually mild and self-limiting. Pulmonary oedema (rare), somnolence, diarrhoea/constipation and increases in serum transaminases.

TTOS REQUIRED

- Anti-emetics appropriate to chemotherapy with high emetogenic potential (day 1) and low emetogenic potential (day 8 and day 15 in 4-weekly schedules).

NOTES FOR PRESCRIBERS

Before each course

- Make sure that you are clear which dosage schedule is being used. Schedules differ between lung and bladder cancer, and other variations have been used elsewhere. Particular care should be taken with patients in clinical trials.
- Make sure that you are aware of which day of the treatment cycle the patient is on – treatment on day 1 differs from that on day 8 and day 15 (where day 15 is given).
- The administration of gemcitabine within 7 days of radiotherapy can lead to serious toxicity because of the radiosensitising action of this drug. Cisplatin is also a radiosensitiser. Therefore this chemotherapy regimen should not normally be combined with radiotherapy. If radiotherapy has been given or is scheduled within 7 days of gemcitabine administration, discuss this with a senior member of the medical team before proceeding.
- Check the FBC prior to giving the go-ahead for chemotherapy. On day 1, seek advice if the neutrophil count is $<1.5 \times 10^9$/L or the platelet count is $<100 \times 10^9$/L. The manufacturer of gemcitabine gives guidance on appropriate dosage adjustments for gemcitabine in the event of myelotoxicity (*see* table below). These adjustments are useful on days when gemcitabine alone is given, but on day 1 allowance must also be made for the contribution of cisplatin. In the study of cisplatin and gemcitabine in bladder cancer by von der Maase *et al.*,[1] day 1 treatment was not given until the WBC had risen to $>3.0 \times 10^9$/L and the platelet count has risen to $>100 \times 10^9$/L, with treatment discontinued if it was delayed by more than 28 days.

Absolute granulocyte count ($\times 10^9$/L)		Platelet count ($\times 10^9$/L)	Percentage of full dose
>1.0	and	>100	100
0.5–1.0	or	50–100	75
<0.5	or	<50	Do not give treatment on this day

[1] Van der Maase H, Hansen SW, Roberts JT *et al.* (2000) Gemcitabine and cisplatin versus methotrexate, vinblastine, doxorubicin and cisplatin in advanced or metastatic bladder cancer: results of a large, randomized, multinational, multicenter Phase III study. *J Clin Oncol.* **18**: 3068–77.

- Renal function should be formally assessed at the start of treatment. Ideally this should be done by EDTA clearance, but estimation using the Cockcroft-Gault equation from serum creatinine levels is acceptable if the patient has a stable creatinine concentration and no confounding factors (e.g. catabolic states):

CrCl (mL/min)

$$= \frac{1.04 \text{ (females) or } 1.23 \text{ (males)} \times (140 - \text{age in years}) \times \text{weight in kg}}{\text{serum creatinine concentration } (\mu\text{mol/L})}.$$

On subsequent cycles the renal function should be reassessed.

Cisplatin doses *must be reduced* if the creatinine clearance drops below 60 mL/min. Consideration should also be given to reducing gemcitabine doses in patients whose CrCl falls below 30 mL/min (*see* Appendix 2 for further guidance).

- Check the serum electrolytes for cisplatin-induced wasting, especially of magnesium, calcium and potassium. Additional supplementation may be required.
- Check the LFTs prior to treatment. No specific guidance is available on dosage modifications, but the manufacturer of gemcitabine recommends caution in patients with severe hepatic impairment.
- Do not forget to prescribe anti-emetics appropriate to highly emetogenic chemotherapy on day 1 and weakly emetogenic chemotherapy on day 8 (and day 15 of 4-week schedules) according to local policy.
- Seek further advice if the patient reports symptoms indicative of neurotoxicity (parasthesias, difficulty with motor control, constipation, jaw pain) or ototoxicity (tinnitus, deafness). These are all side-effects of cisplatin.
- The patients should be warned about the possible side-effects of gemcitabine, some of which are not typical of other chemotherapy drugs. In particular, they should be told not to worry if they develop mild dyspnoea a few hours after treatment, as this will wear off quickly, as will flu-like symptoms (which can be treated with paracetamol). Similarly, moderate swelling as a result of fluid retention or an itchy rash are not a major cause for concern.
- Consider prescribing paracetamol or emollients/mild steroids for patients who experienced flu-like symptoms or rash on earlier courses.
- Review treatment with a view to stopping it if the patient develops adverse pulmonary effects (e.g. pulmonary oedema, interstitial pneumonitis or adult respiratory distress syndrome), which may rarely be caused by gemcitabine.

On the day after each cisplatin dose

For patients who are receiving cisplatin on an inpatient basis, check fluid balance/body weight. In general, if the patient has gained 1.5 L/kg since starting hydration, extra diuresis will be required (e.g. furosemide 20–40 mg by mouth).

NOTES FOR NURSES

- The aim of hydration is to ensure an average urine output of 100 mL/h or more during and for 6–8 h after cisplatin administration. Any patient who is being treated as an inpatient should be on a fluid-balance chart, and daily weights should be recorded. Contact the prescriber if the patient's urine output is inadequate or their body weight increases by 1.5 kg from baseline.

For outpatients, efforts should be made to ensure that urine output is adequate (e.g. by ensuring that the patient has passed 500 mL of urine between the start of IV hydration and the beginning of cisplatin infusion).

Outpatients should also be encouraged to drink 3 L of fluid in the 24 h following each period of IV hydration, and to contact the hospital if this is impossible because of nausea/vomiting or other problems.

- The patient should be warned about the possible side-effects of gemcitabine, some of which are not typical of other chemotherapy drugs. In particular, they should be told not to worry if they develop mild dyspnoea a few hours after treatment, as this will wear off quickly, as will flu-like symptoms (which can be treated with paracetamol). Similarly, moderate swelling as a result of fluid retention or an itchy rash are not a major cause for concern.

NOTES FOR PHARMACISTS

On the day of prescribing

- Make sure that you are clear which dosage schedule is being used. Schedules differ between lung and bladder cancer, and other variations have been used elsewhere. Particular care should be taken with patients in clinical trials.
- Make sure that you are aware of which day of the treatment cycle the patient is on – treatment on day 1 differs from that on day 8 and day 15 (where day 15 is given).
- Check that the FBC has been determined and is within an acceptable range prior to issuing chemotherapy. The manufacturer of gemcitabine gives guidance on appropriate adjustments to gemcitabine doses in the event of myelotoxicity (see Notes for prescribers above). However, allowance must also be made for the contribution of cisplatin on day 1.
- Check that the renal function has been measured/calculated at the start of treatment. Record the CrCl and the corresponding creatinine concentration in any pharmacy patient record (see Appendix 3 for an example). Recalculate the CrCl if the creatinine concentration changes. Doses of cisplatin *must be reduced* if the creatinine clearance drops below 60 mL/min, and consideration should be given to reducing gemcitabine doses if the CrCl falls below 30 mL/min (see Appendix 2 for further guidance).
- Check the serum electrolytes for cisplatin-induced wasting, especially of magnesium, calcium and potassium. Additional supplementation may be required.
- Check the LFTs prior to treatment. No specific guidance is available on dosage modifications, but the manufacturer of gemcitabine recommends caution in patients with severe hepatic impairment.
- Check that anti-emetics appropriate to highly emetogenic (day 1) or weakly emetogenic (days 8 and 15) chemotherapy have been prescribed according to local policy.

On the day after cisplatin administration

- When visiting the ward, check that any inpatient who is receiving cisplatin has not gained more than 1.5 L/kg since the start of treatment. If they have, discuss additional diuresis with the prescriber (if this measure has not already been instituted).

SOURCE MATERIAL

Non-small-cell lung cancer

Many different combinations of cisplatin and gemcitabine are used for non-small-cell lung cancer. The schedule described above uses somewhat less cisplatin than most published trials, but is in line with current UK practice.

3-week schedule

- Cicenas S, Pipiriene T and Burneckis A (2001) Gemcitabine–cisplatin (GC) versus etoposide–cisplatin (EC) in patients with inoperable stage IIIA/IIIB non-small-cell lung cancer (NSCLC) with intermittent radiotherapy: a randomized phase II trial. *Proc Am Soc Clin Oncol.* **20**: 270 (abstract).
- Crino L, De Marinis F, Scagliotti G *et al.* (2001) Neoadjuvant chemotherapy with gemcitabine and platinum in unresectable stage III non-small-cell lung cancer (NSCLC): a phase II experience with a new schedule. *Proc Am Soc Clin Oncol.* **20**: 329 (abstract).

4-week schedule

- Manegold C, Bergman B, Chemaissani A *et al.* (1997) Single-agent gemcitabine *versus* cisplatin–etoposide: early results of a randomised phase II study in locally advanced or metastatic non-small-cell lung cancer. *Ann Oncol.* **8**: 525–9.

Bladder cancer

- Van der Maase H, Hansen SW, Roberts JT *et al.* (2000) Gemcitabine and cisplatin versus methotrexate, vinblastine, doxorubicin and cisplatin in advanced or metastatic bladder cancer: results of a large, randomized, multinational, multicenter, Phase III study. *J Clin Oncol.* **18**: 3068–77.

Ifosfamide (single-agent)

USUAL INDICATION

Malignant thymoma; also used on an ad-hoc basis for the treatment of various sarcomas, especially where doxorubicin-containing combinations are contraindicated.

DOSES

Ifosfamide 1500 mg/m^2 IV on days 1–5
Mesna 400 mg IV bolus prior to each day's ifosfamide infusion
Mesna 1000 mg/m^2 IV on days 1–5

Note: This is the established regimen for ifosfamide in thymoma. In this and other conditions the same total doses have been given empirically over shorter time periods (usually 3 days).

ADMINISTRATION

It is mandatory to give mesna with ifosfamide, to prevent the urothelial toxicity which can be caused by acrolein metabolites of the drug.

A loading dose of mesna is given first as an IV bolus, followed by a short infusion of ifosfamide, followed by an 8-h infusion of mesna. The scheduling is designed to ensure that there is adequate mesna in the bladder throughout the period when ifosfamide metabolites are appearing in the urine. In particular, the long infusion of mesna should not be speeded up to make the regimen shorter.

The modest degree of hydration provided by the fluids in this regimen also increases dilution of toxic ifosfamide metabolites in the bladder and encourages their voiding.

ANTI-EMETICS

High emetogenic potential (see local policy).

CYCLE LENGTH

21 days.

NUMBER OF CYCLES

Usually 6.

SIDE-EFFECTS

Bone-marrow suppression (all blood components are affected), total alopecia, nausea and vomiting, haemorrhagic cystitis leading to bladder fibrosis, encephalopathy during and shortly after the administration period, nephrotoxicity.

BLOOD NADIR

Day 12.

TTOS REQUIRED

Anti-emetics appropriate to highly emetogenic chemotherapy (see local protocol).

NOTES FOR PRESCRIBERS

At the time of prescribing each course

- Check the FBC prior to giving the go-ahead for chemotherapy. Seek advice if the neutrophil count is $<1.5 \times 10^9$/L or the platelet count is $<100 \times 10^9$/L at the time of treatment.
- Ifosfamide encephalopathy (which can be fatal) is an insidious condition that can develop on any treatment course. It presents in a variety of ways, although somnolence and confusion feature strongly in the early stages. Although it is impossible to predict the occurrence of encephalopathy with any accuracy, three factors have been demonstrated to predispose individuals to this problem, namely renal impairment, low serum albumin levels and a large pelvic tumour mass. Therefore renal function should be formally assessed at the start of treatment. Ideally this should be done by EDTA clearance, but estimation from serum creatinine levels using the Cockcroft–Gault equation is acceptable if the patient has a stable creatinine concentration and no confounding factors (e.g. catabolic states):

CrCl (mL/min)

$$= \frac{1.04 \text{ (females) or } 1.23 \text{ (males)} \times (140 - \text{age in years}) \times \text{weight in kg}}{\text{serum creatinine concentration (μmol/L)}}.$$

On subsequent cycles, the renal function should be reassessed if changes in serum creatinine concentration indicate alteration. Ifosfamide is also renally excreted and mildly nephrotoxic, and dosage adjustment is recommended if the CrCl drops below 50 mL/min (see Appendix 2 for further guidance).

- The serum albumin concentration should be checked before each cycle. If the patient has developed a new risk factor for encephalopathy since the previous treatment, discuss this with a senior member of the medical team. In a patient with two of the three risk factors, future treatment should be considered carefully.
- Check the LFTs. If these show severe impairment, dose adjustments may be required (see Appendix 1 for further guidance).
- Liaise with the nurses. The patient should be on a fluid-balance chart (ifosfamide can have an antidiuretic effect) and/or daily weights recorded, urine should be tested for blood (in case of haemorrhagic cystitis), and the nurses should understand the significance of any changes in mental state which may be indicative of encephalopathy.
- If blood is reported in the urine, increasing the mesna dose may help, although it should be noted that the lowest levels of blood detectable with dipstick tests may be of little clinical significance. Consult a senior member of the medical team for advice in this situation.
- If the patient displays changes in mental state which suggest encephalopathy, liaise with a senior member of the medical team immediately. Treatment suspension is strongly advised. Treatment with methylene blue (50 mg IV three times a day) should also be considered. This has been reported to reverse encephalopathy in this situation. Note that mesna has no ability to ameliorate CNS toxicity.
- Prescribe anti-emetics appropriate to a highly emetogenic chemotherapy regimen according to local policy.
- Extensive alopecia is likely with this treatment. If appropriate, liaise with the nursing staff to arrange referral to a wig-fitter early in treatment, before hair loss starts.

NOTES FOR NURSES

- The patient should be on a fluid-balance chart and/or daily weights recorded during ifosfamide treatment. Although hydration is not intensive, ifosfamide can exert an antidiuretic effect, causing fluid retention. A gain of more than 1.5 L/kg from the start of hydration should be reported to the medical team with a view to consideration of diuretic therapy.
- All urine collected on treatment days should be tested for blood because of the possibility of ifosfamide-induced haemorrhagic cystitis, although it should be noted that the lowest levels of blood detectable with dipstick tests may be of little clinical significance. Any haematuria should be reported promptly to the medical team.
- Because of the possibility of ifosfamide-induced CNS toxicity, excessive drowsiness or confusion should be reported promptly to the medical team.
- Extensive alopecia is likely with this treatment. If appropriate, arrange a referral to a wig-fitter early in treatment, before hair loss starts.

NOTES FOR PHARMACISTS

- Check that the FBC has been determined and is within acceptable limits before issuing the chemotherapy.
- Check renal function at the start of treatment. Calculate the CrCl from serum creatinine levels using the Cockroft–Gault equation, and mark this value on any

pharmacy patient record sheet (*see* Appendix 3 for an example), together with the corresponding creatinine concentration. On subsequent courses, recalculate the CrCl if the serum creatinine concentration increases significantly. Poor renal function is a risk factor for ifosfamide encephalopathy, and ifosfamide is also moderately nephrotoxic and renally excreted. A dose reduction should be considered if the CrCl falls below 50 mL/min (*see* Appendix 2 for further advice).

- Check the serum albumin concentration at the start of treatment − a low albumin level is a risk factor for ifosfamide encephalopathy. It is also worth checking on subsequent cycles, especially if the patient has other risk factors for encephalopathy (poor renal function or a large pelvic tumour mass). If the patient has multiple risk factors, especially if these include low albumin (which is often overlooked, as it is not usually an important consideration when deciding whether or not to give chemotherapy), alert the prescriber. Multiple risk factors are not an absolute contraindication to ifosfamide therapy, but where there is a choice of therapy, they may point towards an alternative.
- Check the LFTs. If these show severe impairment, ifosfamide dose adjustment may be required (*see* Appendix 1 for further advice).
- Check that anti-emetics appropriate to highly emetogenic chemotherapy have been prescribed according to local policy.
- Check that mesna has been prescribed and that the dose is appropriate (i.e. if the dose of ifosfamide on the fluid chart has been altered, then the mesna dose should have been altered proportionally).
  Note: Mesna is essentially non-toxic, and considerable rounding up of doses is acceptable to make preparation simpler.
- When visiting the treatment area, check that the patient is not in excessive positive fluid balance (i.e. >1.5 L/kg from the start of treatment). If they are, consult with the medical team about the possibility of prescribing diuretics (if this measure has not already been instituted) (e.g. furosemide 20 mg orally).
- When visiting the ward, check the fluid-balance chart. If any urine sample is described as containing blood, discuss with the prescriber the possibility of increasing the mesna dosage. It is difficult to give guidance on a reasonable increase in the mesna dose, but it is not unreasonable to double the dose in the post-hydration fluid, giving the increased dose in 2 L of fluid instead of 1 L, but over the same time period, thus stimulating diuresis as well.
  Note: Some dipstick urine tests are very sensitive to blood; the lowest levels of positivity may not be clinically significant and do not require intervention.
- Any reports of patients being excessively drowsy or confused should be regarded as indicators of ifosfamide encephalopathy. As this is a progressive condition, liaise with the prescriber urgently with a view to halting treatment immediately and possibly instituting treatment with methylene blue (50 mg IV three times a day). This treatment has been reported to be beneficial but has not been rigorously assessed and should not be relied upon, particularly as a prophylactic measure.

SOURCE MATERIAL

- Highley MS, Underhill CR, Parnis FX *et al.* (1999) Treatment of invasive thymoma with single-agent ifosfamide. *J Clin Oncol.* **17**: 2737–44.

Methylene blue in ifosfamide encephalopathy

- Kupfer A, Aeschlimann C, Wermuth B *et al.* (1994) Prophylaxis and reversal of ifosfamide encephalopathy with methylene blue. *Lancet.* **343**: 763–4.
- Zulian GB, Tullen E and Maton B (1995) Methylene blue for ifosfamide-associated encephalopathy. *NEJM.* **332**: 1239–40.

Irinotecan (CPT-11) (single-agent)

USUAL INDICATION

Second-line treatment of advanced colorectal cancer in patients who fail on a 5-fluorouracil-based regimen.

DOSES

Irinotecan 350 mg/m^2 (maximum 700 mg) IV on day 1

ADMINISTRATION

By IV infusion in 250 mL of 0.9% sodium chloride over a period of 30–90 min.

ANTI-EMETICS

High emetogenic potential (according to local policy).

CYCLE LENGTH

21 days.

NUMBER OF CYCLES

Until progression.

SIDE-EFFECTS

Acute cholinergic syndrome (early diarrhoea, sweating, abdominal cramping, lachrymation, myosis, salivation) at the time of drug infusion, severe diarrhoea starting around 72 h after treatment (dose limiting, together with bone-marrow suppression), bone-marrow suppression, nausea, vomiting.

BLOOD NADIR

10 days.

TTOS REQUIRED

- Anti-emetics appropriate to highly emetogenic chemotherapy.
- Begin loperamide treatment if late-onset diarrhoea starts. The recommended dose is 2 capsules/tablets (4 mg) with the first loose stool, and then 1 capsule/tablet (2 mg) every 2 h for at least 12 h after the last loose stool and for a maximum of 48 h. *This is higher than the standard loperamide dose.*
- A prophylactic course of a broad-spectrum antibiotic (e.g. ciprofloxacin 250 mg twice a day) to be taken if diarrhoea continues for more than 48 h.

Note: Loperamide and antibiotics need not be issued at every course provided that the patient still has an unused supply *and knows where they are.*

NOTES FOR PRESCRIBERS

- Consider the general performance status of the patient. Irinotecan is a toxic treatment and the manufacturer cautions that it should only be used with great circumspection in patients with an ECOG performance status of >2.
- Check the FBC prior to giving the go-ahead for chemotherapy. Irinotecan is contraindicated if the neutrophil count is $<1.5 \times 10^9$/L or the platelet count is $<75 \times 10^9$/L). Patients who experienced febrile neutropenia after a previous cycle or whose neutrophil nadir was $<0.5 \times 10^9$/L (even if they remained well) should have a dose reduction of 15–20% on subsequent cycles.
- Because irinotecan can be quite toxic, the next cycle should not be given until all toxicities have resolved to grade 0 or 1 on the NCIC-CTC grading system and treatment-related diarrhoea is completely resolved. Any patients who experienced grade 3–4 non-haematological toxicity on a previous course should have their dose reduced by 15–20%.
- Check hepatic function. Irinotecan is contraindicated if the bilirubin level is $>1.5 \times$ ULN. If the bilirubin is 1–$1.5 \times$ ULN, the patient should be treated with particular caution (*see* Appendix 1 for further guidance).
- On the first course of treatment, a 300 µg SC dose of atropine should be prescribed 'as required' in case the patient develops an acute cholinergic syndrome. On subsequent courses, atropine should be prescribed charted either as a regular premedication or 'as required', depending on whether it was needed with a previous course.
- Prescribe anti-emetics appropriate to highly emetogenic chemotherapy according to local policy.
- Prescribe loperamide and a broad-spectrum antibiotic as described above, unless you are sure that the patient has adequate unused supplies from their previous course *and knows where they are.*
- Advise the patient on what to do if late diarrhoea develops (i.e. how to take their prescribed medication) and to contact the hospital if diarrhoea persists for more

than 48 h, is not reasonably controlled by loperamide, or is accompanied by vomiting/fever. In such cases the patient should be admitted for IV hydration.

NOTES FOR NURSES

- If the patient develops an acute cholinergic syndrome (stomach cramps, salivation, sweating, pupillary constriction), this should be treated with 300 µg of atropine SC. This should have been prescribed 'as required' or as part of the routine premedication for patients who experienced cholinergic symptoms on earlier courses.
- Advise the patient on what to do if late diarrhoea develops (i.e. how to take their prescribed medication) (see TTO section above) and to contact the hospital if diarrhoea persists for more than 48 h, is not reasonably controlled by loperamide, or is accompanied by vomiting/fever. In such cases the patient should be admitted for IV hydration.

NOTES FOR PHARMACISTS

- Make sure that the FBC has been checked and is within satisfactory limits before issuing the chemotherapy. Irinotecan is contraindicated if the neutrophil count is $<1.5 \times 10^9$/L or the platelet count is $<75 \times 10^9$/L. Check the nadir count where possible. This is one of the few regimens where asymptomatic low nadir neutrophil counts are an indication for treatment modification. Patients with a nadir neutrophil count of $<0.5 \times 10^9$/L should have their next dose reduced by 15–20%, as should patients who experienced febrile neutropenia after the last course.
- Because irinotecan can be quite toxic, the next course should not be given until all of the toxicities from the last course have resolved to grade 0 or 1 on the NCIC-CTC grading system and treatment-related diarrhoea has resolved completely. Any patients who experienced grade 3–4 non-haematological toxicity on a previous course should have their dosage reduced by 15–20%.
- Make sure that hepatic function has been checked. Irinotecan is contraindicated if the bilirubin level is $>1.5 \times$ ULN. If the bilirubin level is 1–$1.5 \times$ ULN, then the patient may be treated, but should be monitored particularly closely. If LFT abnormalities are noted, mark these on any pharmacy patient record (see Appendix 3 for an example) to alert others to be extra vigilant on future courses.
- Make sure that on the first course of treatment a 300 µg SC dose of atropine is prescribed 'as required' in case the patient develops an acute cholinergic syndrome. On subsequent courses, atropine should be charted either as a regular premedication or 'as required', depending on whether it was needed with the first course.
- Make sure that anti-emetics suitable for highly emetogenic chemotherapy have been prescribed according to local policy, and that loperamide and a broad-spectrum antibiotic have been included on the TTO at the appropriate doses (unless you are sure that the patient still has adequate unused supplies from a previous course *and knows where they are*). The TTO will need to be clearly endorsed to ensure that these agents are correctly labelled by non-specialist staff, especially as the loperamide dosing regimen exceeds the normal maximum daily dose.

• Ensure that the patient has been advised on what to do if late diarrhoea develops (i.e. how to take their prescribed medication) and to contact the hospital if diarrhoea persists for more than 48 h, is not controlled by loperamide, or is accompanied by vomiting/fever. In such cases the patient should be admitted for IV hydration.

SOURCE MATERIAL

• Cunningham D, Pyrhonen S, James RD *et al.* (1998) Randomised trial of irinotecan plus supportive care versus supportive care alone after fluorouracil failure for patients with metastatic colorectal cancer. *Lancet.* **352**: 1413–18.

Liposomal daunorubicin (single-agent)

USUAL INDICATION

Advanced HIV-related Kaposi's sarcoma.

DOSES

Liposomal daunorubicin (DaunoXome®) 40 mg/m² IV on day 1

ADMINISTRATION

By infusion in 5% dextrose over a period of 2 h. The infusion time can be extended if infusion-related side-effects (e.g. back pain) are a problem.

ANTI-EMETICS

Low emetogenic potential (see local policy).

CYCLE LENGTH

14 days.

NUMBER OF CYCLES

Continue for as long as disease is controlled and regular cardiac monitoring indicates good cardiac toleration.

SIDE-EFFECTS

Bone-marrow suppression. Liposomal formulations are sometimes associated with infusion-related reactions, including back pain, flushing, chest tightness and hypotension. Risk of dilated cardiomyopathy after high cumulative doses (much less common than with conventional anthracyclines). Low incidence of significant nausea, vomiting or alopecia.

BLOOD NADIR

Because of the short dosage interval, a discrete nadir may not be seen.

TTOS REQUIRED

Anti-emetics appropriate to chemotherapy with low emetogenic potential (see local protocol).

NOTES FOR PRESCRIBERS

- Check the FBC before giving the go-ahead for chemotherapy. In a large trial of this treatment in Kaposi's sarcoma,[1] treatment was delayed if the neutrophil count was $<0.75 \times 10^9$/L or the platelet count was $<75 \times 10^9$/L, although some clinicians are likely to be concerned about giving chemotherapy – even a relatively non-myelotoxic regimen such as this – on such a low neutrophil count. Consult with an experienced prescriber if the neutrophil count is $<1.0 \times 10^9$/L or the platelet count is $<100 \times 10^9$/L. It should be noted that in the trial referred to above,[1] 20% of patients received G-CSF support.
- Patients over 60 years of age, or with a history of heart disease or who have received a cumulative dose of 400 mg/m^2 daunorubicin or equivalent anthracylines (e.g. 450mg/m^2 doxorubicin) should have an echocardiogram or MUGA scan prior to treatment to ensure that there is adequate left ventricular function.
- Monitor the total dose of liposomal daunorubicin administered. The cumulative dose of *conventional* daunorubicin should not exceed 400 mg/m^2 without further consultation, because the risk of anthracycline-induced cardiomyopathy increases rapidly beyond this point. The relationship between dose and cardiotoxicity for *liposomal* daunorubicin is unclear. It is probably less toxic, but a cumulative dose of 320 mg/m^2 should only be exceeded with caution following formal assessment of cardiac function (e.g. a MUGA scan, which should be repeated after every additional 160 mg/m^2). Consideration must be given to previous therapy with other anthracyclines, such as doxorubicin (normal cumulative maximum dose 450 mg/m^2).
- Check the LFTs. If these show serious impairment, then dose reduction may be required (*see* Appendix 1 for further guidance).
- Prior to treatment, hair loss should be discussed with the patient, although the risk of significant alopecia is relatively low. Scalp cooling is likely to be of limited benefit in preventing hair loss because of the prolonged half-life of liposomal daunorubicin.
- If you are administering the drug, it is important to be aware that conventional daunorubicin is vesicant. Although limited evidence suggests that liposomal daunorubicin is much less damaging to tissues, a senior member of the medical team should be contacted in the event of an extravasation. The local extravasation policy should be followed if an extravasation incident has occurred.

[1] Gill PS, Wernz J, Scadden DT *et al.* (1996) Randomized phase III trial of lipsomal daunorubicin versus doxorubicin, bleomycin and vincristine in AIDS-related Kaposi's sarcoma. *J Clin Oncol.* **14**: 2353–64.

NOTES FOR NURSES

- Prior to treatment, hair loss should be discussed with the patient. However, the risk of significant hair loss with this regimen is low, and scalp cooling is unlikely to be of much benefit because of the prolonged circulation of liposomal daunorubicin.
- If you are administering the drug, it is important to be aware that conventional daunorubicin is a vesicant. Although limited evidence suggests that liposomal daunorubicin is much less damaging to tissues, a senior member of the medical team should be contacted in the event of an extravasation. The local extravasation policy should be followed if an incident has occurred.
- Liposomal daunorubicin is incompatible with 0.9% sodium chloride. Intravenous lines should be flushed with 5% dextrose before and after the infusion.
- Infusion-related reactions such as backache, flushing and shortness of breath can be controlled by slowing the infusion rate or temporarily interrupting the drug administration.

NOTES FOR PHARMACISTS

- Check that the FBC has been determined and is within acceptable limits before issuing the chemotherapy.
- Check the LFTs. If these show serious impairment, a dose reduction may be required (see Appendix 1 for further guidance).
- Check that anti-emetics appropriate to chemotherapy of low emetogenic potential have been prescribed according to local protocol.
- Monitor the total dose of liposomal daunorubicin administered. Alert the prescriber if it exceeds $320 \, \text{mg/m}^2$ (unless there is evidence that cardiac function has been checked at this point and is acceptable), and at intervals of $160 \, \text{mg/m}^2$ thereafter. It is especially important when a patient starts a course of treatment to check the pharmacy records and their notes to see whether they have received previous therapy within your hospital or elsewhere. The contribution of other anthracyclines, such as doxorubicin (normal cumulative maximum dose $450 \, \text{mg/m}^2$), should be considered.

SOURCE MATERIAL

- Gill PS, Wernz J, Scadden DT *et al.* (1996) Randomized phase III trial of liposomal daunorubicin versus doxorubicin, bleomycin and vincristine in AIDS-related Kaposi's sarcoma. *J Clin Oncol.* **14**: 2353–64.

Liposomal doxorubicin (pegylated) (Caelyx®; Doxil®) (single-agent)

Note: This monograph refers specifically to the liposomal doxorubicin formulation marketed in the UK as Caelyx® and in the USA as Doxil®. Its content cannot be applied to conventional doxorubicin or to other liposomal preparations that may have very different pharmacokinetic and pharmacodynamic properties. Specifically, it cannot be applied to Myocet®, another liposomal product.

USUAL INDICATION

Advanced ovarian cancer in women who have failed first-line platinum-based chemotherapy; AIDS-related Kaposi's sarcoma (KS) in patients with low CD_4 counts and extensive mucocutaneous or visceral disease.

DOSES

Ovarian cancer

$50 \, mg/m^2$ IV on day 1

Kaposi's sarcoma

$20 \, mg/m^2$ IV on day 1

ADMINISTRATION

By infusion in 5% dextrose. Doses of less than 90 mg should be diluted in 250 mL and those above 90 mg in 500 mL.

Low doses used in Kaposi's sarcoma can be infused over a period of 30 min. The higher doses used for ovarian cancer should be infused no faster than 1 mg/min on the first occasion, but if no infusion reactions are observed, subsequent infusions can be administered over 60 min.

Caelyx® is incompatible with sodium chloride, and the IV line should be flushed before and after infusion with 5% dextrose.

Caelyx® can be introduced (diluted as described above) into the side-arm of a free-running 5% dextrose drip in order to minimise the risk of extravasation or thrombosis.

If infusion reactions are observed (*see* Side-effects section below), the infusion should be suspended (but not discarded), the symptoms treated with an antihistamine (e.g. chlorpheniramine 10–20 mg IV) and/or corticosteroid (e.g. hydrocortisone 100 mg IV), and the infusion then restarted at a slower rate.

Conventional doxorubicin is a powerful vesicant. However, liposomal doxorubicin appears to be less capable of causing severe tissue damage after extravasation. Despite this, reports of exfoliation and sloughing following extravasation have been received, and the drug should still be administered with appropriate precautions to prevent extravasation. If there is any possibility that extravasation has occurred, the infusion should be resited to another vein. The application of ice to the extravasation site is probably sufficient to deal with local pain and stinging, although documentation and follow-up should be in line with the local policy for managing extravasation incidents.

ANTI-EMETICS

Low emetogenic potential (see local policy). Because of the low peak blood levels of free doxorubicin and the sustained low levels of circulating free drug, the pattern of gastrointestinal disturbances is quite different to that seen with conventional doxorubicin.

CYCLE LENGTH

28 days in ovarian cancer; 14–21 days in Kaposi's sarcoma.

NUMBER OF CYCLES

Until disease progression or intolerance in ovarian cancer; for at least 2–3 months to obtain optimum response in Kaposi's sarcoma.

SIDE-EFFECTS

Palmar-plantar erythrodysasthesia ('hand-and-foot' syndrome; may be dose limiing), bone-marrow suppression, alopecia (much less significant than with conventional doxorubicin), nausea and vomiting, mucositis (may be severe), cardiac arrhythmias, dilated cardiomyopathy (especially at cumulative doses in excess of 450 mg/m^2). Allergy-like and anaphylactoid infusion reactions (including flushing, urticaria, chest pain, fever, tachycardia, sweating, shortness of breath, facial oedema, chills, back pain, tightness in the chest and throat). Infusion reactions usually resolve rapidly after treatment interruption, and are rare after the first dose.

BLOOD NADIR

Because of the very prolonged persistence of pegylated liposomal doxorubicin in the circulation, the nadir is likely to be late and ill defined, particularly with the short cycle lengths used for treating Kaposi's sarcoma.

TTOS REQUIRED

- Anti-emetics appropriate to chemotherapy with low emetogenic potential.

NOTES FOR PRESCRIBERS

- Although liposomal doxorubicin may be somewhat less cardiotoxic than the parent drug, caution is still recommended. Therefore, as with conventional doxorubicin, patients over 60 years of age, or with a history of heart disease, must have an echocardiogram or MUGA scan prior to treatment to ensure that there is adequate left ventricular function. The manufacturer of Caelyx$^{®}$ recommends that formal evaluation of left ventricular function follows each dose once the cumulative dose reaches 450 mg/m^2, with endomyocardial biopsies taken as a guide for future treatment, if cardiomyopathy is suspected. However, a typical treatment course will not exceed 450 mg/m^2, and most patients will not experience cardiomyopathy below this cumulative dose. If signs of cardiac dysfunction develop, or a cumulative dose in excess of 450 mg/m^2 is contemplated, the advice of an experienced prescriber should be sought.
- Before starting treatment, check the cumulative dose of doxorubicin and other anthracyclines (e.g. epirubicin, daunorubicin, idarubicin) which the patient may have already received at your hospital or elsewhere. These all contribute to the total lifetime dose of anthracyclines (including liposomal doxorubicin) that can safely be administered.
- Check the LFTs. If the serum bilirubin level exceeds 20 μmol/L, a reduction in starting dose should be considered (see Appendix 1 for further guidance).
- Check the FBC prior to giving the go-ahead for chemotherapy. Because of the different dosage schedules used and the different characteristics of the treated patient groups, the manufacturer of Caelyx$^{®}$ makes different recommendations for dose adjustment for haematological toxicity in the two conditions for which it is approved. For patients who are being treated for Kaposi's sarcoma, it is recommended that treatment is temporarily suspended whenever the absolute neutrophil count is $<1.0 \times 10^9$/L or the platelet count is $<50 \times 10^9$/L, and then resumed, with neutrophil counts supported by haematopoietic growth factors, if this is deemed appropriate (see local policy for haematopoietic growth factor support).

  For ovarian cancer, the following schedule of dose modification is suggested:

Neutrophil count ($\times 10^9$/L)	Platelet count ($\times 10^9$/L)	Dose modification
1.5–1.9	75–150	None required
0.5–1.5	25–75	Delay treatment until neutrophil count is $\geqslant 1.5 \times 10^9$/L and platelet count is $>75 \times 10^9$/L, then resume at full dose
<0.5	<25	Delay treatment until neutrophil count is $\geqslant 1.5 \times 10^9$/L and platelet count is $>75 \times 10^9$, then resume treatment with 25% dose reduction

- Alopecia is relatively uncommon with pegylated liposomal doxorubicin. Because of the prolonged half-life of this drug, scalp cooling is not appropriate as a means of further reducing the risk.
- Prescribe anti-emetics appropriate to chemotherapy of low emetogenic potential (see local policy). Because of the low peak blood levels of free doxorubicin and the sustained low levels of circulating drug, the pattern of gastrointestinal disturbances may be quite different to that seen with conventional doxorubicin.
- Palmar-plantar erythrodysasthesia ('hand-and-foot' syndrome) is often the most troublesome side-effect of pegylated doxorubicin treatment, and can be dose limiting. The manufacturer of Caelyx® makes specific dosage modification recommendations for managing this problem (*see* table below). These recommendations should be followed after a careful assessment of the condition of the patient's hands and feet at each course.

Toxicity grade after prior dose	Week after prior dose		
	Week 4	Week 5	Week 6
1 Mild erythema, swelling or desquamation not interfering with daily activities	*Redose unless* patient has experienced previous Grade 3 or 4 skin toxicity, in which case wait an additional week	*Redose unless* patient has experienced previous Grade 3 or 4 skin toxicity, in which case wait an additional week	*Decrease dose by 25%; return to 4-week dose interval*
2 Erythema, desquamation or swelling interfering with but not precluding normal physical activities; small blisters or ulcerations less than 2 cm in diameter	*Wait an additional week*	*Wait an additional week*	*Decrease dose by 25%; return to 4-week dose interval*
3 Blistering, ulceration or swelling interfering with walking or normal daily activities; cannot wear usual clothing	*Wait an additional week*	*Wait an additional week*	*Withdraw patient*
4 Diffuse or local process causing infectious complications, or a bedridden state or hospitalisation	*Wait an additional week*	*Wait an additional week*	*Withdraw patient*

- Stomatitis can also be a significant problem in patients who are receiving pegylated liposomal doxorubicin, and the following dose modification scheme has been recommended by the manufacturer of Caelyx® as a means of dealing with this:

Toxicity grade after prior dose	Week after prior dose		
	Week 4	Week 5	Week 6
1 Painless ulcers, erythema or mild soreness	Redose *unless* patient has experienced previous Grade 3 or 4 toxicity, in which case wait an additional week	Redose *unless* patient has experienced previous Grade 3 or 4 toxicity, in which case wait an additional week	Decrease dose by 25%; return to 4-week dose interval or withdraw patient according to physician's assessment
2 Painful erythema, oedema or ulcers, but can eat	Wait an additional week	Wait an additional week	Decrease dose by 25%; return to 4-week dose interval or withdraw patient according to physician's assessment
3 Painful erythema, oedema or ulcers and cannot eat	Wait an additional week	Wait an additional week	Withdraw patient
4 Requires parenteral or enteral support	Wait an additional week	Wait an additional week	Withdraw patient

- An antihistamine (e.g. chlorpheniramine 10–20 mg IV) and a corticosteroid (e.g. hydrocortisone 100 mg IV) should be prescribed 'as needed' so that they can be given promptly in the case of significant infusion reactions.
- Pyridoxine (e.g. 50 mg by mouth three times daily) has been used to treat palmar-plantar erythrodysasthesia. However, the evidence to support its use is modest, and it should not be regarded as an alternative to appropriate dose modifications.

NOTES FOR NURSES

- Unlike conventional doxorubicin, pegylated liposomal doxorubicin produces relatively modest hair loss and, because of its prolonged circulation in the blood, scalp cooling is an inappropriate strategy for reducing the risk further.
- Infusion reactions can sometimes be severe and, rarely, life-threatening. If the patient develops signs of infusion reactions, the infusion should be suspended promptly (but left in place) and an antihistamine (e.g. chlorpheniramine 10–20 mg IV) and/or a corticosteroid (e.g. hydrocortisone 100 mg IV) should be

administered. Once the symptoms have abated, the infusion can be restarted at a slower rate (e.g. 0.5 mg/min). Because reactions can sometimes be severe, resuscitation facilities should be available in areas where pegylated doxorubicin is administered. Patients who experience infusion reactions should be reassured that they rarely reoccur on the second or subsequent cycles of treatment.

- Patients who experience hand-and-foot syndrome with pegylated liposomal doxorubicin should be informed of the following measures which may help to minimise the problem: keeping the extremities cool; exposing them to cold water; keeping them unrestricted by tight-fitting gloves, socks or shoes.
- If you are administering the drug, *see* Administration section above for notes on dealing with extravasation.
- Pegylated liposomal doxorubicin is incompatible with sodium chloride, and the infusion line should be flushed with 5% dextrose before and after infusion.

NOTES FOR PHARMACISTS

- Check that the FBC has been determined and is within acceptable limits before issuing the chemotherapy.
- Check the LFTs. If the bilirubin level exceeds 20 μmol/L, a dose reduction is recommended (*see* Appendix 1 for further advice).
- Check that anti-emetics appropriate to weakly emetogenic chemotherapy have been prescribed according to protocol. Note that because of the prolonged serum half-life of pegylated liposomes, symptoms, although moderate, may be prolonged.
- Keep a close eye on the cumulative dose of liposomal doxorubicin and alert the prescriber if it exceeds 450 mg/m². It is especially important when a patient starts a course of treatment to check the pharmacy records and the patient's notes to see whether they have received previous doxorubicin therapy within your hospital or elsewhere. The impact of previous treatment with other anthracyclines (epirubicin, daunorubicin, idarubicin, aclarubicin) must also be considered.
- Check that 'as-required' chlorpheniramine and hydrocortisone have been prescribed to treat infusion reactions if they occur.
- Hand-and-foot syndrome and stomatitis may be dose limiting with this regimen. The manufacturer of the Caelyx® formulation of liposomal doxorubicin makes specific dose-modification recommendations for dealing with these problems (described above). These recommendations should be followed. Note that although pyridoxine (e.g. 50 mg by mouth three times daily) has been used to treat palmar-plantar erythrodysasthesia, the evidence to support its use is modest, and it should not be regarded as an alternative to appropriate dose modifications.

SOURCE MATERIAL

Ovarian cancer

- Gordon AN, Fleagle JT, Guthrie D *et al.* (2001) Recurrent epithelial ovarian carcinoma: a randomised phase III study of pegylated liposomal doxorubicin versus topotecan. *J Clin Oncol.* **19**: 3312–22.

AIDS-related Kaposi's sarcoma

- Northfelt DW, Dezube BJ, Thommes JA *et al.* (1998) Pegylated liposomal doxorubicin versus doxorubicin, bleomycin and vincristine in the treatment of AIDS-related Kaposi's sarcoma: results of a randomised phase III clinical trial. *J Clin Oncol.* **16**: 2445–51.

Mayo regimen (folinic acid plus 5-fluorouracil, 5FU/FA, 5-FU/LV)

USUAL INDICATION

Adjuvant treatment of surgically resected colorectal cancer; first-line palliative treatment of recurrent or inoperable colorectal cancer.

DOSES

> Folinic acid (FA)* 20 mg/m^2 IV
> 5-Fluorouracil (5-FU) 425 mg/m^2 IV

These doses are given on 5 consecutive days in every 28 days, or on 1 day in every 7 days (i.e weekly). The original Mayo Clinic regimen used 5 consecutive days of treatment every month. However, the QUASAR study[1] has demonstrated that, at least in the adjuvant setting, weekly treatment is as effective and possibly better tolerated. Overall, there is no good evidence for the superiority of weekly or monthly treatment, and the final choice should depend on treatment logistics and patient preference.

Note: There are *many* other regimens of 5-FU and FA in use, including the de Gramont and modified de Gramont regimens (*see* separate chapters on those regimens). Make sure that it is clear which regimen is required.

ADMINISTRATION

By IV injection with folinic acid given immediately before 5-FU (its role is to potentiate 5-FU).

ANTI-EMETICS

Very low emetogenic potential (see local policy).

---

* Folinic acid is also known as 'folinate', 'calcium folinate', 'leucovorin' (LV) and 'calcium leucovorin'.

[1] Kerr DJ, Gray RG, McKonkey C *et al.* (2000) Adjuvant chemotherapy (CT) with 5-fluorouracil (FU), L-folinic acid (FA) and levamisole (LEV) for colorectal cancer (CRC): nonrandom comparison of weekly (W) versus monthly (M) schedules. *Proc Am Soc Clin Oncol.* **19**: 258 (abstract).

CYCLE LENGTH

7 or 28 days (*see* Doses section above).

NUMBER OF CYCLES

Adjuvant treatment

Usually 30 doses, as 30 weekly treatments or 6 monthly courses of 5 consecutive days.

Palliative treatment

Until treatment progression, with treatment on 1 day each week or on 5 consecutive days in every 4 weeks.

SIDE-EFFECTS

Bone-marrow suppression, alopecia (usually mild), nausea and vomiting (rare), mucositis (can be dose limiting), diarrhoea (can be dose limiting). A small proportion of patients who are deficient in the 5-FU-metabolising enzyme dihydropyrimidine dehydrogenase (DPD) may experience unexpectedly severe toxicity.

BLOOD NADIR

Around 12 days after the start of 5-day treatment. With weekly treatment, the next dose is given before the nadir is reached, and therefore there is no discrete nadir.

TTOS REQUIRED

- Anti-emetics appropriate to chemotherapy with weakly emetogenic potential.

NOTES FOR PRESCRIBERS

- Make sure that the patient is to receive treatment according to the Mayo protocol, not some other combination of 5-FU and FA.
- Make sure that you are clear whether weekly or monthly treatment is intended. If no decision has yet been made, consult with the patient and the clinic nurses to find the most mutually acceptable solution.
- Check the FBC prior to giving the go-ahead for chemotherapy. Seek advice from a senior member of the medical team if the neutrophil count is $<1.5 \times 10^9$/L or the platelet count is $<100 \times 10^9$/L.

- Prior to prescribing, check the LFTs and renal function for evidence of moderate to severe dysfunction. Consideration should be given to a dose reduction in the case of severe renal dysfunction or moderate hepatic dysfunction (*see* Appendices 1 and 2 for further guidance).

NOTES FOR NURSES

- No special information is needed.

NOTES FOR PHARMACISTS

- Make sure that the patient is to receive treatment according to the Mayo protocol, not some other combination of 5-FU and FA.
- Check that the FBC has been determined and is within acceptable limits before issuing the chemotherapy. However, many patients tolerate this regimen extremely well, and it may be reasonable to prepare weekly treatments or day 1 of monthly treatment ahead of confirmation. This will reduce waiting times but is not likely to lead to significant wastage, as the components of this regimen are relatively inexpensive.
- Check the LFTs and renal function for evidence of moderate to severe dysfunction. Consideration should be given to a dose reduction in the case of severe renal dysfunction or moderate hepatic dysfunction (*see* Appendices 1 and 2 for further guidance).
- This protocol has a low emetogenic potential. Any use of $5HT_3$-antagonists should be questioned. Patients with severe gastrointestinal symptoms may have a psychogenic component to their symptoms which may respond to haloperidol and/or lorazepam.

SOURCE MATERIAL

- Poon MA, O'Connell MJ, Moertel CG *et al.* (1989) Biochemical modulation of fluorouracil: evidence of significant improvement and quality of life in patients with advanced colorectal carcinoma. *J Clin Oncol.* **7**: 1407–18.

Weekly vs. monthly treatment

- Kerr DJ, Gray RG, McKonkey C *et al.* (2000) Adjuvant chemotherapy (CT) with 5-fluorouracil (FU), L-folinic acid (FA) and levamisole (LEV) for colorectal cancer (CRC); non-random comparison of weekly (W) versus monthly (M) schedules. *Proc Am Soc Clin Oncol.* **19**: 258 (abstract).

MCF (mitomycin, cisplatin, 5-fluorouracil)

USUAL INDICATION

Adjuvant and palliative treatment of gastric and oesophageal cancers, especially in patients who are unsuitable for anthracycline treatment, or who have previously been treated with ECF and are therefore unsuitable for MCF.

DOSES

Mitomycin 7 mg/m^2 IV on day 1 (*alternate courses only*)
Cisplatin 60 mg/m^2 IV on day 1
5-Fluorouracil (5-FU) 300 mg/m^2/day IV on days 2–21 by continuous infusion

ADMINISTRATION

Mitomycin

By slow IV injection into the side-arm of a free-running 0.9% sodium chloride drip.

Mitomycin is a powerful vesicant and should be administered with appropriate precautions to prevent extravasation. If there is any possibility that extravasation has occurred, contact a senior member of the medical team immediately and follow local guidance on dealing with extravasation incidents.

Cisplatin

As an infusion in 1 L of saline over a period of 2 h, after pre-hydration with 1 L of 0.9% sodium chloride and followed by post-hydration with a further 1 L of 0.9% sodium chloride. Cisplatin is nephrotoxic, and hydration is mandatory to dilute the drug as it is excreted via the kidneys, to minimise toxicity. The aim of hydration is to maintain a urine output of 100 mL/h during and for 6–8 h after cisplatin administration. Electrolytes are added to compensate for cisplatin-induced electrolyte wasting.

5-FU

By continuous IV infusion via a permanently implanted IV access (PICC, Hickman or Groschong line).

ANTI-EMETICS

High emetogenic potential (see local policy) on day 1 and minimal emetogenic potential on days 2–21.

CYCLE LENGTH

21 days.

NUMBER OF CYCLES

Usually 6.

SIDE-EFFECTS

Nephrotoxicity (dose limiting due to cisplatin), bone-marrow suppression (all blood components are affected), alopecia (moderate and less extensive than with ECF), nausea and vomiting (may be very severe), sensory, motor and autonomic neuropathy (sometimes irreversible, due to cisplatin) including significant potential for ototoxicity, mucositis (especially due to 5-FU), diarrhoea (mainly due to 5-FU), palmar-plantar erythrodysasthesia ('hand-and-foot' syndrome – peeling, soreness and redness of the palms of the hands and soles of the feet, due to 5-FU), diarrhoea (mainly due to 5-FU).

BLOOD NADIR

Around 10 days.

TTOS REQUIRED

- Anti-emetics appropriate to highly emetogenic chemotherapy to cover cisplatin treatment (see local protocol).
- Unless it is contraindicated, low-dose warfarin therapy (1 mg/day) should be instituted once a central venous line (Hickman or Groshong, *not* PICC) is *in situ*, in order to prevent line thrombosis.

NOTES FOR PRESCRIBERS

When considering treatment options

- *Ask yourself whether the patient will really be able to cope with the demands of looking after an infusion pump.* This is important. Home infusion therapy, particularly with an electromechanical pump, requires patients or their immediate carers to take an active part in their treatment. If they are unwilling or unable to do so, other treatment options should be explored. Normally patients should also have access to a telephone in case problems occur at home.

Note: Not all community nursing and medical staff are familiar with home chemotherapy. It cannot be assumed that they will take on responsibility for looking after the patient's pump at home. If this is intended, contact must be made and consent for such an approach obtained at an early stage.

- If your department has a finite number of infusion pumps available, liaise with whoever looks after them to see whether there is a free infusion pump *before* discussing the treatment with the patient. These pumps are often in short supply.
- Liaise in advance with those responsible for setting up the pumps and educating the patient about their treatment. Both processes can be time-consuming, and in a busy department they need to be scheduled in advance.

At the time of prescribing

- Prior to treatment, hair loss should be discussed with the patient. It is likely to be only moderate. Scalp cooling will probably only be partially effective in reducing it further, as it provides little protection against cisplatin-induced hair loss.
- The dose of 5-FU in this regimen is quite high, particularly since it is used in combination. Especially in frail patients, it may be prudent to start at 200 mg/m²/day (which most patients will tolerate) and increase the dose stepwise to 300 mg/m²/day on successive cycles, if it is well tolerated (say 250, 275 then 300 mg/m²/day).
- Unless it is contraindicated, prescribe low-dose warfarin (*see* TTO section) and ensure that arrangements are made for either the GP or the hospital to check the INR about 1 week after starting therapy to ensure that the patient is not hypersensitive to the drug. Communicate to the GP that this dose of warfarin is not intended to alter the INR significantly and should not be increased.
- The patient's renal function should be formally assessed at the start of treatment. Ideally this should be done by EDTA clearance, but estimation from the serum creatinine level using the Cockcroft–Gault equation is acceptable if the patient has a stable creatinine concentration and no confounding factors (e.g. catabolic states):

CrCl (mL/min)

$$= \frac{1.04 \text{ (females) or } 1.23 \text{ (males)} \times (140 - \text{age in years}) \times \text{weight in kg}}{\text{serum creatinine concentration (}\mu\text{mol/L)}}.$$

On subsequent cycles the renal function should be reassessed.

Cisplatin doses *must be reduced* if the creatinine clearance drops below 60 mL/min, and consideration should be given to a mitomycin dose adjustment if the CrCl falls below 50 mL/min (*see* Appendix 2 for further guidance).

- Check the serum electrolytes for cisplatin-induced wasting, especially of magnesium, calcium and potassium. Additional supplementation may be required.
- Prescribe anti-emetics appropriate to highly emetogenic chemotherapy according to local policy.

- Check the FBC prior to giving the go-ahead for chemotherapy. Seek advice if the neutrophil count is $<1.5 \times 10^9$/L or the platelet count is $<100 \times 10^9$/L.
- The LFTs should be checked before treatment. Consideration should be given to reducing the 5-FU and mitomycin doses in cases of severe hepatic impairment (*see* Appendix 1 for further guidance).
- Seek further advice if the patient reports symptoms indicative of neurotoxicity (parasthesias, difficulty with motor control) or ototoxicity (tinnitus, deafness).
- If you are administering the drugs, *see* Administration section above for notes on the vesicant nature of mitomycin.
- This treatment has unusual toxicities associated with the 5-FU infusion ('hand-and-foot' syndrome, mucositis, diarrhoea). If these are causing more than mild discomfort, this is an indication for a treatment break. Hand-and-foot syndrome, mucositis and diarrhoea all resolve very rapidly (within 5–7 days) after stopping treatment. Empirical dose reductions should be of the order 25–30% if they are to be worthwhile.
  Note: Some individuals lack the 5-FU-metabolising enzyme dihydropyrimidine dehydrogenase (DPD) and may therefore be particularly sensitive to the effects of 5-FU.
- Prescribe 5-FU supplies for a suitable period depending on local arrangements. For example, is the patient returning to the hospital periodically for pump reservoir changes? Or are they having this done in the community by a visiting nurse or doing it themselves? However long this period is, it is recommended that the patient is seen 10–14 days after starting treatment in order to review any problems.

On the day after each cisplatin dose (if the patient is an inpatient)

- Monitor the fluid balance/body weight. If the patient has gained 1.5 L/kg or more from the start of hydration, extra diuresis will be required (e.g. furosemide 20–40 mg by mouth).

NOTES FOR NURSES

- Discuss possible hair loss with the patient. Note that with this regimen hair loss will probably be only moderate and scalp cooling is likely to be of limited value in reducing it further, because of the prolonged exposure to cisplatin.
- Patients with home infusion pumps will need support at home, including advice on side-effects, the patient's pump and their venous access. They are also likely to need practical help with dressing venous line insertion sites, changing infusion reservoirs and flushing unused lumens on the venous line in accordance with local policies. Local arrangements for this support should be formalised and robust. District and practice nurses may be unfamiliar with this type of treatment. *It should not be assumed that they will be willing to support patients* – liaise with them first.
- Details of setting up pumps, etc., are beyond the scope of this book. If this is being undertaken by nursing staff, it should be the subject of robust and formal local procedures.

- If pharmacy staff set up infusion pumps, and if the patient's dose has been adjusted, ensure as far as possible that the infusion rate on any variable-rate infusion pump (where the dose is governed by the infusion rate) has been reset to deliver the correct dose.
- The aim of hydration is to ensure an average urine output of 100 mL/h or more during and for 6–8 h after cisplatin administration. Any patient who is being treated as an inpatient should be on a fluid-balance chart, and daily weights should be recorded. Contact the prescriber if the patient's urine output is inadequate or their body weight increases by 1.5 kg from baseline.

    For outpatients, efforts should be made to ensure that urine output is adequate (e.g. by ensuring that the patient has passed 500 mL of urine between the start of IV hydration and the beginning of cisplatin infusion).

    Outpatients should also be encouraged to drink 3 L of fluid in the 24 h following each period of IV hydration, and to contact the hospital if this is impossible because of nausea/vomiting or other problems.
- If you are administering mitomycin, *see* Administration section above for notes on the vesicant nature of this drug.

NOTES FOR PHARMACISTS

- Check that the FBC has been determined and is within acceptable limits before issuing the chemotherapy.
- Check that the creatinine clearance has been measured/calculated at the start of treatment. Record the CrCl and the corresponding creatinine concentration on any pharmacy patient record (*see* Appendix 3 for an example). Recalculate the CrCl if the creatinine concentration changes. A cisplatin dose reduction is needed if the CrCl drops below 60 mL/min. Consideration should also be given to a mitomycin dose adjustment if the CrCl drops below 50 mL/min (*see* Appendix 2 for further guidance).
- Check that anti-emetics appropriate to highly emetogenic chemotherapy have been prescribed according to local protocol to cover cisplatin treatment.
- At the start of treatment, make sure that the patient's LFTs have been checked, and note any abnormalities on the pharmacy patient record. Consideration should be given to 5-FU and mitomycin dose reductions in cases of severe hepatic impairment (*see* Appendix 1 for further guidance).
- Details of setting up 5-FU pumps, etc., are beyond the scope of this book. If this is being undertaken by pharmacy staff, it should be the subject of robust and formal local procedures.
- If pharmacy staff set up infusion pumps, and if the patient's 5-FU dose has been adjusted, ensure that the infusion rate on any variable-rate infusion pump (where the dose is governed by the infusion rate) is reset to deliver the correct dose.
- When calculating 5-FU requirements for a given period of time, remember to allow enough overage to ensure that the patient will not run out before their next supply is due. The overage required will depend on the type of pump being used.
- If the patient is an inpatient, when you are visiting the ward the day after chemotherapy, check that they have not gained more than 1.5 L/kg since the start of treatment. If they have, discuss additional diuresis (e.g. furosemide 20–40 mg by mouth) with the prescriber (if this measure has not already been instituted).

- If the patient is not prescribed low-dose warfarin at the start of treatment, check whether this is needed (it is not required if the patient has a PICC line). If it is contraindicated, mark this clearly on the patient's pharmacy record sheet to prevent future prescribing.

SOURCE MATERIAL

- Ross P, Cunningham D, Scarffe H *et al.* (1999) Results of a randomised trial comparing ECF with MCF in advanced oesophago-gastric cancer. *Proc Am Soc Clin Oncol.* **18**: 272.

Melphalan (IV intermediate-dose) plus dexamethasone

USUAL INDICATION

First-line treatment of multiple myeloma.

DOSES

Melphalan 25 mg/m^2 IV on day 1
Dexamethasone 40 mg by mouth once daily on days 1–4

Note: There are many combinations of melphalan and steroids in use. This one is used at the author's hospital, but the reader should be aware that there are other regimens in use. The guidance given here is *not* appropriate to high-dose regimens that require stem-cell support.

ADMINISTRATION

Melphalan is given as a short (15–20 min) intravenous infusion in 0.9% sodium chloride. Dexamethasone is given orally. The highest strength of dexamethasone tablet available in the UK is 2 mg, so patients on this regimen will need to take 20 dexamethasone tablets each day.

Although it is not always regarded as a vesicant, melphalan can cause serious tissue damage if extravasated, and should therefore be administered with appropriate precautions to prevent extravasation. If there is any possibility that extravasation has occurred, contact a senior member of the medical team immediately and follow the local procedure for managing extravasation incidents.

ANTI-EMETICS

High emetogenic potential on day 1 (see local policy). Note that this regimen incorporates large doses of dexamethasone, so additional steroids are not required for anti-emesis.

CYCLE LENGTH

28 days.

NUMBER OF CYCLES

Until the patient enters complete remission or paraprotein levels stabilise.

SIDE-EFFECTS

Bone-marrow suppression and long-term impairment of bone-marrow function, nausea and vomiting, mucositis, skin rashes and nailbed pigmentation. The high doses of dexamethasone used in this regimen may produce typical steroid side-effects, including impaired glucose tolerance, euphoria, insomnia and other mental disturbances, sodium and water retention, electrolyte loss and proximal myopathy.

BLOOD NADIR

2 to 3 weeks after treatment.

TTOS REQUIRED

- Anti-emetics appropriate to highly emetogenic chemotherapy (excluding additional steroids; see above) plus dexamethasone.
- It may be appropriate to prescribe an H_2-antagonist or other gastroprotective agent on the days of dexamethasone therapy if gastritis is a problem or the patient has a history of gastrointestinal ulceration. Ranitidine is preferred to cimetidine, which has been reported to increase melphalan elimination.

NOTES FOR PRESCRIBERS

- Check the FBC prior to giving the go-ahead for chemotherapy. Seek advice if the neutrophil count is $<1.5 \times 10^9$/L or the platelet count is $<100 \times 10^9$/L at the time of treatment.
- Although the relationship between renal function and melphalan clearance is controversial, dosage reduction in renal impairment has been suggested. Therefore it is recommended that at the start of treatment an estimation of renal function is made from the serum creatinine concentration using the Cockcroft–Gault equation, assuming that the patient has no confounding factors (e.g. catabolic states):

CrCl (mL/min)

$$= \frac{1.04 \text{ (females) or } 1.23 \text{ (males)} \times (140 - \text{age in years}) \times \text{weight in kg}}{\text{serum creatinine concentration } (\mu\text{mol/L})}.$$

In the case of significant renal impairment, a dosage reduction should be considered. In patients who tolerate a reduced dose well, doses can be increased on subsequent courses if appropriate (see Appendix 2 for further information).

On subsequent cycles the renal function should be reassessed.

- Prescribing the dexamethasone to be taken early in the day may help to prevent problems with night-time wakefulness.
- Make sure that it is stated clearly on any prescription or in any communication with the patient's GP that the dexamethasone is a short course of 4 days only. *Fatalities have resulted from the inadvertent continuation of short courses of steroids.*
- It may be appropriate to prescribe an H_2-antagonist or other gastroprotective agent on the days of dexamethasone treatment if gastritis is a problem or the patient has a history of gastrointestinal ulceration. Ranitidine is preferred to cimetidine, which has been reported to increase melphalan elimination.
- If you are administering melphalan, *see* Administration section above for notes on the dangers of melphalan extravasation.
- The highest strength of dexamethasone tablet available in the UK is 2 mg, so patients on this regimen will need to take 20 dexamethasone tablets each day. Some patients may find this alarming, so they should be reassured that this is a 'normal' dose. Other patients may find the tablets difficult to swallow. Unfortunately, there is no other suitable oral formulation routinely available. However, the tablets can be fairly readily made into a slurry with water immediately before use.

NOTES FOR NURSES

- If you are administering melphalan, *see* Administration section above for notes on the dangers of melphalan extravasation.
- The highest strength of dexamethasone tablet available in the UK is 2 mg, so patients on this regimen will need to take 20 dexamethasone tablets each day. Some patients may find this alarming, so they should be reassured that this a 'normal' dose. Other patients may find the tablets difficult to swallow. Unfortunately, there is no other suitable oral formulation routinely available. However, the tablets can be fairly readily made into a slurry with water immediately before use.
- Ensure that any diabetic patients are aware of the need to be extra vigilant about monitoring their blood sugar levels during treatment with dexamethasone, and advise them to contact their doctor if they have problems with the control of their blood sugar levels.
- Encourage patients to take their dexamethasone tablets early in the day, as this may help to prevent problems with night-time wakefulness.
- If you are issuing dexamethasone tablets to patients, explain to them that these should be taken for 4 days only, and that they should not attempt to obtain further supplies from their GP. *Fatalities have resulted from the inadvertent continuation of short courses of steroids.*

NOTES FOR PHARMACISTS

- Check that the FBC has been determined and is within acceptable limits before issuing the chemotherapy.
- Although the relationship between renal function and melphalan clearance is controversial, dosage reduction in renal impairment has been suggested. Therefore it is recommended that at the start of treatment an estimation of the renal

function is made from the serum creatinine concentration using the Cockcroft–Gault equation. In the presence of confounding factors (e.g. catabolic states), a more formal measure of renal function may be required.

In the case of significant renal impairment, a dosage reduction should be considered. In patients who tolerate a reduced dose well, the doses can be increased on subsequent cycles if appropriate (*see* Appendix 2 for further information). The patient's creatinine concentration and corresponding CrCl should be recorded on any pharmacy patient record (*see* Appendix 3 for an example), and the CrCl should be recalculated on subsequent courses if the creatinine concentration has changed significantly.

- Check that anti-emetics appropriate to chemotherapy with low emetogenic potential have been prescribed according to protocol. Note that no additional steroids are required for anti-emesis, since the regimen contains significant doses of dexamethasone.
- The highest strength of dexamethasone tablet available in the UK is 2 mg, so patients on this regimen will need to take 20 dexamethasone tablets each day. Some patients may find this alarming, so they should be reassured that this a 'normal' dose. Other patients may find the tablets difficult to swallow. Unfortunately, there is no other suitable oral formulation routinely available. However, the tablets can be fairly readily made into a slurry with water immediately before use.
- Make sure that it is clearly stated on any discharge prescription or prescription being sent elsewhere for dispensing that the dexamethasone is for a short course of 4 days only. *Fatalities have resulted from the inadvertent continuation of short courses of steroids.* Dexamethasone should not be continued by the GP, nor is routine 'tailing off' of doses necessary.
- It may be appropriate to prescribe an H_2-antagonist or other gastroprotective agent on the days of dexamethasone treatment if gastritis is a problem or the patient has a history of gastrointestinal ulceration. Ranitidine is preferred to cimetidine, which has been reported to increase melphalan elimination.

SOURCE MATERIAL

Schey SA, Kazmi M, Ireland R and Lakhani A (1998) The use of intravenous intermediate-dose melphalan and dexamethasone as induction treatment in the management of *de novo* multiple myeloma. *Eur J Haematol.* **61**: 306–10.

MIC (mitomycin, ifosfamide, cisplatin)

USUAL INDICATION

Non-small-cell lung cancer (NSCLC).

DOSES

> Mitomycin C 6 mg/m^2 IV on day 1
> Ifosfamide 3000 mg/m^2 IV plus mesna 1500 mg/m^2 IV on day 1
> plus mesna 1500 mg/m^2 IV infused over 4 h after ifosfamide infusion
> is complete
> Cisplatin 50 mg/m^2 IV on day 1

Note: There are several variants on the MIC regimen, which vary particularly in the degree and scheduling of hydration. The above schedule, first described by Cullen *et al.*,[1] is typical of current UK practice and is suitable for both inpatient and outpatient use. Variants incorporating much higher cisplatin doses (e.g. that described by Crino *et al.*[2]) are not widely used in the UK, require much more intensive hydration and are unsuitable for outpatient use.

ADMINISTRATION

Ifosfamide and mesna

Mesna administration is mandatory with ifosfamide, to prevent the urothelial toxicity that can be caused by acrolein metabolites of the drug.

Ifosfamide is infused concurrently with mesna. This is followed, after a 1-h break for cisplatin infusion, by a 4-h infusion of mesna alone. This scheduling is designed to ensure that there is adequate mesna in the bladder throughout the period when ifosfamide metabolites are appearing in the urine. Therefore the administration rate of the mesna infusion should not be increased in order to shorten the regimen.

---

[1] Cullen MH, Woodroffe CM, Billingham LJ *et al.* (1997) Mitomycin, ifosfamide and cisplatin (MIC) in non-small-cell lung cancer (NSCLC). 2. Results of a randomised trial in patients with extensive disease. *Lung Cancer.* **18** (**Supplement 1**): 5.

[2] Crino L, Clerici M, Figoli F *et al.* (1995) Chemotherapy of advanced non-small-cell lung cancer: a comparison of three active regimens. A randomized trial of the Italian Oncology Group for Clinical Research (GOIRC). *Ann Oncol.* **6**: 347–53.

Mitomycin

By slow IV injection into the side-arm of a free-running 0.9% sodium chloride drip. *Mitomycin is a powerful vesicant* and should be administered with appropriate precautions to prevent extravasation. If there is any possibility that extravasation has occurred, contact a senior member of the medical team and follow local guidance on dealing with cytotoxic extravasation.

Cisplatin

As an infusion in 500 mL of 0.9% sodium chloride over 1 h, immediately after the combined mesna and ifosfamide infusion. Cisplatin is nephrotoxic, and hydration is mandatory to dilute the drug as it is excreted via the kidneys and thus minimise toxicity. Typically another 1 L of 0.9% sodium chloride is administered after the cisplatin. The aim of hydration is to maintain a urine output of 100 mL/h during and for 6–8 h after cisplatin administration. Electrolytes are added to compensate for cisplatin-induced electrolyte wasting.

ANTI-EMETICS

High emetogenic potential (according to local policy).

CYCLE LENGTH

21 days.

NUMBER OF CYCLES

Usually 6.

SIDE-EFFECTS

Bone-marrow suppression (all blood components are affected), total alopecia, haemorrhagic cystitis leading to bladder fibrosis, encephalopathy during the administration period, nephrotoxicity, vomiting (may be very severe), sensory, motor and occasionally autonomic (sometimes irreversible) neuropathy (including significant potential for ototoxicity), mucositis.

BLOOD NADIR

Day 12.

TTOS REQUIRED

- Anti-emetics appropriate to highly emetogenic chemotherapy (according to local protocol).

NOTES FOR PRESCRIBERS

At the time of prescribing each course

- Check the FBC prior to giving the go-ahead for chemotherapy. Seek advice if the neutrophil count is $<1.5 \times 10^9$/L or the platelet count is $<100 \times 10^9$/L at the time of treatment.
- Cisplatin is highly nephrotoxic, and the creatinine clearance should be formally assessed at the start of treatment. Ideally this should be done by EDTA clearance, but estimation from serum creatinine levels using the Cockcroft–Gault equation is acceptable if the patient has a stable creatinine concentration and no confounding factors (e.g. catabolic states):

CrCl (mL/min)

$$= \frac{1.04 \text{ (females) or } 1.23 \text{ (males)} \times (140 - \text{age in years}) \times \text{weight in kg}}{\text{serum creatinine concentration (}\mu\text{mol/L)}}.$$

On subsequent cycles the renal function should be reassessed.

Doses of cisplatin *must be reduced* if the creatinine clearance drops below 60 mL/min. Adjustment of the dose of mitomycin, which is renally excreted and can also be nephrotoxic, should also be considered if the CrCl falls below 60 mL/min (*see* Appendix 2 for further guidance).

- Poor renal function is not only a contraindication to cisplatin and mitomycin therapy, but is also (together with a low serum albumin level and a large pelvic tumour mass) a risk factor for the development of ifosfamide encephalopathy. This is an insidious condition which can develop on any treatment course and which presents in a variety of ways, although somnolence and confusion feature strongly in the early stages. It can be fatal. Therefore, as well as close monitoring of renal function, serum albumin levels should be checked on each course. If a patient has two or more risk factors, particularly if these have developed since previous treatment, discuss this with an experienced prescriber.
- Check electrolytes for cisplatin-induced wasting, especially of magnesium, calcium and potassium. Additional supplementation may be required.
- Ifosfamide and possibly mitomycin are also contraindicated in patients with significant hepatic dysfunction (*see* Appendix 1 for further guidance).
- Ensure that anti-emetics appropriate to a highly emetogenic regimen have been prescribed according to local protocol.
- Liaise with the nurses who are looking after the patient. Any patient who is staying in hospital during their chemotherapy should have their urine tested for blood (in case they have haemorrhagic cystitis). Nurses should also understand the significance of any changes in mental state which may be indicative of encephalopathy.
- If blood is reported in the urine, then increasing the mesna dose may help. Macroscopic evidence of haematuria should always be acted upon, but some test strips are very sensitive and may give a positive result when there are clinically insignificant traces of blood in the urine. Consult a senior member of the medical team for advice if drug-induced haematuria is suspected.
- If the patient displays changes in mental state which suggest encephalopathy, liaise with a senior member of the medical team immediately. *Treatment suspension*

is strongly advised. Treatment with methylene blue (50 mg IV three times a day) should also be considered. This has been reported to reverse encephalopathy in this situation. Note that mesna has no ability to ameliorate CNS toxicity.

- If administering the treatment, *see* Administration section above for notes on the vesicant nature of mitomycin.

On the day after each cisplatin dose (if the patient is an inpatient)

- Check the patient's fluid balance. If the patient has gained more than 1.5 L/kg since the start of hydration, extra diuresis should be provided (e.g. furosemide 20–40 mg by mouth).

NOTES FOR NURSES

- The aim of hydration is to ensure an average urine output of 100 mL/h or more during and for 6–8 h after cisplatin administration. Any patient who is being treated as an inpatient should be on a fluid-balance chart, and daily weights should be recorded. Contact the prescriber if the patient's urine output is inadequate or their body weight increases by 1.5 kg from baseline.

  For outpatients, efforts should be made to ensure that urine output is adequate (e.g. by checking that the patient has passed 500 mL of urine between the start of IV hydration and the beginning of cisplatin infusion).

  Outpatients should also be encouraged to drink 3 L of fluid in the 24 h following each period of IV hydration, and to contact the hospital if this is impossible because of nausea/vomiting or other problems.
- Where possible (i.e. for inpatients), once the ifosfamide infusion has commenced all urine should be tested for blood because of the possibility of ifosfamide-induced haemorrhagic cystitis. Some dipstick tests are very sensitive and may indicate the presence of clinically insignificant amounts of blood. Nevertheless, the presence of any amount of blood, however small, should be drawn to the attention of the medical team promptly, as the patient may require extra prophylactic mesna.
- Because of the possibility of ifosfamide-induced CNS toxicity, any excessive drowsiness or confusion should be reported promptly to the medical team. Patients, and also the carers of patients who are being treated in the day-case unit, should be encouraged to report any unusual CNS symptoms, although they should also be reassured that such problems are rare.
- If administering the drugs, *see* Administration section above for notes on the vesicant nature of mitomycin.

NOTES FOR PHARMACISTS

- Check that the FBC has been determined and is within an acceptable range before issuing the chemotherapy.

- Check that renal function is satisfactory at the start of treatment. If no formal measure of renal function is available, and provided that the patient's serum creatinine concentration is stable (i.e. there are no catabolic states or similar confounding factors), calculate the CrCl from the serum creatinine levels using the Cockroft–Gault equation, and mark this value on any pharmacy patient record sheet (*see* Appendix 3 for an example), together with the corresponding serum creatinine concentration. On subsequent courses, recalculate the CrCl if the serum creatinine concentration increases significantly. Poor renal function is a risk factor for ifosfamide encephalopathy, and both cisplatin and (to a lesser extent) ifosfamide and mitomycin are nephrotoxic. A reduction in cisplatin dose is required if the CrCl is <60 mL/min. A reduction in mitomycin and ifosfamide doses should also be considered if the CrCl falls to <60 mL/min and <50 mL/min, respectively (*see* Appendix 2 for further guidance).
- Check the serum albumin concentration at the start of treatment. Low albumin levels are another risk factor for ifosfamide encephalopathy. It is also worth checking on subsequent cycles, especially if the patient has other risk factors for encephalopathy (e.g. poor renal function or a large pelvic tumour mass). If the patient has multiple risk factors, especially if these include low albumin levels (which are often overlooked, as they are not routinely checked prior to most other chemotherapy regimens), alert the prescriber. Multiple risk factors are not an absolute contraindication to ifosfamide therapy, but if there is a choice of therapy they may point towards an alternative.
- Check the LFTs before treatment is commenced. Ifosfamide and possibly mitomycin are contraindicated in patients with significant hepatic dysfunction (*see* Appendix 1 for further guidance).
- Check that anti-emetics appropriate to highly emetogenic chemotherapy have been prescribed according to local protocol.
- Check that mesna has been prescribed and that the dose is appropriate (i.e. if the dose of ifosfamide has been altered, then the mesna dose should be altered proportionally).

Note: Mesna is essentially non-toxic, and considerable rounding up of doses is acceptable to make preparation simpler.

- If the patient is an inpatient, when you are visiting the ward check that they are not in excessive positive fluid balance (i.e. that they have not gained more than 1.5 L/kg from the start of hydration, and that urine output is maintained at a level above 100 mL/h during and for 6–8 h after cisplatin infusion). If there is excessive fluid retention, consult with the medical team about the possibility of extra diuretics being prescribed (if this measure has not already been instituted) (e.g. furosemide 20–40 mg by mouth).

    In addition, if any urine sample is described as showing macroscopic or dipstick-detected traces of blood, discuss with the prescriber the possibility of increasing the mesna dosage, although it should be noted that some dipstick tests are very sensitive, and that the lowest levels of blood detected with them may not require intervention. It is difficult to give guidance on a suitable increase in the mesna dose, but it is not unreasonable to double the dose.
- Any reports of patients being excessively drowsy or confused should be regarded as indicators of ifosfamide encephalopathy. As this is a progressive condition, liaise with the prescriber urgently with a view to halting treatment

immediately, and possibly instituting treatment with methylene blue (50 mg IV three times a day). This treatment has been reported to be beneficial, but it has not been rigorously assessed and should not be relied upon, particularly as a prophylactic measure.

SOURCE MATERIAL

- Cullen MH, Woodroffe CM, Billingham LJ *et al.* (1997) Mitomycin, ifosfamide and cisplatin (MIC) in non-small-cell lung cancer (NSCLC). 2. Results of a randomised trial in patients with extensive disease. *Lung Cancer.* **18** (**Supplement 1**): 5.

- Crino L, Clerici M, Figoli F *et al.* (1995) Chemotherapy of advanced non-small-cell lung cancer: a comparison of three active regimens. A randomized trial of the Italian Oncology Group for Clinical Research (GOIRC). *Ann Oncol.* **6**: 347–53.

Methylene blue in the management of ifosfamide encephalopathy

- Kupfer A, Aeschlimann C, Wermuth B *et al.* (1994) Prophylaxis and reversal of ifosfamide encephalopathy with methylene blue. *Lancet.* **343**: 763–4.
- Zulian GB, Tullen E and Maton B (19695) Methylene blue for ifosfamide-associated encephalopathy. *NEJM.* **332**: 1239–40.

MMM (mitomycin, methotrexate, mitoxantrone)

USUAL INDICATION

Breast cancer, usually second-line therapy in advanced disease, but may be used earlier as adjuvant treatment or first-line therapy for advanced disease, especially if chemotherapy-induced hair loss is a major concern (this is relatively modest with MMM).

DOSES

Mitomycin 7 mg/m^2 IV on day 1
Methotrexate 35 mg/m^2 IV (maximum dose 50 mg) on days 1 and 21
Mitoxantrone 7 mg/m^2 IV on days 1 and 21

ADMINISTRATION

By slow IV injection into the side-arm of a free-running 0.9% sodium choride drip. The sequence of drug administration is not critical. *Mitomycin is vesicant*, and mitoxantrone may also cause tissue damage if extravasated, so it should be administered with appropriate precautions to prevent extravasation. If there is any possibility that extravasation has occurred, contact a senior member of the medical team immediately and follow your local policy for dealing with extravasation incidents.

ANTI-EMETICS

Moderate emetogenic potential (according to local policy).

CYCLE LENGTH

42 days.

NUMBER OF CYCLES

Usually 3.

SIDE-EFFECTS

Bone-marrow suppression, nausea and vomiting, mucositis. The risk of alopecia is relatively modest. Cardiotoxicity has been reported after mitoxantrone administration, but it is less common than with anthracyclines. It seems to be more likely to occur at cumulative doses in excess of $160 \, mg/m^2$, or $100 \, mg/m^2$ after previous anthracycline therapy.

BLOOD NADIR

There is no discrete nadir because the drugs within this combination give rise to differential patterns of myelotoxicity which combine to produce a pattern of chronic suppression of blood counts.

TTOS REQUIRED

- Anti-emetics appropriate to moderately emetogenic chemotherapy (according to local policy).
- Folinic acid (calcium folinate/calcium leucovorin) 'rescue' is not routinely required with the doses of methotrexate used in MMM. If it is used because of unexpected toxicity on previous courses or because the patient has a 'third-space' fluid collection or severe renal impairment, a reasonable dose is 15 mg by mouth 6-hourly for 6 doses (prior toxicity) or 12 doses (reduced clearance) *starting 24 h after methotrexate*. Starting the 'rescue' earlier negates the effects of chemotherapy.

NOTES FOR PRESCRIBERS

- Make sure it is clearly stated what chemotherapy regimen the patient is due to receive. The MMM acronym is used for at least two chemotherapy regimens, and yet another regimen, MM (mitoxantrone plus mitomycin), is also used for breast cancer.
- Make sure it is clearly understood whether the patient is on day 1 or day 21 of their treatment cycle. Mitomycin is only administered on day 1.
- Renal function should be assessed before the start of treatment and before each course. Mitomycin is nephrotoxic, and both mitomycin and methotrexate are renally excreted, so dose modifications are necessary if the GFR is <60 mL/min (*see* Appendix 2 for further guidance). Formal assessment of renal function is not generally required. For patients with a stable serum creatinine concentration and no confounding factors (e.g. catabolic states), it is reasonable to calculate the creatinine clearance using the Cockcroft–Gault equation:

CrCl (mL/min)

$$= \frac{1.04 \, (\text{females}) \text{ or } 1.23 \, (\text{males}) \times (140 - \text{age in years}) \times \text{weight in kg}}{\text{serum creatinine concentration } (\mu mol/L)}.$$

Formal measurement of renal function should be reserved for patients in whom the latter is known to be significantly impaired.

- Mitoxantrone is extensively metabolised in the liver, and a dosage reduction may be necessary in cases of significant hepatic impairment (*see* Appendix 1 for further guidance).
- Check the FBC prior to giving the go-ahead for chemotherapy. Seek advice if the neutrophil count is $<1.5 \times 10^9$/L, or the platelet count is $<100 \times 10^9$/L. In the original description of this regimen,[1] treatment was only given if the WBC was $>3.0 \times 10^9$/L and the platelet count was $>100 \times 10^9$/L. Doses were reduced by 25% after two dose delays or an incident of neutropenic infection, and by 50% after four dose delays.
- If the patient has a 'third-space' fluid collection (ascites, effusion or extensive oedema) or significant renal impairment, the elimination of methotrexate may be prolonged, enhancing its toxicity. Consider folinic acid rescue in such cases (discuss this with an experienced prescriber first). If folinic acid is to be used, make sure it is charted to start 24 h after methotrexate, as earlier administration will negate the effect of methotrexate as well as its toxicity.
- If administering the drugs, *see* Administration section above for notes on the vesicant nature of mitomycin and mitoxantrone.
- Mitomycin treatment rarely induces haemolytic uraemic syndrome. The risk of this disorder is increased by concurrent tamoxifen therapy, and tamoxifen and MMM should not be given together.
- It is unlikely that, at the doses of mitoxantrone used in MMM, cumulative cardiac toxicity will be a problem (*see* Side-effects section above). However, great care should be exercised in patients with pre-existing cardiac dysfunction, including that induced by previous anthracyclines.

NOTES FOR NURSES

- If administering the drugs, *see* Administration section above for notes on the vesicant nature of mitomycin and mitoxantrone.
- If the patient is prescribed folinic acid (calcium folinate/calcium leucovorin), it should be prescribed to start 24 h after methotrexate, as starting any earlier will negate the effect of methotrexate as well as its toxicity. If it is charted to start 24 h after methotrexate, *do not* administer it before this time. If the start time is not specified, check with the prescriber. If you are issuing folinic acid to a patient, make sure that they know when to take this medication.

NOTES FOR PHARMACISTS

- Make sure it is clear what chemotherapy regimen the patient is due to receive. The MMM acronym is used for at least two chemotherapy regimens, and yet another regimen, MM (mitoxantrone plus mitomycin), is also used for breast cancer.

---

[1] Smith IE and Powles TJ (1993) MMM (Mitomycin/Mitoxantrone/Methotrexate): an effective new regimen in the treatment of metastatic breast cancer. *Oncology*. **50** (**Supplement 1**): 9–15.

- Make sure it is clearly understood whether the patient is on day 1 or day 21 of their treatment cycle. Mitomycin is only administered on day 1.
- When a patient starts treatment, block out the mitomycin box on any pharmacy record sheet (*see* Appendix 3 for an example) for each alternate course to avoid inadvertent administration.
- Both methotrexate and mitomycin are renally excreted, and mitomycin can be nephrotoxic. Dose modifications may be required for both drugs if the CrCl is <60 mL/min (*see* Appendix 2 for further guidance). On the first cycle of treatment, renal function should be measured or assessed using the Cockcroft–Gault equation. Enter the CrCl value along with the corresponding serum creatinine concentration on any pharmacy patient record sheet. On subsequent courses, the CrCl should be remeasured/recalculated if there is a significant change in serum creatinine concentration.
- Mitoxantrone is extensively metabolised in the liver, and a dosage reduction may be necessary in cases of significant hepatic impairment (*see* Appendix 1 for further guidance).
- Check that the FBC has been determined and is within acceptable limits before issuing the chemotherapy.
- Folinic acid (calcium folinate/calcium leucovorin) rescue is not routinely required. However, when it is used (e.g. in patients with unexpected toxicity on a previous course, 'third-space' fluid collection or significant renal impairment), it should be prescribed to start 24 h after methotrexate. Starting the rescue any earlier will negate the effect of methotrexate as well as its toxicity. If it is charted to start 24 h after methotrexate, block out any earlier spaces on the drug chart to prevent it being given before, endorse any TTO clearly and/or add this instruction to the pack label. If the start time is not specified, check this with the prescriber. If a patient does receive folinic acid with MMM, make a note of this (with the reason) on any pharmacy patient record sheet to ensure that this is included in future courses if necessary.
- 'Third-space' fluid collections (ascites, effusions, gross oedema) and significant renal impairment prolong the half-life of methotrexate, enhancing its toxicity. If it is known that a patient has such problems, ask the prescriber whether folinic acid rescue is required (*see* TTOs section above).
- It is unlikely that, at the doses of mitoxantrone used in MMM, cumulative cardiac toxicity will be a problem (*see* Side-effects section above). However, great care should be exercised in patients with pre-existing cardiac dysfunction, including that induced by previous anthracyclines.

SOURCE MATERIAL

- Smith IE and Powles TJ (1993) MMM (Mitomycin/Mitoxantrone/Methotrexate): an effective new regimen in the treatment of metastatic breast cancer. *Oncology*. **50** (**Supplement 1**): 9–15.

MOPP (chlormethine [mustine], vincristine [Oncovin®], prednisolone, procarbazine)

USUAL INDICATION

Hodgkin's disease, usually in relapse.

DOSES

Chlormethine (mustine) 6 mg/m² IV on days 1 and 8
Vincristine 1.4 mg/m² (maximum 2 mg*) IV on days 1 and 8
Prednisolone† 40 mg/m² by mouth on days 1–14
Procarbazine 100 mg/m² by mouth on days 1–14

ADMINISTRATION

Chlormethine and vincristine

By slow IV injection into the side-arm of a free-running 0.9% sodium chloride drip.
Chlormethine and vincristine are powerful vesicants and should be administered with appropriate precautions to prevent extravasation. If there is any possibility that extravasation has occurred, contact a senior member of the medical team immediately and follow the local guidance on management of extravasation incidents.

Procarbazine and prednisololone

These drugs are only available as oral preparations. Procarbazine is only available as 50 mg capsules, which cannot be divided, so individual doses must be calculated to the nearest 50 mg. Intermediate doses can be achieved by administering unequal doses on successive days.

ANTI-EMETICS

High emetogenic potential (see local policy, although note that because of the high dose of prednisolone on days 1–14, no additional steroids are needed).

---

* The 2 mg cap was not imposed in the original description of this regimen,[1] but is now universally applied to prevent excessive neurotoxicity.

† In the original description of this regimen, prednisone was used. This is no longer readily available in the UK, and is replaced by prednisolone at the same dose.

[1] DeVita VT Jr, Serpick AA and Carbone PP (1970) Combination chemotherapy in the treatment of advanced Hodgkin's disease. *Ann Intern Med.* **73**: 881–95.

CYCLE LENGTH

28 days.

NUMBER OF CYCLES

Complete remission plus a further two cycles, unless consolidation with high-dose chemotherapy and stem-cell transplantation is intended, in which case only two courses may be used as a test of disease chemosensitivity.

SIDE-EFFECTS

Bone-marrow suppression, alopecia, nausea and vomiting, mucositis. Peripheral neuropathy from vincristine. Procarbazine is a weak inhibitor of MAO and can lead to CNS side-effects such as somnolence, hallucinations, ataxia, headache and insomnia, especially when administered with tyramine-rich foods, alcohol or interacting medications.

The high doses of prednisolone used in this regimen can produce a variety of steroid side-effects, including euphoria/depression, epigastric discomfort, insomnia, glucose intolerance, psychosis, sodium and water retention, potassium loss and proximal myopathy.

BLOOD NADIR

Because of the dose scheduling, with cytotoxic drugs administered on days 1 and 8, and the relatively late nadir (14–18 days) which follows chlormethine treatment, the time to nadir is difficult to predict for MOPP, but is likely to fall within the 14 days following day 8 treatment.

TTOS REQUIRED

- Anti-emetics appropriate to highly emetogenic chemotherapy (according to local policy), but without additional steroids (the prednisolone in the regimen should be sufficient).
- Sufficient procarbazine and prednisolone to finish the course of treatment (i.e. the complete 14 days if treatment is being given on an outpatient basis).
- Allopurinol, 300 mg each morning (reduce the dose in cases of renal impairment), should be prescribed to prevent tumour lysis syndrome, especially early in treatment when there is a large tumour bulk.
- Consideration should be given to the prescription of a gastroprotective agent (e.g. an H_2-antagonist) to provide cover during courses of prednisolone.

NOTES FOR PRESCRIBERS

- Make sure that it is clearly understood whether the patient is due day 1 or day 8 treatment. On day 1, the full 14-day course of oral medications should normally be prescribed, so that on day 8 only IV medication is required.

- Check the FBC prior to giving the go-ahead for chemotherapy. Seek advice from a senior member of the medical team if the neutrophil count is $<1.5 \times 10^9$/L or the platelet count is $<100 \times 10^9$/L. Note that because treatment is being given with curative intent, it may proceed on a lower count than would be acceptable for palliative regimens. The following schedule of dosage adjustments for low blood counts on the day of treatment was used in the original published study[1] of this regimen, if dose delays of up to 7 days failed to permit full-dose treatment. It should be noted that this study was published more than 30 years ago, and that this approach to treatment would now be considered by most to be somewhat conservative for a curable condition.

WBC on treatment day $(\times 10^9$/L)	Dosage (% of planned)
>4	100% of all drugs
3.0–3.999	100% of vincristine and prednisolone, 50% of chlormethine and procarbazine
2.0–2.999	100% of vincristine and prednisolone, 25% of chlormethine and procarbazine
1.0–1.999	100% of prednisolone, 50% of vincristine, 25% of chlormethine and procarbazine
<0.999	No treatment

Platelet count on treatment day $(\times 10^9$/L)	Dosage (% of planned)
>100	100% of all drugs
50–100	100% of vincristine and prednisolone, 25% of chlormethine and procarbazine
<50	No treatment

- Check the serum creatinine concentration. The procarbazine dosage may require adjustment in cases of significant renal impairment. The manufacturer recommends a 50% dose reduction in patients with a serum creatinine concentration of >177 µmol/L.
- Check the LFTs. Dose adjustments should be considered for both procarbazine and vincristine in cases of significant hepatic impairment (see Appendix 1 for further advice).
- Check that the maximum 2 mg dose for vincristine has not been exceeded. Note that a 2 mg capped dose was not applied originally, but is now almost universally adhered to in an attempt to prevent excessive neurotoxicity. Some clinicians use a lower limit (typically 1.5 mg in patients over 70 years of age) in elderly patients who are perceived to be at increased risk of neurotoxicity, although this is not evidence based.
- This is a potentially curative treatment, and it is important to maintain dose intensity. Dose delays should be avoided if at all possible. The use of haematopoietic growth factors to support neutrophil numbers may be justified (see local policy on the use of haematopoietic growth factors for a suitable

dosage). Note that asymptomatic low nadir counts that recover prior to the next treatment day are *not* a reason to institute growth factor support.

- Vincristine can cause peripheral neuropathy. The patient should be questioned about abnormal sensations, jaw pain or constipation, any of which may be indicative of neuropathy. Discuss such symptoms with a senior member of the medical team with a view to dose modification or switching to vinblastine, which appears to be more myelosuppressive but less neurotoxic.

- Lymphomas are very sensitive to chemotherapy, and massive tumour lysis is possible at the start of chemotherapy. This can result in the generation of large amounts of insoluble uric acid, which is capable of precipitating in the kidneys, causing renal damage. To prevent this, allopurinol 300 mg once daily (reduce the dose in cases of renal impairment) should be commenced the day before starting cytotoxic therapy and continued for as long as a significant tumour bulk remains and cytotoxic therapy continues.

- Prior to treatment, hair loss should be discussed with the patient. Scalp cooling may be of benefit in preventing hair loss in patients who are concerned about this problem. Liaise with the nurses with regard to referral to a wig-fitter at the start of treatment, and before alopecia is evident, if this is required.

- If administering the treatment, *see* Administration section above for notes on the vesicant nature of chlormethine and vincristine.

- All prescriptions and communications with the patient's GP should make it clear that procarbazine and prednisolone are given as discrete courses. Further supplies should not be sought or prescribed via the patient's GP. Lack of clarity with regard to this matter may result in inadvertent continuation of oral therapy with cytotoxics/steroids. *Inadvertent continuation of short courses of oral cytotoxics or steroids has resulted in fatalities.*

- Because procarbazine is a weak MAOI, it has the *potential* to cause CNS side-effects and to interact with those foods and medications which are known to cause problems with MAOIs. Although full dietary restrictions and discontinuation of existing interacting medications are not justified, this problem should be considered if the patient presents with headache or CNS side-effects. Because it has a weak disulfiram-like effect, procarbazine may also cause adverse reactions to alcohol. Therefore the patient should be counselled about this and advised to avoid alcoholic drink.

- Procarbazine is only available in 50 mg capsules, which cannot be divided. If rounding off the daily dose to the nearest 50 mg is unacceptable, a closer approach to the calculated dose may be achieved by giving uneven doses on successive days (e.g. a calculated daily dose of 175 mg could be given as 200 mg and 150 mg on alternate days).

NOTES FOR NURSES

- Prior to treatment, hair loss should be discussed with the patient. Scalp cooling may be of benefit. If appropriate, referral to a wig-fitter should be made at the start of treatment, and before alopecia is evident.

- If administering the drugs, *see* Administration section above for notes on the vesicant properties of vincristine and chlormethine.

- If you are involved in counselling the patient about their oral medication, explain clearly that the procarbazine and prednisolone are intended to be taken for 14 days at a time only. A full course should normally be issued at the time of day 1 IV treatment. The patient should not seek additional supplies from their GP. On day 8, check that the patient still has a 1-week supply remaining and has not run out/been issued with a further 14 days' supply.
- Because procarbazine has a weak disulfiram-like effect, it may cause adverse reactions to alcohol. Therefore the patient should be counselled about this and advised to avoid alcoholic drink.
- Ensure that any diabetic patients are aware of the need to be extra vigilant about monitoring their blood sugar levels during treatment with prednisolone, and advise them to contact their doctor if they experience problems with the control of their blood sugar levels.

NOTES FOR PHARMACISTS

- Make sure that you clearly understand whether the patient is due day 1 or day 8 treatment. Normally on day 1 the full 14-day course of oral medications should be prescribed, so that on day 8 only the IV medication is required. Record the issue of oral medications on any pharmacy patient record (see Appendix 3 for an example), and on day 8 check that a 14-day supply was dispensed on day 1.
- Check that the FBC has been determined and is within acceptable limits before issuing the chemotherapy. Because this is a potentially curative treatment, it is reasonable to treat on a somewhat lower neutrophil/platelet count than would be considered acceptable for a palliative regimen.
- Check the serum creatinine concentration. The procarbazine dosage may require adjustment in cases of significant renal impairment. The manufacturer recommends a 50% dose reduction in patients with a serum creatinine concentration of >177 μmol/L.
- Check the LFTs. Dose adjustments should be considered for both procarbazine and vincristine in cases of significant hepatic impairment (see Appendix 1 for further guidance).
- This is a potentially curative treatment, and it is important to maintain dose intensity. Dose delays should be avoided if at all possible. The use of haematopoietic growth factors to support neutrophil numbers may be justified. Consult your local policy on haematopoietic growth factors for further advice. Note that asymptomatic low nadir counts that recover before chemotherapy is next due are not an indication for growth factor treatment.
- Check that the maximum 2 mg dose for vincristine has not been exceeded. Note that a 2 mg cap was not applied originally, but is now almost universally adhered to in an attempt to prevent excessive neurotoxicity. Some clinicians use a lower limit (typically 1.5 mg for patients over 70 years of age) in elderly patients who are perceived to be at increased risk of neurotoxicity, although this is not evidence based.
- Check that appropriate anti-emetics have been prescribed according to local protocol. However, because MOPP incorporates 14 days of high-dose prednisolone, additional steroids are not required.

- Lymphomas are very sensitive to chemotherapy, and massive tumour lysis is possible at the start of chemotherapy. This can result in the generation of large amounts of insoluble uric acid, which is capable of precipitating in the kidneys, causing renal damage. To prevent this, allopurinol 300mg once daily (reduced in cases of renal impairment) should be commenced the day before starting cytotoxic therapy and continued for as long as a significant tumour bulk remains.
- Make sure that it is clearly stated on any TTO or prescription that is being sent elsewhere for dispensing that the prednisolone is a short course of 14 days only. It should not be continued by the GP, nor is tailing off of doses necessary. Similarly, ensure that procarbazine prescriptions and TTOs state clearly that this agent should be continued for 14 days only. *Fatalities have resulted from the inadvertent continuation of short courses of oral cytototoxics or steroids by GPs.*
- Because procarbazine is a weak MAOI, it has the *potential* to cause CNS side-effects and to interact with those foods and medications which are known to cause problems with MAOIs. Although full dietary restrictions and discontinuation of existing interacting medications are not justified, this problem should be considered if patients present with headache or CNS side-effects. Because it has a weak disulfiram-like effect, procarbazine may also cause adverse reactions to alcohol. Therefore the patient should be counselled about this and advised to avoid alcoholic drink.
- Procarbazine is only available in 50 mg capsules, which cannot be divided. If rounding off the daily dose to the nearest 50 mg is unacceptable, a closer approach to the calculated dose may be achieved by giving uneven doses on sucessive days (e.g. a calculated dose of 175 mg could be given as 200 mg and 150 mg on alternate days).

SOURCE MATERIAL

- DeVita VT Jr, Serpick AA and Carbone PP (1970) Combination chemotherapy in the treatment of advanced Hodgkin's disease. *Ann Intern Med.* **73**: 881–95.

MV (mitomycin, vinblastine)

USUAL INDICATION

Metastatic breast cancer previously treated with chemotherapy.

DOSES

Mitomycin 12 mg/m^2 IV on day 1
Vinblastine 6 mg/m^2 IV on days 1 and 21

Note: There are many published and unpublished variations on these doses. This is one of the best characterised schedules, having been used as the control arm of a large comparative randomised trial.[1]

ADMINISTRATION

Mitomycin and vinblastine

By slow IV injection into the side-arm of a free-running 0.9% sodium chloride drip. *Mitomycin and vinblastine are powerful vesicants*, and should be administered with appropriate precautions to prevent extravasation. If there is any possibility that extravasation has occurred, contact a senior member of the medical team immediately and follow local guidance on dealing with extravasation incidents.

ANTI-EMETICS

Low emetogenic potential (see local policy).

CYCLE LENGTH

42 days.

---

[1] Nabholtz J-M, Senn HJ, Bezwoda WR *et al.* (1999) Prospective randomised trial of docetaxel versus mitomycin plus vinblastine in patients with metastatic breast cancer progressing despite previous anthracycline-containing chemotherapy. *J Clin Oncol.* **17**: 1413–24.

NUMBER OF CYCLES

Until disease progression.

SIDE-EFFECTS

Bone-marrow suppression (all blood components are affected), alopecia (usually very moderate hair loss), nausea and vomiting (usually very modest), mucositis, haemolytic uraemic syndrome secondary to mitomycin, peripheral neurotoxic side-effects due to vinblastine (e.g. tingling in the extremities and constipation).

BLOOD NADIR

Unpredictable because of the prolonged myelosuppression produced by mitomycin.

TTOS REQUIRED

- Anti-emetics appropriate to weakly emetogenic chemotherapy (see local protocol).

NOTES FOR PRESCRIBERS

At the time of prescribing each course

- Check the FBC prior to giving the go-ahead for chemotherapy. Seek advice if the neutrophil count is $<1.5 \times 10^9$/L or the platelet count is $<100 \times 10^9$/L. In the randomised study of this regimen compared with docetaxel in relapsed breast cancer,[1] mitomycin doses were reduced from $12\,mg/m^2$ to $8\,mg/m^2$ and from $8\,mg/m^2$ to $5\,mg/m^2$, and vinblastine doses were reduced from $6\,mg/m^2$ to $4\,mg/m^2$ in the event of severe haematological or other toxicities (other than anaemia and alopecia), although precise definitions of severe toxicity were not given.
- Make sure it is clearly understood which treatment week the patient is due. Mitomycin is only given every 6 weeks and vinblastine every 3 weeks.
- Check the patient's renal function at the start of therapy. Estimation from the serum creatinine level using the Cockcroft–Gault equation is acceptable if the patient has a stable serum creatinine concentration and no confounding factors (e.g. catabolic states):

CrCl (mL/min)

$$= \frac{1.04\ (\text{females}) \text{ or } 1.23\ (\text{males}) \times (140 - \text{age in years}) \times \text{weight in kg}}{\text{serum creatinine concentration (}\mu\text{mol/L)}}.$$

On subsequent cycles the renal function should be reassessed.

Mitomycin doses *should normally be reduced* if the creatinine clearance drops below 60 mL/min (*see* Appendix 2 for further advice).

- Check the LFTs. Doses of vinblastine and possibly mitomycin should be reduced in cases of significant hepatic impairment (*see* Appendix 1 for further advice).
- Prescribe anti-emetics appropriate to weakly emetogenic chemotherapy according to standard policy.
- If administering the drugs, *see* Administration section above for notes on the vesicant nature of mitomycin and vinblastine.

NOTES FOR NURSES

- If administering the drugs, *see* Administration section above for notes on the vesicant nature of mitomycin and vinblastine.
- Make sure it is clearly understood which treatment week the patient is due. Mitomycin is only given every 6 weeks and vinblastine every 3 weeks.

NOTES FOR PHARMACISTS

- Check that the FBC has been determined and is within acceptable limits before issuing the chemotherapy.
- Check the renal function at the start of treatment. If this has not been formally measured, calculate it from the serum creatinine levels using the Cockroft–Gault equation. Record the CrCl and the corresponding creatinine concentration on any pharmacy patient record sheet (*see* Appendix 3 for an example). On subsequent courses, recalculate the CrCl if the serum creatinine concentration increases significantly. Mitomycin is renally excreted, and a reduction in dose should be considered if the CrCl falls below 60 mL/min (*see* Appendix 2 for further advice).
- Check the LFTs. Doses of vinblastine and possibly mitomycin should be reduced in cases of significant hepatic impairment (*see* Appendix 1 for further advice).
- Check that anti-emetics appropriate to weakly emetogenic chemotherapy have been prescribed according to local protocol.
- Remember that mitomycin is given only every 6 weeks and vinblastine every 3 weeks. When the first course is prescribed, block out the mitomycin-dose column for even-numbered cycles or otherwise endorse any pharmacy patient record sheet (*see* Appendix 3 for an example), in order to prevent inadvertent administration.

SOURCE MATERIAL

- Nabholtz J-M, Senn HJ, Bezwoda WR *et al.* (1999) Prospective randomised trial of docetaxel versus mitomycin plus vinblastine in patients with metastatic breast cancer progressing despite previous anthracycline-containing chemotherapy. *J Clin Oncol.* **17**: 1413–24.

MVAC (methotrexate, vinblastine, doxorubicin ['Adriamycin'], cisplatin)

USUAL INDICATION

Bladder cancer.

DOSES

Methotrexate 30 mg/m^2 IV on days 1, 15 and 22
Doxorubicin 30 mg/m^2 IV on day 2
Vinblastine 3 mg/m^2 IV on days 2, 15 and 22
Cisplatin 70 mg/m^2 IV on day 2

Note: This is a highly myelosuppressive regimen, and the original investigators recognised that day 15 and day 22 doses may not be possible because of low blood counts (see below).

ADMINISTRATION

Methotrexate

By IV bolus injection.

Doxorubicin and vinblastine

By slow IV injection into the side-arm of a free-running 0.9% sodium chloride drip. *Doxorubicin and vinblastine are powerful vesicants*, and should be administered with appropriate precautions to prevent extravasation. If there is any possibility that extravasation has occurred, contact a senior member of the medical team immediately and follow local guidance on dealing with extravasation incidents.

Cisplatin

As an infusion in 1 L of 0.9% sodium chloride over a period of 3 h, after pre-hydration with 2 L of 0.9% sodium chloride and followed by intensive post-hydration with a further 2 L of intravenous fluid. This may be reduced to 1 L to facilitate outpatient treatment provided that the patient drinks 3 L of fluid in the 24 h after completing intravenous therapy. Cisplatin is nephrotoxic, and hydration is mandatory to dilute the drug as it is excreted via the kidneys, and thus to minimise toxicity. The aim of hydration is to maintain a urine output of 100 mL/h during and for 6–8 h after cisplatin administration. Mannitol is usually also given to ensure that urine output is brisk. Electrolytes are added to compensate for cisplatin-induced electrolyte wasting.

ANTI-EMETICS

Anti-emetics appropriate to chemotherapy with high emetogenic potential (follow local policy) on day 2 and appropriate to chemotherapy with low emetogenic potential (follow local policy) on days 1, 15 and 22.

CYCLE LENGTH

28 days.

NUMBER OF CYCLES

Usually 6.

SIDE-EFFECTS

Nephrotoxicity (dose limiting due to cisplatin), bone-marrow suppression (all blood components are affected), alopecia (extensive), nausea and vomiting (may be very severe), sensory, motor and occasionally autonomic neuropathy (sometimes irreversible and due to cisplatin and vinblastine) including significant potential for ototoxicity, mucositis, dilated cardiomyopathy (due to doxorubicin, especially if the cumulative dose exceeds $450 \, \text{mg/m}^2$). Rarely, methotrexate-induced pneumonitis.

BLOOD NADIR

With this protocol, repeated chemotherapy is given before the nadir from previous courses is reached. Therefore there is no clear-cut nadir, but a pattern of chronic myelosuppression.

TTOS REQUIRED

- Anti-emetics appropriate to highly emetogenic chemotherapy according to protocol for day 2/3 of each cycle, and appropriate to weakly emetogenic regimen for days 1, 15 and 22.
- Folinic acid (calcium folinate/calcium leucovorin) 'rescue' is not routinely required at the doses of methotrexate used in MVAC. If it is used because of unexpected toxicity on previous courses or because the patient has a 'third-space' fluid collection or renal impairment, a reasonable dose is 15 mg by mouth 6-hourly for 6–12 doses *starting 24 h after methotrexate*. Starting folinic acid earlier negates the effects of the methotrexate.

NOTES FOR PRESCRIBERS

At the time of prescribing the first course

- Patients over 60 years of age or with a history of heart disease must have had an echocardiogram or MUGA scan prior to treatment to ensure that there is adequate left ventricular function. If they have received previous treatment with doxorubicin and the planned treatment course will take their cumulative doxorubicin dose above 450 mg/m^2, discuss the treatment plan with a senior member of the medical team. Once this cumulative dose is exceeded, the risk of drug-induced cardiac damage increases sharply. Prior treatment with other anthracyclines (epirubicin, daunorubicin, idarubicin, aclarubicin) should also be considered.
- Prior to treatment, hair loss should be discussed with the patient. Scalp cooling is unlikely to be completely effective as it provides little protection against cisplatin- or vinblastine-induced hair loss, and it should only be used with doxorubicin. If appropriate, liaise with the nursing staff with regard to referral to a wig-fitter at the start of treatment, before alopecia is evident.

At the time of prescribing each course

- Make sure it is clearly understood where the patient is in their treatment course. Day 1 and 2 treatment differs from that on days 15 and 22. In addition, treatment on days 15 and 22 should not be delayed if the blood count is too low – it should be omitted altogether. The aim is to give day 1 treatment every 28 days, even if day 15 and/or day 22 drugs have been omitted.
- Renal function should be formally assessed at the start of treatment. Ideally this should be done by an EDTA clearance test, but estimation by the Cockcroft–Gault equation from the serum creatinine levels is acceptable if the patient has a stable creatinine concentration and no confounding factors (e.g. catabolic states):

CrCl (mL/min)

$$= \frac{1.04 \text{ (females) or } 1.23 \text{ (males)} \times (140 - \text{age in years}) \times \text{weight in kg}}{\text{serum creatinine concentration (μmol/L)}}.$$

On subsequent cycles, the renal function should be reassessed on day 1 (i.e. prior to cisplatin prescribing).

Cisplatin doses *should normally be reduced* if the creatinine clearance drops below 60 mL/min. In addition, consideration should be given to reducing the methotrexate doses if the CrCl falls below 80 mL/min (*see* Appendix 2 for further advice). Doxorubicin doses also need reduction in cases of severe renal impairment, although in such cases MVAC is unlikely to be a treatment option because of the problems with administering cisplatin and methotrexate.

- Check the LFTs. Doses of doxorubicin, vinblastine and methotrexate should all be reviewed in cases of significant hepatic impairment (*see* Appendix 1 for advice).
- If the patient has a 'third-space' fluid collection (ascites, effusion or extensive oedema), the elimination of methotrexate may be prolonged, enhancing its toxicity. Consider folinic acid rescue in such cases (discuss this with an experienced

prescriber). If folinic acid is to be used, make sure it is charted to start 24 h after methotrexate. If it is given any earlier it will negate the effect of methotrexate as well as its toxicity.

- Check serum electrolytes for cisplatin-induced wasting, especially of magnesium, calcium and potassium. Additional supplementation may be required.
- Ensure that anti-emetics appropriate to highly emetogenic chemotherapy have been prescribed on day 2 and anti-emetics appropriate to weakly emetogenic treatment on days 1, 15 and 22. Prescribing should be in accordance with local policy.
- Seek further advice if the patient reports symptoms indicative of neurotoxicity (parasthesias, difficulty with motor control) or ototoxicity (tinnitus, deafness).
- Check the FBC prior to giving the go-ahead for chemotherapy. On day 1, seek advice if the neutrophil count is $<1.5 \times 10^9/L$ or the platelet count is $<100 \times 10^9/L$. On days 15 and 22 doses should normally be omitted if the WBC is $<2.5 \times 10^9/L$ or the platelet count is $<100 \times 10^9/L$, as in the major trial of this regimen administered without G-CSF.[1] G-CSF has been shown to allow closer adherence to the intended dosage schedule. However, haematopoietic growth factor treatment should not be instituted without consulting local policies on growth factor use. In particular, where this regimen is being used with palliative intent, a degree of dose reduction may be appropriate as an alternative to growth factor support.
- If administering doxorubicin and vinblastine, *see* Administration section above for notes on their vesicant nature.
- Any unexplained breathlessness should be investigated, as it may indicate the onset of methotrexate-induced pneumonitis.

On the day after each cisplatin dose (if the patient is an inpatient)

- Monitor the fluid balance/body weight. If the patient has gained more than 1.5 L/kg since the start of hydration, extra diuresis should be considered (e.g furosemide 20 mg by mouth).

NOTES FOR NURSES

- Discuss hair loss with the patient and refer them to a wig-fitter at the start of treatment, before alopecia is a problem, if this is appropriate. Scalp cooling may reduce hair loss caused by doxorubicin, but is unlikely to have much impact on the lesser degrees of hair loss induced by the other drugs in this regimen. The technique, if adopted, should only be used with doxorubicin.
- If you are administering doxorubicin or vinblastine, *see* Administration section above for notes on their vesicant nature.
- The aim of hydration is to ensure an average urine output of 100 mL/h or more during and for 6–8 h after cisplatin administration. Any patient who is being treated as an inpatient should be on a fluid-balance chart and daily weights should

---

[1] Sternberg CN, Yagoda A, Scherr HI *et al.* (1989) Methotrexate, vinblastine, doxorubicin and cisplatin for advanced transitional-cell carcinoma of the urothelium. *Cancer.* **64**: 2448–58.

be recorded. Contact the prescriber if the patient's urine output is inadequate or their body weight increases by 1.5 kg from baseline.

For outpatients, efforts should be made to ensure that urine output is adequate (e.g. by checking that the patient has passed 500 mL of urine between the start of IV hydration and the beginning of cisplatin infusion).

Outpatients should also be encouraged to drink 3 L of fluid in the 24 h following each period of IV hydration, and to contact the hospital if this is impossible because of nausea/vomiting or other problems.

- The gap between day 1 methotrexate and day 2 drugs is important. Make sure that a full day has passed between methotrexate administration and the start of day 2 treatment.
- If the patient is prescribed folinic acid (calcium folinate/calcium leucovorin), the latter should be prescribed to start 24 h after methotrexate. If it is given any earlier it will negate the effect of methotrexate as well as its toxicity. If it is charted to start 24 h after methotrexate, *do not* give it before. If the start time is not specified, check with the prescriber.

NOTES FOR PHARMACISTS

- Make sure that you know where the patient is in their treatment course. Pharmacy patient records will facilitate this (*see* Appendix 3 for an example). Day 1 and 2 treatment is different to that on days 15 and 22. In addition, treatment on days 15 and 22 should not be delayed if the blood count is too low – it is omitted altogether. The aim is to give day 1 treatment every 28 days, even if day 15 and/or day 22 drugs have been omitted.
- At the start of treatment, check the pharmacy and patient records to see whether the patient has received previous anthracyclines. If they have received prior treatment with doxorubicin, and the planned treatment course will take their cumulative doxorubicin dose above 450 mg/m^2, discuss the treatment plan with the prescriber. Once this cumulative dose is exceeded, the risk of drug-induced cardiac damage increases sharply. Previous treatment with other anthracyclines (epirubicin, daunorubicin, idarubicin, aclarubicin) should also be considered. For previously treated patients, any pharmacy patient record should be annotated to alert future pharmacists and prescribers to the cumulative dose received.
- Check that the FBC has been determined and is within acceptable limits before issuing the chemotherapy. On day 1, seek advice if the neutrophil count is $<1.5 \times 10^9$/L or the platelet count is $<100 \times 10^9$/L. Day 15 and day 22 doses should be omitted if the WBC is $<2.5 \times 10^9$/L or the platelet count is $<100 \times 10^9$/L. These doses are omitted completely, and day 1 of the next treatment cycle is given on time, provided that the blood count has recovered sufficiently. G-CSF has been shown to allow closer adherence to the intended dosage schedule. However, treatment with haematopoietic growth factors should not be instituted without consulting the local haematopoietic growth factor policy. In particular, where this regimen is being used with palliative intent, a degree of dose reduction may be appropriate.
- Check that the renal function has been measured or calculated at the start of treatment. Record the CrCl and the corresponding creatinine concentration on any patient pharmacy record sheet, and recalculate the CrCl if the creatinine

concentration changes. A cisplatin dose reduction is essential if the CrCl drops below 60 mL/min. A methotrexate dose reduction should also be considered if the CrCl drops below 80 mL/min. In addition, doxorubicin requires a dose reduction, but only at levels of renal impairment that are likely to preclude the use of MVAC (*see* Appendix 2 for further guidance).

- Check the LFTs. Doses of doxorubicin, vinblastine and methotrexate should all be reviewed in cases of significant hepatic impairment (*see* Appendix 1 for advice).

- Ensure that, on day 2, anti-emetics appropriate to highly emetogenic chemotherapy have been prescribed according to local anti-emetic policy. For day 1, 15 and 22 methotrexate and vinblastine, minimal anti-emetics are required. Any gastrointestinal symptoms are quite likely to be at least in part psychogenic (especially if patients have been nauseated on previous cisplatin treatment) and may be more amenable to lorazepam/haloperidol than to other anti-emetics.

- If the patient is an inpatient, when you are visiting the ward the day after cisplatin chemotherapy check that the individual has not gained more than 1.5 L/kg since the start of hydration. If they have, discuss additional diuresis (e.g. furosemide 20 mg by mouth) with the prescriber (if this measure has not already been instituted).

- Folinic acid (calcium folinate/calcium leucovorin) rescue is not routinely required. However, when it is used (e.g. in patients with unexpected toxicity on a previous course or 'third-space' fluid collection), it should be prescribed to start 24 h after methotrexate. Starting folinic acid any earlier will negate the effect of methotrexate as well as its toxicity. If it is charted to start 24 h after methotrexate, block out any earlier spaces on the drug chart to prevent it being given before, endorse any TTO clearly and/or add this instruction to the bottle label. If the start time is not specified, and the administration time for methotrexate is unclear, check with the prescriber. If a patient *does* receive folinic acid with their MVAC, make a note of this (with the reason) on their pharmacy record sheet, to ensure that they do not miss out on future courses, if it is still required.

- 'Third-space' fluid collections (ascites, effusions, gross oedema) significantly prolong the half-life of methotrexate, enhancing its toxicity. If it is known that a patient has such a fluid collection, ask the prescriber whether folinic acid rescue is required (*see* TTO section above for further details).

SOURCE MATERIAL

- Gabrilove JL, Jakubowski A, Scherr H *et al.* (1988) Effect of granulocyte-colony-stimulating factor on neutropenia and associated morbidity due to chemotherapy for transitional-cell carcinoma of the urothelium. *NEJM.* **318**: 1414–22.
- Sternberg CN, Yagoda A, Scherr HI *et al.* (1989) Methotrexate, vinblastine, doxorubicin and cisplatin for advanced transitional-cell carcinoma of the urothelium. *Cancer.* **64**: 2448–58.

MVP (mitomycin, vinblastine, cisplatin)

USUAL INDICATION

Non-small-cell lung cancer (NSCLC).

DOSES

Mitomycin 8 mg/m^2 IV on day 1 *Alternate courses only*
Vinblastine 6 mg/m^2 IV (maximum 10 mg) on day 1
Cisplatin 50 mg/m^2 IV on day 1

ADMINISTRATION

Mitomycin and vinblastine

By slow IV injection into the side-arm of a free-running 0.9% sodium chloride drip. *Mitomycin and vinblastine are powerful vesicants,* and should be administered with appropriate precautions to prevent extravasation. If there is any possibility that extravasation has occurred, contact a senior member of the medical team immediately and follow local guidance on dealing with extravasation incidents.

CISPLATIN

As an infusion in 1 L of 0.9% sodium chloride over 2 h, after pre-hydration with 1.5 L of 0.9% sodium chloride and followed by post-hydration with 1 L of 0.9% sodium chloride. Cisplatin is nephrotoxic, and hydration is mandatory to dilute the drug as it is excreted via the kidneys, and thus minimise toxicity. The aim of hydration is to maintain a urine output of 100 mL/h during and for 6–8 h after cisplatin administration. Electrolytes are added to compensate for cisplatin-induced electrolyte wasting.

ANTI-EMETICS

High emetogenic potential (see local policy).

CYCLE LENGTH

21 days (but mitomycin is given on cycles 1, 2, 4 and 6 only).

NUMBER OF CYCLES

Usually 6.

SIDE-EFFECTS

Bone-marrow suppression (all blood components are affected), alopecia (usually moderate), nephrotoxicity, vomiting (may be very severe), sensory and motor neuropathy (sometimes irreversible due to cisplatin and vinblastine) including significant potential for ototoxicity, mucositis and haemolytic uraemic syndrome secondary to mitomycin.

BLOOD NADIR

Unpredictable because of the prolonged myelosuppression produced by mitomycin.

TTOS REQUIRED

- Anti-emetics appropriate to highly emetogenic chemotherapy (see local protocol).

NOTES FOR PRESCRIBERS

At the time of prescribing each course

- Check the FBC prior to giving the go-ahead for chemotherapy. Seek advice if the neutrophil count is $<1.5 \times 10^9$/L or the platelet count is $<100 \times 10^9$/L at the time of treatment.
- Make sure it is clearly understood which course of treatment the patient is on. Mitomycin is only given on alternate courses.
- Question the patient about any symptoms of neuropathy (e.g. parasthesias, tinnitus, constipation, jaw pain, diarrhoea or difficulty with fine motor control), and seek advice if they report such symptoms.
- Cisplatin is highly nephrotoxic, as (to a lesser degree) is mitomycin. Both drugs are renally excreted. Renal function should be formally assessed at the start of treatment. Ideally this should be done by an EDTA clearance test, but estimation from the serum creatinine level using the Cockcroft–Gault equation is acceptable if the patient has a stable creatinine concentration and no confounding factors (e.g. catabolic states):

CrCl (mL/min)

$$= \frac{1.04 \text{ (females) or } 1.23 \text{ (males)} \times (140 - \text{age in years}) \times \text{weight in kg}}{\text{serum creatinine concentration } (\mu\text{mol/L})}.$$

On subsequent cycles the renal function should be reassessed.

Doses of cisplatin and mitomycin *should be reduced* if the creatinine clearance drops below 60 mL/min (*see* Appendix 2 for further advice).

- Check serum electrolytes for cisplatin-induced wasting, especially of magnesium, calcium and potassium. Additional supplementation may be required.
- Check the LFTs. Doses of vinblastine and possibly mitomycin should be reduced in cases of significant hepatic impairment (*see* Appendix 1 for further advice).
- Prescribe anti-emetics appropriate to chemotherapy with a highly emetogenic regimen, according to local policy.
- Liaise with the nurses who are looking after the patient. If the latter is being treated as an inpatient, they should have a fluid-balance chart and daily weights should be recorded. If they are being treated as an outpatient, they should be advised to drink at least 3 L of fluid over the following 24 h, and to contact the hospital if vomiting prevents them from consuming this amount of fluid.
- If administering the drugs, *see* Administration section above for notes on the vesicant nature of mitomycin and vinblastine.

On the day after each dose of cisplatin

- For inpatients, check the fluid balance. If the patient has gained 1.5 L/kg or more since the start of hydration, extra diuresis will be required (e.g. furosemide 20–40 mg by mouth).

NOTES FOR NURSES

- The aim of hydration is to ensure an average urine output of 100 mL/h or more during and for 6–8 h after cisplatin administration. Any patient who is being treated as an inpatient should be on a fluid-balance chart, and daily weights should be recorded. Contact the prescriber if the patient's urine output is inadequate or their body weight increases by 1.5 kg from baseline.

  For outpatients, efforts should be made to ensure that urine output is adequate (e.g. by checking that the patient has passed 500 mL of urine between the start of IV hydration and the beginning of cisplatin infusion).

  Outpatients should also be encouraged to drink 3 L of fluid in the 24 h following each period of IV hydration, and to contact the hospital if this is impossible because of nausea/vomiting or other problems.
- If administering the drugs, *see* Administration section above for notes on the vesicant nature of mitomycin and vinblastine.

NOTES FOR PHARMACISTS

- Check that the FBC has been determined and is within acceptable limits before issuing the chemotherapy.
- Check the renal function at the start of treatment. If this has not been formally measured, calculate the CrCl from the serum creatinine concentration using the Cockroft–Gault equation. Record the CrCl and the corresponding creatinine

concentration on any pharmacy patient record (*see* Appendix 3 for an example). On subsequent courses, recalculate the CrCl if the serum creatinine concentration increases significantly. Cisplatin and to a lesser extent mitomycin are nephrotoxic, and both drugs are renally excreted. A reduction in cisplatin and mitomycin doses should be considered if the CrCl falls below 60 mL/min (*see* Appendix 2 for further guidance).

- Check the LFTs. Doses of vinblastine and possibly mitomycin should be reduced in cases of significant hepatic impairment (*see* Appendix 1 for further advice).
- Check that anti-emetics appropriate to highly emetogenic chemotherapy have been prescribed according to the local anti-emetic protocol.
- Remember that mitomycin is given on alternate cycles only. When the first course is prescribed, block out the mitomycin dose column for cycles 3 and 5 on any pharmacy patient record sheet to prevent inadvertent administration.
- When you are visiting the ward, check that patients who are receiving MVP as inpatients are not in excessive positive fluid balance (i.e. have not gained more than 1.5 L/kg since the start of hydration). Ensure that the urine output is maintained at a level above 100 mL/h during and for 6–8 h after cisplatin infusion. If there is excessive fluid retention, consult with the medical team about the possibility of extra diuretics being prescribed (if this measure has not already been instituted) (e.g. furosemide 20–40 mg by mouth).

SOURCE MATERIAL

- Ellis PA, Smith IE, Hardy JR *et al.* (1995) Symptom relief with MVP (mitomycin C, vinblastine and cisplatin) chemotherapy in advanced non-small-cell lung cancer. *Br J Cancer.* **71**: 366–70.

NP (vinorelbine [Navelbine®] plus cisplatin)

USUAL INDICATION

First-line treatment of non-small-cell lung cancer.

DOSES

Vinorelbine 30 mg/m^2 (maximum 60 mg) IV on days 1 and 8
Cisplatin 80 mg/m^2 by IV infusion on day 1

Note: There are many variations on this regimen. These doses represent common UK practice.

ADMINISTRATION

Day 1

After pre-hydration with 1 L of 0.9% sodium chloride (containing 20 mmol of potassium chloride), vinorelbine is administered as a slow IV bolus diluted to 20 mL with 0.9% sodium chloride and injected into a free-running saline drip. Vinorelbine should be flushed in with 250 mL of 0.9% sodium chloride.

Cisplatin is then administered as an IV infusion in 1 L of 0.9% sodium chloride (containing 20 mmol of potassium chloride) over a period of 2 h, followed by a minimum of a further 1 L of 0.9% sodium chloride (with 20 mmol of potassium chloride) as post-hydration. The patient should be instructed to drink a further 3 L of fluid in the 24 h following the end of IV hydration. The aim of hydration is to maintain a urine output of 100 mL/h during and for 6–8 h after cisplatin administration.

Day 8

Vinorelbine is administered as a slow IV bolus diluted to 20 mL with 0.9% sodium chloride and injected into a free-running saline drip. It should then be flushed in with 250 mL of 0.9% sodium chloride.

Vinorelbine is a powerful vesicant, and should be administered with appropriate precautions to prevent extravasation. If there is any possibility that extravasation has occurred, contact a senior member of the medical team immediately and follow local guidance on dealing with extravasation incidents.

ANTI-EMETICS

Day 1

High emetogenic potential (see local policy).

Day 8

Low emetogenic potential (see local policy).

CYCLE LENGTH

21 days.

NUMBER OF CYCLES

Usually 6.

SIDE-EFFECTS

Nephrotoxicity (dose limiting), bone-marrow suppression (all blood components are affected, but seldom dose limiting), alopecia (rarely extensive), nausea and vomiting (may be very severe), sensory motor and autonomic neuropathy (sometimes irreversible) including significant potential for ototoxicity and constipation (due to both vinorelbine and cisplatin), mucositis (not usually serious), phlebitis (due to vinorelbine).

BLOOD NADIR

This is difficult to predict. Because of the administration of vinorelbine on days 1 and 8, a clear nadir may not emerge.

TTOS REQUIRED

- Anti-emetics appropriate to highly emetogenic chemotherapy (day 1) and weakly emetogenic chemotherapy (day 8).

NOTES FOR PRESCRIBERS

Before each course

- Be sure that it is clearly understood what dosage schedule is being used. Schedules other than that described above have been used.
- No single dose of vinorelbine should exceed 60 mg.

- Check the FBC prior to giving the go-ahead for chemotherapy. Seek advice if the neutrophil count is $<2.0 \times 10^9$/L or the platelet count is $<75 \times 10^9$/L. In a study by Depierre et al.[1] of a similar combination of vinorelbine and cisplatin to that described here (but with additional vinorelbine administered on day 15), treatment was delayed for 7 days if the neutrophil count was $<1.0 \times 10^9$/L or the platelet count was $<75 \times 10^9$/L, and full doses were administered if the neutrophil count was $>1.5 \times 10^9$/L and the platelet count was $>100 \times 10^9$/L. In patients with intermediate blood counts, vinorelbine doses were reduced by 50%. The manufacturer of vinorelbine recommends withholding treatment until counts return to these levels.
- If administering vinorelbine, see Administration section above for notes about its vesicant properties. However, extravasation should be distinguished from phlebitis tracking along the vein used for injection. The latter can be minimised by liberal flushing of the vein during and after injection.
- Renal function should be formally assessed at the start of treatment. Ideally this should be done by an EDTA clearance test, but estimation from the serum creatinine level using the Cockcroft–Gault equation is acceptable if the patient has a stable serum creatinine concentration and no confounding factors (e.g. catabolic states):

CrCl (mL/min)

$$= \frac{1.04 \text{ (females) or } 1.23 \text{ (males)} \times (140 - \text{age in years}) \times \text{weight in kg}}{\text{serum creatinine concentration } (\mu\text{mol/L})}.$$

On subsequent cycles the renal function should be reassessed.

Doses of cisplatin should normally be reduced if the creatinine clearance drops below 60 mL/min. Consideration should also be given to withholding vinorelbine in patients with a significantly elevated serum creatinine concentration (see Appendix 2 for further advice).

- Check the serum electrolytes for cisplatin-induced wasting, especially of magnesium, calcium and potassium. Additional supplementation may be required.
- Check the LFTs at the time of prescribing. A vinorelbine dose reduction should be considered in cases of significant hepatic impairment or very extensive metastatic liver disease (see Appendix 1 for further advice).
- Prescribe anti-emetics appropriate to highly emetogenic chemotherapy (day 1) and weakly emetogenic chemotherapy (day 8) according to local policy.
- Seek further advice if the patient reports symptoms indicative of neurotoxicity (parasthesias, difficulty with motor control, constipation, jaw pain) or ototoxicity (tinnitus, deafness).

On the day after each cisplatin dose

- For patients who are receiving cisplatin on an inpatient basis, check the fluid balance/body weight. In general, if the patient has gained 1.5 L/kg or more since starting hydration, extra diuresis will be required (e.g. furosemide 20–40 mg by mouth).

---

[1] Depierre A, Chastang C, Quoix E et al. (1994) Vinorelbine versus vinorelbine plus cisplatin in advanced non-small-cell lung cancer: a randomized trial. Ann Oncol. **5**: 37–42.

NOTES FOR NURSES

- The aim of hydration is to ensure an average urine output of 100 mL/h or more during and for 6–8 h after cisplatin administration. Any patient who is being treated as an inpatient should be on a fluid-balance chart, and daily weights should be recorded. Contact the prescriber if the patient's urine output is inadequate or their body weight increases by 1.5 kg or more from baseline.

  For outpatients, efforts should be made to ensure that urine output is adequate (e.g. by checking that the patient has passed 500 mL of urine between the start of IV hydration and the beginning of cisplatin infusion).

  Outpatients should also be encouraged to drink 3 L of fluid in the 24 h following each period of IV hydration, and to contact the hospital if this is impossible because of nausea/vomiting or other problems.

- If administering vinorelbine, *see* Administration section above for notes about its vesicant properties. However, extravasation should be distinguished from phlebitis tracking along the vein used for injection. The latter can be minimised by liberal flushing of the vein during and after injection.

NOTES FOR PHARMACISTS

Day of prescribing

- Be sure that it is clearly understood what dosage schedule is being used. Schedules other than that described above have been used.
- No single dose of vinorelbine should exceed 60 mg.
- Check that the FBC has been determined and is within acceptable limits before issuing the chemotherapy. The manufacturer of vinorelbine recommends withholding the drug if the neutrophil count is $<2.0 \times 10^9/L$ or the platelet count is $<75 \times 10^9/L$.
- Check that the renal function has been measured/calculated at the start of treatment. Record the CrCl and the corresponding creatinine concentration in any pharmacy patient record (*see* Appendix 3 for an example), and recalculate the CrCl if the creatinine concentration changes. Doses of cisplatin *should normally be reduced* if the creatinine clearance drops below 60 mL/min. Consideration should also be given to withholding vinorelbine in patients with a significantly elevated serum creatine concentration (*see* Appendix 2 for further advice).
- Check the LFTs. A vinorelbine dose reduction should be considered in cases of significant hepatic impairment or very extensive metastatic liver disease (*see* Appendix 1 for further advice).
- Check that anti-emetics appropriate to highly emetogenic chemotherapy (day 1) and weakly emetogenic chemotherapy (day 8) have been prescribed according to local protocol.

The day after cisplatin chemotherapy

- When you are visiting the ward, check that any inpatient who is receiving cisplatin has not gained more than 1.5 L/kg since the start of treatment. If they have, discuss additional diuresis with the prescriber (e.g. furosemide 20–40 mg by mouth) (if this measure has not already been instituted).

SOURCE MATERIAL

Many different combinations of cisplatin and vinorelbine have been used, and virtually no two research groups have used the same one. The regimen described in this chapter is widely used in the UK and is currently being used in the LU22 and Big Lung trials. However, to our knowledge it has not formed the basis of any published paper. The earliest use of this combination was probably in the study by Berthaud et al. (see below). The closest to that described in this chapter was probably that reported by Depierre et al. (see below), and the study with the greatest clinical impact was probably that by Le Chevalier et al. (see below).

- Berthaud P, Le Chevalier T, Ruffie P et al. (1992) Phase I–II study of vinorelbine (Navelbine) plus cisplatin in advanced non-small-cell lung cancer. *Eur J Cancer.* **28A**: 1863–5.
- Depierre A, Chastang C, Quoix E et al. (1994) Vinorelbine versus vinorelbine plus cisplatin in advanced non-small-cell lung cancer: a randomized trial. *Ann Oncol.* **5**: 37–42.
- Le Chevalier T, Brisgand D, Douillard JY et al. (1994) Randomized study of vinorelbine and cisplatin versus vindesine and cisplatin versus vinorelbine alone in advanced non-small cell lung cancer: results of a European multicenter trial including 612 patients. *J Clin Oncol.* **12**: 360–7.

Paclitaxel (Taxol®) (single-agent)

USUAL INDICATION

Platinum (carboplatin, cisplatin)-resistant ovarian cancer and anthracycline (epirubicin, doxorubicin)-resistant breast cancer.

DOSES

175 mg/m^2 IV every 21 days

or

80–100 mg/m^2 IV every 7 days

Note: Although weekly treatment is becoming increasingly widely used, and may possibly be more effective than 3-weekly treatment, it is outside the current Marketing Authorisation for the drug.

ADMINISTRATION

3-weekly treatment

By IV infusion in 5% dextrose or 0.9% sodium chloride over a period of 3 h using a PVC-free administration system with a 0.22-μm in-line filter after *mandatory* premedication with steroids and H$_1$- and H$_2$-antihistamines.

The following combination is widely used.

Dexamethasone 20 mg by slow IV injection immediately prior to chemotherapy (the UK package insert currently recommends a regimen with oral steroids, but this is rather inconvenient and requires good patient compliance. Intravenous steroid regimens are now widely used, and show good evidence of safety and efficacy).

Ranitidine 50 mg by slow IV injection immediately prior to chemotherapy.

Chlorpheniramine 10 mg IV immediately prior to chemotherapy.

Weekly treatment

By IV infusion over a period of 1 h in 5% dextrose or 0.9% sodium chloride using a PVC-free administration system with a 0.22-μm in-line filter. On the first cycle, premedication should be as described for 3-weekly administration. In the case of patients who show no signs of hypersensitivity on the first course, consideration may be given to reducing or withdrawing premedication on subsequent courses.

This has been investigated with weekly treatment because of the problems associated with high cumulative steroid doses, and several centres have found it to be achievable.

ANTI-EMETICS

Low emetogenic potential (see local policy).

CYCLE LENGTH

21 or 7 days.

NUMBER OF CYCLES

Usually 6 (3-weekly) or 18 (weekly).

SIDE-EFFECTS

Bone-marrow suppression (mainly neutropenia), total alopecia, nausea and vomiting, myalgia, sensory neuropathy, hypersensitivity, mucositis.

BLOOD NADIR

Day 10 for 3-weekly treatment; no clear-cut nadir for weekly treatment.

TTOS REQUIRED

- Anti-emetics appropriate to weakly emetogenic chemotherapy, according to local policy.
- If local policy requires oral dexamethasone as premedication, ensure that it is prescribed for the next course of chemotherapy. Prescriptions should direct the patient to 'Take 20 mg (10 × 2 mg tablets) 12 h and 6 h before the next paclitaxel (Taxol®) treatment'.

NOTES FOR PRESCRIBERS

- Make sure that it is clearly understood whether the patient is due to receive weekly or 3-weekly paclitaxel.
- Check the FBC prior to giving the go-ahead for chemotherapy. Seek further advice if the neutrophil count is $<1.5 \times 10^9$/L or the platelet count is $<100 \times 10^9$/L. The manufacturer of the drug states that paclitaxel is contraindicated in patients with blood counts below these levels. They also recommend dose reductions in

patients who experienced profound neutropenia on previous courses (neutrophil count $<0.5 \times 10^9$/L for 7 days or longer).

- Check the LFTs before starting treatment. Consideration should be given to a dose reduction if the bilirubin level is more than 1.25 times the normal value (*see* Appendix 1 for further guidance).
- Question the patient about abnormal sensations, as these may indicate neuropathy requiring dose modification. Seek advice from an experienced prescriber if such symptoms are reported.
- Make sure that the patient has been prescribed appropriate premedication to prevent hypersensitivity reactions (unless a decision has been made to stop such treatment in patients who have received at least one cycle of weekly paclitaxel without experiencing problems).

NOTES FOR NURSES

- Make sure that the patient has been prescribed and has received appropriate premedication to prevent hypersensitivity reactions (unless a documented decision has been made to stop such treatment in patients who have received at least one cycle of weekly paclitaxel without experiencing problems)
- Patients should be closely observed during the first few minutes of drug infusion, especially on the first cycle. Serious hypersensitivity reactions can occur, usually on the first cycle.
- Inform the prescriber if the patient reports any abnormal sensations, as these may be indicative of drug-induced neuropathy.
- Try not to agitate bags or bottles of paclitaxel infusion too much, as this causes foaming which can trigger 'air-in-line' alarms on infusion pumps.

NOTES FOR PHARMACISTS

- Make sure it is clearly understood whether the patient is due to receive weekly or 3-weekly paclitaxel.
- Check that the FBC has been determined and is within acceptable limits before issuing the chemotherapy.
- Check the LFTs before starting treatment. Consideration should be given to a dose reduction if the bilirubin level is more than 1.25 times the normal value (*see* Appendix 1 for further guidance).
- Make sure that appropriate premedications have been prescribed (unless a documented decision has been made to stop such treatment in patients who have received at least one cycle of weekly paclitaxel without experiencing problems).
- If local policy requires oral dexamethasone as premedication, ensure that it is prescribed for the next course of chemotherapy. Prescriptions should direct the patient to 'Take 20 mg (10 × 2 mg tablets) 12 h and 6 h before the next paclitaxel (Taxol®) treatment'.
- Try not to agitate bags or bottles of paclitaxel infusion too much, as this causes foaming which can trigger 'air-in-line' alarms on infusion pumps.
- Use PVC-free bags/glass bottles for all paclitaxel infusions.

SOURCE MATERIAL

3-weekly paclitaxel

- Eisenhauer EA, ten Bokkel Huinink WW, Sweneton KD *et al.* (1994) European–Canadian randomized trial of paclitaxel in relapsed ovarian cancer: high-dose versus low-dose and long versus short infusion. *J Clin Oncol.* **12**: 2654–66.
- Peretz T, Sulkes A, Chollet P *et al.* (1995) A multicenter, randomized study of two schedules of paclitaxel (PTX) in patients with advanced breast cancer (ABC). *Eur J Cancer.* **31A (Supplement 5)**: S75.

Weekly paclitaxel

- Seidman AD, Hudis CA, Albanel J *et al.* (1998) Dose-dense therapy with weekly 1-hour paclitaxel infusions in the treatment of metastatic breast cancer. *J Clin Oncol.* **16**: 3353–61.
- Perez EA, Irwin DH, Patel R *et al.* (1999) A large phase II trial of paclitaxel administered as a weekly one-hour infusion in patients with metastatic breast cancer. *Proc Am Soc Clin Oncol.* **18**: 126 (abstract).

IV premedication regimens

- Ellerton JA and Rowan N (1996) Single-dose i.v. dexamethasone one hour before infusion as pre-treatment for paclitaxel. *Proc Am Soc Clin Oncol.* **15**: 548 (abstract).

Paclitaxel (Taxol®) plus trastuzumab (Herceptin®)

USUAL INDICATION

Metastatic breast cancer over-expressing HER2 at the 3+ level by immunohisto-chemistry (IHC) or exhibiting gene amplification by fluorescence *in situ* hybridisation (FISH) testing.

DOSES

Paclitaxel 175 mg/m^2 IV on day 2 of the first cycle, then every 21 days on the same day as trastuzumab

or

90 mg/m^2 IV on day 2 of the first cycle, then every 7 days on the same day as trastuzumab (note that although weekly treatment is becoming increasingly widely used, and may possibly be more effective than 3-weekly treatment, it is outside the current Marketing Authorisation for the drug)

Trastuzumab* 4 mg/kg IV on day 1 of the first cycle, then 2 mg/kg IV once weekly thereafter

ADMINISTRATION

3-weekly treatment

Trastuzumab is administered first as an IV infusion in 250 mL of 0.9% sodium chloride (it is incompatible with dextrose) over a period of 90 min for the first infusion, or 30 min for subsequent courses.

Trastuzumab is followed by paclitaxel administered by IV infusion in 5% dextrose or 0.9% sodium chloride over a period of 3 h using a PVC-free administration system with a 0.22-μm in-line filter after *mandatory* premedication with steroids and H$_1$- and H$_2$-antihistamines.

---

* A recent study by Verma *et al.* with trastuzumab has suggested that an 8 mg/kg loading dose followed by 6 mg/kg IV every 3 weeks is as effective and more convenient than the weekly schedule, although this dosage schedule is outside the product's current Marketing Authorisation in the UK. Verma S, Leyland-Jones B, Ayoub J-P *et al.* (2001) Efficacy and safety of three-weekly Herceptin with paclitaxel in women with HER2-positive metastatic breast cancer: preliminary results of a phase II trial. *Eur J Cancer.* **37** (**Supplement 6**): S146.

The following combination is convenient and widely used.

Dexamethasone 20 mg by slow IV injection immediately prior to chemotherapy (the package literature supplied with paclitaxel suggests the use of oral steroids, but this is inconvenient and also requires good patient compliance).

Ranitidine 50 mg by slow IV injection immediately prior to chemotherapy.

Chlorpheniramine 10 mg IV immediately prior to chemotherapy.

The manufacturer of trastuzumab recommends that the patient should be kept under observation for 6 h from the start of the first infusion and 2 h from the start of subsequent infusions.

Weekly treatment

Trastuzumab is administered first as an IV infusion in 250 mL of 0.9% sodium chloride (it is incompatible with dextrose) over a period of 90 min for the first infusion, or 30 min for subsequent courses.

Paclitaxel is then administered as an IV infusion over a period of 1 h in 5% dextrose or 0.9% sodium chloride using a PVC-free administration system with a 0.22-μm in-line filter. On the first cycle, paclitaxel premedication should be as described for 3-weekly administration. For patients who show no signs of hypersensitivity on the first course, consideration may be given to reducing or withdrawing premedication on subsequent courses. This has been investigated with weekly treatment because of the problems with high cumulative steroid doses, and several centres have found this approach to be feasible.

The manufacturer of trastuzumab recommends that the patient should be kept under observation for 6 h from the start of the first infusion and 2 h from the start of subsequent infusions.

ANTI-EMETICS

Days with paclitaxel treatment

Low emetogenic potential (see local policy).

Days with trastuzumab treatment alone

Minimal emetogenic potential; no routine anti-emesis is required.

CYCLE LENGTH

21 or 7 days.

NUMBER OF CYCLES

Usually 6 (3-weekly) or 18 (weekly) cycles of combined therapy, followed by continuation of weekly trastuzumab as a single agent in patients who show a good response. Trastuzumab may be continued until disease progression.

SIDE-EFFECTS

As a consequence of paclitaxel

Bone-marrow suppression (mainly neutropenia), total alopecia, nausea and vomiting, myalgia, sensory neuropathy, hypersensitivity, mucositis.

As a consequence of trastuzumab

Infusion reactions, including dyspnoea, hypotension, wheezing, bronchospasm, tachycardia, reduced oxygen saturation, anaphylaxis, respiratory distress, urticaria and angioedema. Infusion reactions are usually mild to moderate in intensity, and most such reactions occur within 2.5 h of starting the first infusion. Rarely they are severe or even life-threatening and may develop up to 6 h or even longer after the start of infusion. Very rarely fatalities have been reported, which seem to be particularly associated with patients who are experiencing dyspnoea at rest as a result of advanced malignancy.

Other side-effects include cardiac failure (particularly when the drug is administered in conjunction with anthracyclines), diarrhoea (not usually severe) and an increase in non-life-threatening infections.

BLOOD NADIR

Day 10 for 3-weekly treatment; no clear-cut nadir for weekly treatment; continuation treatment with trastuzumab (single-agent) is not myelosuppressive.

TTOS REQUIRED

- Anti-emetics appropriate to weakly emetogenic chemotherapy on paclitaxel treatment days. None on trastuzumab-only days.

NOTES FOR PRESCRIBERS

- On the *first* cycle only, paclitaxel should be given on the day after trastuzumab administration. From the *second* cycle onwards, paclitaxel can be given on the same day as the weekly trastuzumab dose.
- A prolonged 6-h observation period is required after the first dose of trastuzumab, so treatment appointments should be made early enough in the day for this to be completed during the normal opening hours of the treatment area.
- Check the FBC prior to giving the go-ahead for paclitaxel treatment. Seek further advice if the neutrophil count is $<1.5 \times 10^9$/L or the platelet count is $<100 \times 10^9$/L. The manufacturer of the drug states that paclitaxel is contraindicated in patients with blood counts below these levels. They also recommend dose reductions in patients who experienced profound neutropenia on previous courses (neutrophil count $<0.5 \times 10^9$/L for 7 days or longer).

Trastuzumab is non-myelosuppressive, and treatment can proceed on a lower blood count than is acceptable for chemotherapy.

- Check the LFTs before starting treatment. Consideration should be given to a paclitaxel dose reduction if the bilirubin level is more than 1.25 times the normal value (*see* Appendix 1 for further advice).
- Question the patient about abnormal sensations, as these may indicate paclitaxel-induced neuropathy that requires a dose modification. Seek advice from a senior member of the medical team if such symptoms are reported.
- Make sure that the patient has been prescribed appropriate IV premedication prior to paclitaxel administration, in order to prevent hypersensitivity reactions (unless a documented decision has been made to stop such treatment in patients who have received at least one cycle of weekly paclitaxel without experiencing problems).
- Antihistamines, paracetamol and hydrocortisone should be prescribed on an 'as-required' basis when trastuzumab is being given alone, in order to allow swift treatment of infusion reactions. On days when trastuzumab is being given with paclitaxel, the standard paclitaxel premedication contains steroids and antihistamines, but 'as-required' paracetamol should also be prescribed. Even if treatment is required for reactions to the first infusion, it should not be routinely administered on a prophylactic basis for subsequent trastuzumab infusions, since infusion reactions are generally much less frequent and severe on subsequent infusions.
- Cardiac function should be assessed by means of history, physical examination, ECG, echocardiogram and/or MUGA scan in patients for whom trastuzumab therapy is being considered. In patients who show evidence of compromised cardiac function, especially if they have a history of anthracycline therapy, a careful risk–benefit assessment should be conducted before proceeding with treatment. In patients who are receiving trastuzumab, cardiac function should be monitored regularly (e.g. every 3 months, or more regularly (e.g. every 6–8 weeks) in patients with asymptomatic cardiac impairment). Discuss any patient with symptomatic cardiac dysfunction or worsening asymptomatic dysfunction with a senior member of the medical team with a view to discontinuation of treatment.
- Staff who are administering trastuzumab should be instructed to interrupt treatment if infusion reactions occur. Treatment should be suspended until such symptoms have resolved, at which point it can be cautiously restarted.
- Although *3-weekly* trastuzumab treatment cannot yet be recommended for routine use, it may be appropriate for patients who will be unable to attend the hospital on a weekly basis because of holidays or similar commitments.
- If a patient misses a single *trastuzumab* dose, the next dose should be given without modification. If two or more doses are missed, a second loading dose of 4 mg/kg should be used. No attempt should be made to catch up on missed doses of paclitaxel.

NOTES FOR NURSES

- On days when patients are due to receive paclitaxel as well as trastuzumab, make sure that they receive the appropriate IV premedication prior to both paclitaxel and trastuzumab administration. Steroid and antihistamine premedication is mandatory to prevent hypersensitivity reactions to paclitaxel (unless a documented decision has been made to stop such treatment in patients who have received at least one cycle of weekly paclitaxel without experiencing problems). However, by giving it prior to trastuzumab as well, it may also reduce the incidence and severity of trastuzumab infusion reactions.

- If the patient develops an infusion reaction during trastuzumab infusion (these are much more common with the first infusion), treatment should be interrupted but the infusion left in place. It is normally possible to continue the infusion once the symptoms have resolved. Paracetamol and antihistamines are appropriate for treating most infusion-related symptoms.

- Prophylactic use of drugs to prevent infusion reactions to trastuzumab cannot be recommended, even in patients who experienced such reactions during their first infusion. Such patients are much less likely to experience problems on their second infusion.

- For trastuzumab, a 6-h observation period is required from the start of treatment for the first infusion, and a 2-h period is needed for subsequent infusions. This means that treatments should be scheduled sufficiently early in the day to allow such observations during the normal opening hours of the treatment area. The observation period is recommended in case late infusion reactions occur, and the need for it should be explained to patients, who may not understand why they are being kept waiting for such a long time.

- In-line filters should not be used with trastuzumab, although they are mandatory for paclitaxel, as there is insufficient information about trastuzumab binding to such devices.

- Inform the prescriber if the patient reports any abnormal sensations, as these may be indicative of paclitaxel-induced neuropathy.

- Try not to agitate bags or bottles of paclitaxel infusion too much, as this causes foaming which can trigger 'air-in-line' alarms on infusion pumps.

NOTES FOR PHARMACISTS

- Make sure it is clearly understood whether the patient is due to receive weekly or 3-weekly paclitaxel/trastuzumab.

- On days when paclitaxel is scheduled, check that the FBC has been determined and is within acceptable limits before issuing chemotherapy. Trastuzumab is not myelosuppressive, and can be given on a low blood count.

- Check the LFTs before starting paclitaxel treatment. Consideration should be given to a dose reduction if the bilirubin level is more than 1.25 times the normal value (see Appendix 1 for further advice).

- Make sure that standard IV premedications for paclitaxel and 'as-required' items to accompany trastuzumab have been prescribed (unless a documented decision has been made to stop such treatment in patients who have received at least one cycle of weekly paclitaxel without experiencing problems).

- Try not to agitate bags or bottles of paclitaxel infusion too much, as this causes foaming which can trigger 'air-in-line' alarms on infusion pumps.

- Use PVC-free bags/glass bottles for all paclitaxel infusions.

- Although 3-weekly trastuzumab treatment (see Doses section above) cannot yet be recommended for routine use, it may be appropriate for patients who will be unable to attend the hospital on a weekly basis because of holidays or similar commitments.

- If a patient misses a single *trastuzumab* dose, the next dose should be given without modification. If two or more doses are missed, a second loading dose of 4 mg/kg should be used. No attempt should be made to catch up on missed doses of paclitaxel.
- Trastuzumab is not a conventional cytotoxic agent, so it can reasonably be manipulated in any aseptic dispensing facility. However, as it is being used for patients with advanced malignancy who have received or are receiving chemotherapy, it is also reasonable to handle it in any area that is set aside for cytotoxic drugs.

SOURCE MATERIAL

Three-weekly paclitaxel plus trastuzumab

- Slamon DJ, Leyland-Jones B, Shak S *et al.* (2001) Use of chemotherapy plus a monoclonal antibody against HER2 for metastatic breast cancer that overexpresses HER2. *NEJM.* **344**: 783–92.

Weekly paclitaxel plus trastuzumab

- Fornier M, Seidman AD, Esteva FJ *et al.* (1999) Weekly (W) Herceptin (H) + 1 hour Taxol (T): phase II study in HER2 overexpressing (H2+) and non-overexpressing (H2−) metastatic breast cancer (MBC). *Proc Am Soc Clin Oncol.* **18**: 126 (abstract).

Three-weekly trastuzumab administration

- Verma S, Leyland-Jones B, Ayoub J-P *et al.* (2001) Efficacy and safety of three-weekly Herceptin with paclitaxel in women with HER2-positive metastatic breast cancer: preliminary results of a phase II trial. *Eur J Cancer.* **37** (**Supplement 6**): S146.

IV paclitaxel premedication regimens

- Ellerton JA and Rowan N (1996) Single-dose i.v. dexamethasone one hour before infusion as pre-treatment for paclitaxel. *Proc Am Soc Clin Oncol.* **15**: 548 (abstract).

PCV (procarbazine, lomustine [CCNU®], vincristine)

USUAL INDICATION

Brain tumours.

DOSES

Lomustine* 110 mg/m^2 by mouth on day 1
Procarbazine† 60 mg/m^2 by mouth on days 0–21
Vincristine 1.4 mg/m^2 (maximum 2 mg) IV on days 8 and 29

ADMINISTRATION

Vincristine

By slow IV injection into the side-arm of a free-running 0.9% sodium chloride drip.

Vincristine is a powerful vesicant, and should be administered with appropriate precautions to prevent extravasation. If there is any possibility that extravasation has occurred, contact a senior member of the medical team immediately and follow local guidance on dealing with extravasation incidents.

Procarbazine and lomustine

These drugs are only available as oral preparations. Procarbazine is only available as 50 mg capsules, which cannot be divided, so individual doses must be calculated to the nearest 50 mg. Intermediate doses can be achieved by administering unequal doses on subsequent days.

Lomustine is only available as 40 mg capsules, which cannot be divided, so considerable rounding off of doses may be needed. Rounding down rather than up is often done, due to the highly myelosuppressive nature of lomustine.

---

*Lomustine is only available as 40 mg capsules. These are unsuitable for cutting or breaking, so doses should be rounded off to the nearest 40 mg.

†Procarbazine is only available in 50 mg capsules. These are unsuitable for cutting or breaking, so daily doses should be rounded off to the nearest 50mg. However, note that a closer approximation to any calculated doses may be achieved by using unequal doses on alternate days, effectively allowing a dose increment of 25 mg.

ANTI-EMETICS

Day 1

High emetogenic potential (see local protocol). This may be overstating the emetogenic potential of lomustine, but in view of the importance of preventing vomiting after the single oral dose of the latter, a cautious approach is suggested. Note that many patients with brain tumours will already be taking significant doses of oral steroids to reduce cerebral oedema. In such cases, additional steroids are not required for anti-emesis.

Days 8 to 21 plus day 29

Low emetogenic potential.

CYCLE LENGTH

6–8 weeks (as blood counts allow).

NUMBER OF CYCLES

For 1 year or until tumour progression.

SIDE-EFFECTS

Bone-marrow suppression (late and sometimes prolonged with lomustine), alopecia (this regimen is commonly used after cranial irradiation, which is already likely to have caused hair loss, so this may not be an issue), nausea and vomiting, mucositis. Peripheral neuropathy due to vincristine. Procarbazine is a weak inhibitor of MAO, and can lead to CNS side-effects such as somnolence, hallucinations, ataxia, headache and insomnia, especially when administered with tyramine-rich foods, alcohol or interacting medications. It also has a weak disulfiram-like effect and may lead to alcohol intolerance. Lomustine can cause pulmonary dysfunction (shortness of breath, decreased diffusion capacity, fibrosis) after high cumulative doses (lifetime treatment doses should not exceed $1100-1400\,\mathrm{mg/m^2}$).

BLOOD NADIR

This is somewhat difficult to predict. The nadir from procarbazine is likely to fall 2–3 weeks after finishing the 14-day course, and that from lomustine is likely to fall 4–6 weeks after treatment, with a slow recovery over a period of 1–2 weeks, so that the time of highest risk is a period around 35–42 days after the start of the treatment cycle.

TTOS REQUIRED

- Anti-emetics appropriate to highly emetogenic (day 1) and weakly emetogenic (days 8–21 and 29) chemotherapy (according to local protocol).
- A single dose of lomustine plus sufficient procarbazine to finish the cycle of treatment.

NOTES FOR PRESCRIBERS

- Check the FBC prior to giving the go-ahead for chemotherapy on day 1. Seek advice from a senior member of the medical team if the neutrophil count is $<1.5 \times 10^9$/L or the platelet count is $<100 \times 10^9$/L. The blood count must be taken late enough to be after the delayed nadir that follows lomustine treatment. The manufacturer of lomustine recommends that the WBC should be $>4 \times 10^9$/L and the platelet count $>100 \times 10^9$/L before further lomustine is administered. A blood count prior to starting procarbazine and giving vincristine on day 8 is not likely to be informative, since the myelosuppressive effects of day 1 treatment will not have fully developed. Vincristine has little bone-marrow toxicity, and adjustments of the vincristine dose for blood counts are probably unnecessary.
- Check the renal function before prescribing. Estimation from the serum creatinine level using the Cockcroft–Gault equation is appropriate if the patient has a stable serum creatinine concentration and no confounding factors (e.g. catabolic states):

CrCl (mL/min)

$$= \frac{1.04 \text{ (females) or } 1.23 \text{ (males)} \times (140 - \text{age in years}) \times \text{weight in kg}}{\text{serum creatinine concentration } (\mu\text{mol/L})}.$$

On subsequent cycles renal function should be reassessed.

Lomustine doses should be reviewed in patients with a CrCl of <60 mL/min, and procarbazine doses may require adjustment in patients with significant renal impairment (*see* Appendix 2 for further advice).
- Check the LFTs. Dose adjustment should be considered for procarbazine, vincristine and possibly lomustine in cases of significant hepatic impairment (*see* Appendix 1 for further advice).
- Check that the maximum 2 mg dose for vincristine has not been exceeded. The purpose of this cap is to try to prevent excessive neurotoxicity. Some clinicians use a lower limit (typically 1.5 mg in patients over 70 years of age) in elderly patients who are perceived to be at increased risk of neurotoxicity, although this is not evidence based.
- Vincristine can cause peripheral neuropathy. Patients should be questioned about abnormal sensations, jaw pain or constipation, any of which may be indicative of neuropathy. If such symptoms are reported, discuss them with a senior member of the medical team with a view to dose modification.
- Lomustine can cause lung dysfunction. This is rare at cumulative doses of <1100 mg/m^2, but this dose should only be exceeded with caution, and a dose

of 1400 mg/m^2 should not normally be exceeded. Monitor the total dose care-
- fully and investigate unexplained pulmonary symptoms thoroughly, even in patients who have received lower cumulative doses.
- If administering the treatment, *see* Administration section above for notes on the vesicant nature of vincristine.
- All prescriptions and communications with the patient's GP should clearly state that procarbazine is given as a discrete course and lomustine is given as a single dose per cycle. Further supplies should not be sought from or prescribed by the GP. Lack of clarity with regard to this matter may result in inadvertent continuation of oral therapy with cytotoxics. *Inadvertent continuation of short courses of oral cytotoxics has resulted in fatalities.*
- Because procarbazine is a weak MAOI, it has the *potential* to cause CNS side-effects and to interact with those foods and medications which are known to cause problems with MAOIs. Although full dietary restrictions and discontinuation of existing interacting medications are not justified, this problem should be considered if the patient presents with headache or CNS side-effects. Because procarbazine also has a weak disulfiram-like effect, it may in addition cause adverse reactions to alcohol. Therefore the patient should be counselled about this and advised to avoid alcoholic drink.
- Procarbazine is only available in 50 mg capsules, which cannot be divided. If rounding off of the daily dose to the nearest 50 mg is unacceptable, a closer approach to the calculated dose may be achieved by giving uneven doses on successive days (e.g. a calculated daily dose of 175 mg could be given as 200 mg and 150 mg on alternate days). Similarly, lomustine capsules cannot be divided, and lomustine doses should be rounded off to the nearest 40 mg. Doses are often rounded *down* because of the profoundly myelosuppressive nature of lomustine.

NOTES FOR NURSES

- If administering the drugs, *see* Administration section above for notes on the vesicant nature of vincristine.
- If you are involved in counselling the patient about their oral medication, explain clearly that lomustine is given as a single dose at the beginning of each cycle, and that procarbazine is intended to be taken for 10 days at a time only. A full course will normally be issued at the time of IV treatment, and the patient should not seek additional supplies from their GP. *Inadvertent continuation of short courses of oral cytotoxics has resulted in fatalities.*
- Because procarbazine has a weak disulfiram-like effect, it may cause adverse reactions to alcohol. Therefore the patient should be counselled about this and advised to avoid alcoholic drink.

NOTES FOR PHARMACISTS

- Check that the FBC has been determined and is within acceptable limits before issuing the chemotherapy. It must be clear that the blood count has been taken after the late nadir induced by lomustine treatment.

- Lomustine can cause lung dysfunction. This is rare at cumulative doses of $<1100 \, mg/m^2$, but this dose should only be exceeded with caution, and a dose of $1400 \, mg/m^2$ should not normally be exceeded. At the start of treatment, pharmacy and patient records should be checked for evidence of previous lomustine therapy, and the cumulative dose from any previous treatment should be clearly endorsed on any pharmacy patient record (*see* Appendix 3 for an example). Thereafter the cumulative dose should be monitored and the prescriber alerted if it exceeds $1100 \, mg/m^2$. In addition, any unexplained new prescriptions for respiratory drugs should be investigated as possible indicators of lomustine toxicity.

- Check the renal function at the start of treatment. Lomustine doses should be reviewed in patients with a CrCl of $<60 \, mL/min$, and the procarbazine dosage may also require adjustment in cases of significant renal impairment. If the patient has a stable serum creatinine concentration and lacks confounding factors (e.g. significant renal impairment or catabolic states), calculation of the CrCl from serum creatinine levels using the Cockcroft–Gault equation is acceptable. The patient's CrCl should be recorded on any pharmacy patient record, together with the corresponding creatinine concentration. The CrCl should be recalculated if there is a significant change in creatinine concentration (*see* Appendix 2 for further advice).

- Check the LFTs. Dose adjustments should be considered for all three drugs in this regimen in cases of significant hepatic impairment (*see* Appendix 1 for further advice).

- Check that the maximum 2 mg dose for vincristine has not been exceeded. This cap is applied in an attempt to prevent excessive neurotoxicity. Some clinicians use a lower limit (typically 1.5 mg in patients over 70 years of age) in elderly patients who are perceived to be at increased risk of neurotoxicity, although this is not evidence based.

- Check that anti-emetics appropriate to highly emetogenic chemotherapy have been prescribed according to local protocol on day 1. A vigorous approach is appropriate in an attempt to prevent vomiting on day 1, when it could interfere with the absorption of the single lomustine dose in each cycle.

- Make sure that it is clearly stated on any TTO or prescription being sent elsewhere that the lomustine is a single dose only, and that the procarbazine is a short course of 14 days only that should not be continued by the GP. *Fatalities have resulted from the inadvertent continuation of short courses of oral cytototoxics or steroids by GPs.*

- Because procarbazine is a weak MAOI, it has the *potential* to cause CNS side-effects and to interact with those foods and medications which are known to cause problems with MAOIs. Although full dietary restrictions and discontinuation of existing interacting medications are not justified, this problem should be considered if patients present with headache or CNS side-effects. Because procarbazine also has a weak disulfiram-like effect, it may in addition cause adverse reactions to alcohol. Therefore the patient should be counselled about this and advised to avoid alcoholic drink.

- Procarbazine is only available in 50 mg capsules, which cannot be divided. If rounding off of the daily dose to the nearest 50 mg is unacceptable, a closer approach to the calculated dose may be achieved by giving uneven doses on sucessive days (e.g. a calculated dose of 175 mg could be given as 200 mg and 150 mg on alternate days). Similarly, lomustine is only available in 40 mg capsules. These cannot be broken, and considerable rounding off of doses may be required. Doses are often rounded *down* because of the profoundly myelosuppressive nature of lomustine.

SOURCE MATERIAL

- Levin VA, Silver P and Hannigan MS (1990) Superiority of post-radiotherapy adjuvant chemotherapy with CCNU, procarbazine and vincristine (PCV) over BCNU for anaplastic gliomas: NCOG 6G61 final report. *Int J Radiat Oncol Biol Phys.* **18**: 321–4.

PE (cisplatin plus etoposide)

Note: This regimen is sometimes alternated with the CAV regimen to form the hybrid regimen CAV/PE.

USUAL INDICATION

Small-cell lung cancer, and occasionally other rarer small-cell and neuroendocrine tumours.

DOSES

Cisplatin 80 mg/m^2 IV on day 1
Etoposide 100 mg/m^2 IV on days 1–3

Note: There are *many* variations on this protocol. This is one of the more widely used schedules.

ADMINISTRATION

Both IV drugs are given as an infusion in 0.9% sodium chloride. Etoposide is given in 500 mL of 0.9% sodium chloride on day 1. This forms part of the pre-hydration regimen for cisplatin.

Cisplatin is nephrotoxic, and hydration is mandatory to dilute the drug as it is excreted via the kidneys, and thus to minimise toxicity. The aim of hydration is to maintain a urine output of 100 mL/h during and for 6–8 h after cisplatin administration. Typically, hydration consists of 3 L of IV 0.9% sodium chloride (1 L over a period of 2 h before cisplatin, 1 L over 3 h containing cisplatin and 1 L over 2 h after cisplatin). This is less intensive than some hydration regimens that were formerly used, and it permits outpatient therapy. The patient should be instructed to drink at least 3 L of fluid in the 24 h after the completion of IV hydration. Potassium and magnesium are usually added to the hydration fluids to compensate for cisplatin-induced electrolyte loss.

ANTI-EMETICS

High emetogenic potential (see local policy).

CYCLE LENGTH

21 days (or 42 days if alternating with CAV).

NUMBER OF CYCLES

Usually 6 (or 3 if alternating with CAV).

SIDE-EFFECTS

Nephrotoxicity (dose limiting), bone-marrow suppression (all blood components are affected), alopecia (often total), nausea and vomiting (may be severe), mucositis (not usually severe), sensory, motor and occasionally autonomic neuropathy (sometimes irreversible) including significant potential for ototoxicity.

TTOS REQUIRED

- Anti-emetics appropriate to highly emetogenic chemotherapy (see local policy).

NOTES FOR PRESCRIBERS

Before each course

- Make sure that it is clearly understood which PE regimen is required, especially if the patient is enrolled in a clinical trial. There are many variants on this regimen that utilise different schedules and doses of both etoposide and cisplatin, including some with day 2 and 3 etoposide given orally. If a regimen with oral etoposide is being used, it must be prescribed in such a way that it is absolutely clear to the pharmacist, the patient and anyone else involved in the care of the patient, such as the GP, that a short course is intended and that this should *not* be continued. *Fatalities have resulted from the inappropriate continuation of short courses of oral cytotoxic drugs.*
- Check the FBC prior to giving the go-ahead for chemotherapy. Seek advice if the neutrophil count is $<1.5 \times 10^9$/L or the platelet count is $<100 \times 10^9$/L at the time of treatment.
- Renal function should be formally assessed at the start of treatment. Ideally this should be done by EDTA clearance, but estimation from the serum creatinine level using the Cockcroft–Gault equation is acceptable if the patient has a stable creatinine concentration and no confounding factors (e.g. catabolic states):

CrCl (mL/min)

$$= \frac{1.04 \text{ (females) or } 1.23 \text{ (males)} \times (140 - \text{age in years}) \times \text{weight in kg}}{\text{serum creatinine concentration } (\mu\text{mol/L})}.$$

On subsequent cycles the renal function should be reassessed.

Cisplatin doses *should normally be reduced* if the creatinine clearance drops below 60 mL/min. Consideration should also be given to an etoposide dose reduction in cases of renal impairment (*see* Appendix 1 for further guidance).

- Check the LFTs at the start of treatment. Consideration should be given to an etoposide dose reduction in cases of significant hepatic impairment (*see* Appendix 1 for further guidance).
- Check electrolytes for cisplatin-induced wasting, especially of magnesium, calcium and potassium. Additional supplementation may be required.
- Ensure that anti-emetics appropriate to highly emetogenic chemotherapy have been prescribed in accordance with local policy.
- Seek further advice if the patient reports symptoms indicative of neurotoxicity (parasthesias, difficulty with motor control) or ototoxicity (tinnitus, deafness).

On the day after each cisplatin dose (for inpatients)

- Check the patient's fluid balance and body weight. If they have gained more than 1.5 L/kg from the start of hydration, extra diuresis will be required (e.g. furosemide 20–40 mg by mouth).

NOTES FOR NURSES

- The aim of hydration is to ensure an average urine output of 100 mL/h or more during and for 6–8 h after cisplatin administration. Any patient who is being treated as an inpatient should be on a fluid-balance chart, and daily weights should be recorded. Contact the prescriber if the patient's urine output is inadequate or their body weight increases by 1.5 kg from baseline.

  For outpatients, efforts should be made to ensure that urine output is adequate (e.g. by checking that the patient has passed 500 mL of urine between the start of IV hydration and the beginning of cisplatin infusion).

  Outpatients should also be encouraged to drink 3 L of fluid in the 24 h following each period of IV hydration, and to contact the hospital if this is impossible because of nausea/vomiting or other problems.
- If a variant on this regimen is being used where etoposide is given by mouth, make sure that the patient understands that the etoposide should be taken for a short course only, and that they should not approach their GP for a further supply of the drug. *Fatalities have resulted from the inappropriate continuation of short courses of oral cytotoxic drugs.*

NOTES FOR PHARMACISTS

On the day of prescribing

- Check that the FBC has been determined and is within acceptable limits before issuing the chemotherapy.
- Check that the renal function has been measured or calculated at the start of treatment. Record the CrCl and the corresponding creatinine concentration on any

pharmacy patient record sheet (*see* Appendix 3 for an example). Recalculate the CrCl if the creatinine concentration changes. A cisplatin dose reduction is needed if the CrCl drops to <60 mL/min, and an etoposide dose reduction should also be considered in cases of significant renal impairment (*see* Appendix 2 for further guidance).

- Check the LFTs at the start of treatment. Consideration should be given to an etoposide dosage reduction in cases of significant hepatic impairment (*see* Appendix 1 for further guidance).
- Check that anti-emetics appropriate to highly emetogenic chemotherapy have been prescribed according to local policy.

On the day after cisplatin chemotherapy

- Check that any patient who is receiving PE as an inpatient has not gained more than 1.5 L/kg since the start of hydration. If they have, discuss additional diuresis with the prescriber (e.g. furosemide 20–40 mg by mouth) (if this measure has not already been instituted).

If using a variant regimen in which day 2 and 3 etoposide is administered orally

- Make sure that whoever dispenses the treatment understands that the oral etoposide is to be taken for 2 days only, and that this is clearly labelled on the pack. *Fatalities have resulted from the inappropriate continuation of short courses of oral cytotoxic drugs.*
- Etoposide capsules are large, and supplying 50 mg (rather than 100 mg) capsules may help if the patient has difficulty swallowing. If the patient cannot swallow capsules at all, then the injection concentrate can be given by mouth, although the dose should be reduced to 80% to compensate for its superior bioavailability when administered via this route. Individual doses should be loaded into syringes prior to dispensing. The injection concentrate should be mixed with a suitably strongly flavoured soft drink (e.g. cola) to mask its taste.
- Giving unequal individual doses may help you to get closer to a calculated dose based on BSA than is possible using increments of 50 mg (the smallest capsule size).

Note: Because of the poor oral absorption of etoposide, oral and IV doses are *not interchangeable*.

SOURCE MATERIAL

This is one of the earlier reports of PE using a regimen similar to that described here, but with etoposide administered on days 1, 3 and 5, rather than on days 1–3.

- Fukuoka M, Furuse K, Saijo N *et al.* (1991) Randomized trial of cyclophosphamide, doxorubicin and vincristine versus cisplatin and etoposide versus alternation of these regimens in small-cell lung cancer. *J Natl Cancer Inst.* **12**: 855–61.

PMB (cisplatin, methotrexate, bleomycin)

USUAL INDICATION

Cervical cancer.

DOSES

Bleomycin 30 000 U (30 old units, 30 mg) IV on day 1
Methotrexate 300 mg/m² IV on day 1
Cisplatin 60 mg/m² IV on day 2
Folinic acid (calcium folinate, calcium leucovorin) 15 mg by mouth every 6 h for
    8 doses, starting 24 h from the commencement of methotrexate infusion
Sodium bicarbonate 600 mg by mouth 6 times daily for 96 h, starting 48 h before
    the start of methotrexate infusion.

Note: There are many variations on this regimen. The above doses are typical of
those widely used.

ADMINISTRATION

All three drugs are given as IV infusions in saline. There are pharmacokinetic/
pharmacodynamic interactions between the drugs in this regimen, so the schedule
and timing of the standard protocol should be adhered to.

Methotrexate

This is administered first as a 12-h infusion in 0.9% sodium chloride.

Bleomycin

This is administered immediately after methotrexate as two infusions each of
15 000 U of bleomycin in 1 L of 0.9% sodium chloride.

Cisplatin

Cisplatin is nephrotoxic, and hydration is mandatory to dilute the drug as it is
excreted via the kidneys, and thus to minimise toxicity. If it is administered immediately after the completion of bleomycin infusion, no further pre-hydration is

required, although 100 mL of 20% mannitol are often administered IV, immediately before cisplatin, in order to stimulate diuresis.

Cisplatin is then administered as a 4-h infusion in 1 L of 0.9% sodium chloride and followed by a further 2 L of 0.9% sodium chloride, each infused over a period of 6 h. The aim of hydration is to maintain a urine output of 100 mL/h during and for 6–8 h after cisplatin administration.

Electrolytes are added to the hydration fluid to compensate for cisplatin-induced electrolyte wasting – typically 20 mmol potassium chloride in each 4 L of saline and 1 g of magnesium in each 2 L of saline (magnesium sulphate and potassium chloride can be added to the same infusion solution).

ANTI-EMETICS

Low emetogenic potential on day 1 and high emetogenic potential on day 2 (see local policy).

CYCLE LENGTH

21 days.

NUMBER OF CYCLES

Usually 6.

SIDE-EFFECTS

Nephrotoxicity (dose limiting due primarily to cisplatin but also to methotrexate), bone-marrow suppression (all blood components are affected), alopecia, nausea and vomiting (may be severe), sensory and motor neuropathy (sometimes irreversible) including significant potential for ototoxicity, mucositis, lung fibrosis (bleomycin induced, but rare at cumulative doses lower than 300 000 U), rigors and other allergic reactions due to bleomycin.

TTOS REQUIRED

- Anti-emetics appropriate to highly emetogenic chemotherapy (see local protocol).
- The high dose of methotrexate in this protocol requires folinic acid (calcium folinate/leucovorin/folinate) 'rescue' to be administered (normally 15 mg by mouth, 6-hourly for 8 doses beginning 24 h after the start of the methotrexate infusion). If this has not been completed by the time the patient leaves hospital, enough tablets must be added to their TTO prescription to finish the treatment course.

- Oral sodium bicarbonate 600 mg six times daily to start 48 h before the next chemotherapy admission to alkalinise the urine prior to methotrexate treatment.

NOTES FOR PRESCRIBERS

Before each course

- Check the FBC prior to giving the go-ahead for chemotherapy. Seek advice if the neutrophil count is $<1.5 \times 10^9$/L or the platelet count is $<100 \times 10^9$/L at the time of treatment.
- Renal function should be formally assessed at the start of treatment. Ideally this should be done by an EDTA clearance test, but estimation from the serum creatinine level using the Cockcroft–Gault equation is acceptable if the patient has a stable serum creatinine concentration and no confounding factors (e.g. catabolic states):

CrCl (mL/min)

$$= \frac{1.04 \text{ (females) or } 1.23 \text{ (males)} \times (140 - \text{age in years}) \times \text{weight in kg}}{\text{serum creatinine concentration } (\mu\text{mol/L})}.$$

On subsequent cycles, renal function should be reassessed if the creatinine concentration changes.

Consideration should be given to reducing the doses of all three drugs in cases of renal impairment. Cisplatin and methotrexate doses *must normally be reduced* if the creatinine clearance drops to <60 mL/min, and consideration should be given to reducing the bleomycin doses if the CrCl falls to <50 mL/min (*see* Appendix 2 for further advice.)

- Check the serum electrolytes for cisplatin-induced wasting, especially of magnesium, calcium and potassium. Additional supplementation may be required.
- Check the LFTs before starting treatment. Consideration should be given to reducing the doses of bleomycin and methotrexate in cases of significant hepatic impairment (*see* Appendix 1 for further advice).
- Prescribe anti-emetics appropriate to weakly emetogenic chemotherapy (day 1) and highly emetogenic chemotherapy (day 2) according to local policy.
- Hydrocortisone 100 mg IV and chlorpheniramine 10–20 mg IV should be prescribed 'as needed' to allow reactions to bleomycin to be treated promptly, should they occur. If such reactions have occurred on previous courses, prophylactic treatment should be considered. Consideration should also be given to prescribing pethidine (50 mg IV as required) to allow prompt treatment of bleomycin-induced rigors.
- Ask the patient about symptoms indicative of neurotoxicity (parasthesias, difficulty with motor control) or ototoxicity (tinnitus, deafness). Seek further advice if they report such symptoms, which may indicate cisplatin toxicity.
- Ask the patient about breathlessness. If they report this symptom, consult a senior member of the medical team about the need for respiratory function tests. Respiratory symptoms may indicate bleomycin-induced lung fibrosis or, even more rarely, methotrexate-induced pneumonitis.
- To prevent retention of methotrexate and unnecessary toxicity, the urinary pH must be alkaline (> pH 7) before starting methotrexate treatment, and for the

duration of each IV chemotherapy regimen. To achieve this, continue oral sodium bicarbonate (which should have been started prior to admission) 600 mg six times a day, and prescribe 'as-required' IV sodium bicarbonate to be given if the urinary pH falls. A suitable dose is 50 mmol — this equates to 50 mL of 8.4% solution, although it should be noted that this concentration of bicarbonate is very hypertonic and can only be administered via a central line. Dilution is necessary prior to administration via a peripheral line. Liaise with the nursing staff to ensure that the patient is on a fluid-balance chart, all urine is tested for pH and the nursing staff know what action to take if the urinary pH falls.

- To prevent methotrexate toxicity, folinic acid 'rescue' needs to be prescribed — 15 mg, 6-hourly for eight doses starting 24 h after the *start* of methotrexate infusion. Once the starting time of the methotrexate is known, write up the folinic acid on the drug chart and block out doses which would fall before the 24-h point is reached, as giving folinic acid sooner than 24 h after starting methotrexate will negate its activity as well as removing its toxicity. As far as possible, the dose interval for folinic acid should be 6 h (i.e. not just four times a day with a 12-h gap between doses overnight). Because of the importance of folinic acid, it should be written 'oral/IV' on the inpatient chart so that it can be given IV if the patient is vomiting after cisplatin administration.

- Methotrexate excretion is prolonged in patients with 'third-space' fluid collections (ascites, effusions, severe oedema) or renal impairment, and in those taking non-steroidal anti-inflammatory drugs (NSAIDs). In such cases, discuss the possibility of extended folinic acid rescue with a senior member of the medical team. If possible, NSAIDs should be stopped for at least 72 h from the start of treatment. Alternatively, give prolonged folinic acid rescue.

On the day after each cisplatin dose

- Check the fluid balance/body weight. If the patient has gained more than 1.5 L/kg since the start of hydration, extra diuresis will be required (e.g. furosemide 20–40 mg by mouth).

NOTES FOR NURSES

- The patient should be on a fluid-balance chart and daily weights recorded during chemotherapy. The aim of hydration in this regimen is to maintain an average urine output of 100 mL/h or more during and for 6–8 h after cisplatin administration. Contact the prescriber if the urine output is inadequate or body weight increases by more than 1.5 kg from the start of hydration. While the IV regimen is in progress, all urine should be tested for pH. If the urinary pH falls below 7, then 'as-required' IV bicarbonate should be administered. The medical team should be contacted if no 'as-required' bicarbonate is prescribed, or if its administration fails to alkalinise the urine. Note that the usual dose of 'as-required' bicarbonate is 50 mmol IV, which is equivalent to 50 mL of 8.4% solution. However, this strength of bicarbonate is extremely hypertonic and should only be given undiluted via a central line. Dilution is necessary prior to infusion via a peripheral line.

- Timing is important in this regimen, and every effort should be made to keep to the prescribed schedule. Liaise with the medical team if there are any problems with this (e.g. venous access failure).
- Folinic acid (folinate/calcium folinate/calcium leucovorin) needs to be administered to start 24 h after the *start* of the methotrexate. Look at the time the methotrexate was started before commencing folinic acid administration. Do not give it *less* than 24 h after the start of the methotrexate infusion, as this will counteract the antitumour effects of methotrexate. If folinic acid has not been prescribed, remind the medical team. As far as possible, folinic acid should be administered at regular 6-h intervals.
- If you are issuing TTOs to patients, explain the importance of completing the short course of folinic acid (if it was not completed before discharge) and the importance of taking the tablets at regular intervals. Also explain that folinic acid treatment is a short course only, and that further supplies of tablets will not be needed from the patient's GP. In addition, it should be explained that any sodium bicarbonate which is prescribed for use before the next admission should be started 2 days before the planned treatment, and that failure to do this may delay future treatment.

NOTES FOR PHARMACISTS

On the day of prescribing

- Check that the FBC has been determined and is within acceptable limits before issuing the chemotherapy.
- Check that the renal function has been measured or calculated at the start of treatment. Record the CrCl and the corresponding creatinine concentration on any pharmacy patient record sheet (*see* Appendix 3 for an example), and recalculate the CrCl if the creatinine concentration changes. The doses of cisplatin and methotrexate should be reduced if the CrCl drops to <60 mL/min, and bleomycin dose adjustments should be considered if the CrCl falls to <50 mL/min (*see* Appendix 2 for further guidance).
- Check serum electrolytes for cisplatin-induced wasting, especially of magnesium, calcium and potassium. Additional supplementation may be required.
- Check the LFTs before starting treatment. Consideration should be given to reducing the doses of bleomycin and methotrexate in cases of significant hepatic impairment (*see* Appendix 1 for further guidance).
- Check that anti-emetics appropriate to highly emetogenic chemotherapy have been prescribed according to local policy.
- Check that sodium bicarbonate (600 mg six times daily regularly by mouth and 50 mL of 8.4% (50 mmol) IV as required) has been prescribed to maintain the urinary pH above 7 throughout the IV chemotherapy administration period. Endorse the prescription chart to indicate that 8.4% sodium bicarbonate solution must be either diluted prior to infusion or administered via a central line because of its hypertonicity. Also check that oral sodium bicarbonate has been prescribed to start 48 h before the next admission for chemotherapy.
- Check that folinic acid (folinate/calcium folinate/calcium leucovorin) has been prescribed to start 24 h after the *start* of methotrexate infusion. Block out any

spaces on the drug chart between the time of prescribing and the time when folinic acid treatment is due to start, to avoid it being given too soon. If the patient leaves hospital before folinic acid treatment is completed, ensure that the end of the course is added to their TTO. If you are counselling a patient about their discharge medication, make sure that they understand the importance of taking folinic acid doses at regular intervals and completing the course. Explain that the folinic acid treatment (like their anti-emetics) is a short treatment course and that further supplies are not routinely required from their GP.

- Methotrexate excretion is prolonged in patients with 'third-space' fluid collections (ascites, effusions, severe oedema) or renal impairment and in those taking non-steroidal anti-inflammatory drugs (NSAIDs). Discuss the possibility of extended folinic acid rescue in such patients with the medical team. If possible, NSAIDs should be stopped for at least 72 h from the start of treatment, although in some patients the loss of pain control that results from this is unacceptable, and prolonged folinic acid rescue should be considered as an alternative.

- When you are visiting the ward, check that the patient has not gained more than 1.5 L/kg since the start of hydration. If they have, discuss additional diuresis with the prescriber (e.g. furosemide 20–40 mg by mouth) (if this measure has not already been instituted). In addition, check that all urine has been tested for pH. It should be above pH 7 at the start of methotrexate infusion, and the pH should be maintained above 7 for the duration of the IV regimen. Check that if the pH has fallen at any point, appropriate corrective action has been taken (i.e. administration of IV bicarbonate until the pH rises again).

SOURCE MATERIAL

Note: There are many variations on this regimen. In the paper cited below it is unclear whether flat doses or m^2 doses were used. The above doses are typical of those widely used.

- Hoskin PJ and Blake PR (1991) Cisplatin, methotrexate and bleomycin (PMB) for carcinoma of the cervix: the influence of presentation and previous treatment upon response. *Int J Gynecol Cancer*. **1**: 75–80.

PMitCEBO (prednisolone, mitoxantrone, cyclophosphamide, etoposide, bleomycin, vincristine [Oncovin®])

USUAL INDICATION

High-grade non-Hodgkin's lymphoma.

DOSES

Prednisolone 50 mg (total dose) by mouth on days 1–28, *then* on alternate days on days 29–56
Mitoxantrone 7 mg/m^2 IV on days 1, 15, 29 and 43
Cyclophosphamide 300 mg/m^2 IV on days 1, 15, 29 and 43
Etoposide 150 mg/m^2 IV on days 1, 15, 29 and 43
Bleomycin 10 000 units (10 old units; 10 mg)/m^2 IV on days 8, 22, 36 and 50
Vincristine 1.4 mg/m^2 (maximum 2 mg) IV on days 8, 22, 36 and 50

ADMINISTRATION

Vincristine

By slow IV injection into the side-arm of a free-running saline drip.

Cyclophosphamide, bleomycin and mitoxantrone

By short IV infusion in 100 mL of 0.9% sodium chloride over a period of 15–20 min. Although the manufacturer recommends that mitoxantrone should be administered as an IV bolus, it is widely given as a short infusion.

Etoposide

By infusion in 500 mL of 0.9% sodium chloride over a period of 1 h.

Vincristine is a powerful vesicant, and should be administered with appropriate precautions to prevent extravasation. Mitoxantrone and (to a lesser extent) etoposide may also cause tissue damage if extravasated. If there is any possibility that extravasation has occurred, contact a senior member of the medical team and follow the local guidance on dealing with such incidents.

Note: On a given day the order of administration of the IV drugs in this regimen is not critical.

ANTI-EMETICS

Days 1, 15, 29 and 43 (cyclophosphamide, mitoxantrone, etoposide)

Moderate emetogenic potential (treat according to local protocol). Because oral prednisolone is given throughout the treatment course, additional *oral* steroids are not required. However, after day 28, additional *IV* dexamethasone may be prudent on days when cyclophosphamide, mitoxantrone and etoposide are given, since the scheduling of prednisolone is such that patients will not necessarily receive prednisolone on these specific days.

Days 8, 22, 36 and 50 (vincristine, bleomycin)

Low emetogenic potential. Treat according to standard local protocol. Remember that this regimen already incorporates significant doses of oral steroids, so additional steroids are unlikely to be appropriate, even in patients who are experiencing nausea/vomiting.

CYCLE LENGTH

IV portions of the treatment are repeated every 14 days. However, oral steroids are continuous, but with a change from daily to alternate daily dosing after 4 weeks.

NUMBER OF CYCLES

Usually four cycles delivered at 2-week intervals (i.e. 4 treatment days with mitoxantrone, cyclophosphamide and etoposide, and 4 treatment days with bleomycin and vincristine, with oral prednisolone throughout).

SIDE-EFFECTS

Bone-marrow suppression, alopecia (generally hair thinning rather than total loss), nausea and vomiting, mucositis. Cardiotoxicity has been reported after mitoxantrone, but it is less common than with anthracyclines. It seems to be more likely at cumulative doses in excess of $160 \, mg/m^2$ or $100 \, mg/m^2$ and with previous anthracycline therapy (i.e. at doses considerably in excess of those achieved here).

Peripheral neuropathy, constipation, jaw pain, diarrhoea and postural hypotension as a result of vincristine neurotoxicity (rare at the total doses used here). Lung fibrosis due to bleomycin (very rare at the doses used here). Cyclophosphamide *can* cause haemorrhagic cystitis at high doses. However, the doses used in PMitCEBO are not likely to cause this problem, so prophylactic mesna or hydration are not required.

The high doses of prednisolone used in this regimen can produce a variety of steroid side-effects, including euphoria/depression, epigastric discomfort, glucose intolerance, insomnia and psychosis, sodium and water retention, potassium loss and proximal myopathy.

BLOOD NADIR

10 days.

TTOS REQUIRED

- Anti-emetics appropriate to moderately (mitoxantrone, etoposide, cyclophospha-mide days) or weakly (vincristine and bleomycin days) emetogenic chemotherapy. In practice, because of the contribution of the oral steroids that patients receive in any case, it may be simpler and more effective to give a short course of a regular dopamine antagonist (domperidone or metoclopramide) after each IV chemother-apy treatment.
- Allopurinol 300 mg (reduced dose in renal impairment) each morning for the first 4 weeks of treatment to prevent tumour lysis syndrome.
- Prophylactic co-trimoxazole during and for 2 weeks after the end of treatment (480 mg by mouth twice daily on alternate days was used by Mainwaring et al.[1]).
- Consideration may be given to the use of a gastroprotective agent (e.g. an H_2-antagonist) during prolonged prednisolone therapy, especially in patients with a low platelet count.

NOTES FOR PRESCRIBERS

- Check which treatment week the patient is on. This regimen consists of two alternating IV chemotherapy schedules.
- This treatment requires each IV chemotherapy treatment to be scheduled 2 weeks after the last one.
- Ensure that the steroid dose is reduced to alternate days after the first 4 weeks of treatment. Note that the prednisolone dose in this protocol is not to be multi-plied by the patient's body surface area − the dose given above is the *total* dose.
- Check the FBC prior to giving the go-ahead for chemotherapy. On days when mitoxantrone, cyclophosphamide and etoposide are given, it is recommended that treatment is deferred for 7 days if the neutrophil count is $<0.5 \times 10^9$/L, and that doses are reduced by 35% if the neutrophil count is between 0.5×10^9/L and 1.0×10^9/L. No reductions or dose delays are recommended for low neutro-phil counts on days when only vincristine and bleomycin are due, nor are doses amended or delayed because of low platelet counts, although platelet support is recommended for patients with symptomatic thrombocytopenia and a platelet count of $<40 \times 10^9$/L, or a platelet count of $<10 \times 10^9$/L, even if asymptomatic. These dose modifications were used with satisfactory outcomes in the trial of this regimen reported by Mainwaring et al.[1]
- It is unlikely that, at the doses of mitoxantrone used in PMitCEBO, cumulative cardiac toxicity will be a problem (*see* Side-effects section above). However, great care should be exercised in patients with pre-existing cardiac dysfunction, includ-ing that induced by anthracyclines.

---

[1] Mainwaring PN, Cunningham D, Gregory W *et al.* (2001) Mitoxantrone is superior to doxorubicin in a multi-agent weekly regimen for patients older than 60 with high-grade lymphoma: results of a BNLI randomized trial of PAdriaCEBO versus PMitCEBO. *Blood.* **97**: 2991–7.

- Check the LFTs. If these show serious impairment, a reduction in mitoxantrone and vincristine doses may be required (*see* Appendix 1 for further guidance).
- Check the renal function. Reductions in etoposide and bleomycin doses should be considered in patients with a CrCl of <60 mL/min and <50 mL/min, respectively. A cyclophosphamide dose reduction should also be considered in cases of severe renal impairment (*see* Appendix 2 for further guidance). Formal assessment of renal function is not generally required. For patients with a stable serum creatinine concentration and no confounding factors (e.g. catabolic states), it is reasonable to calculate the creatinine clearance using the Cockcroft–Gault equation:

$$\text{CrCl (mL/min)} = \frac{1.04 \text{ (females) or } 1.23 \text{ (males)} \times (140 - \text{age in years}) \times \text{weight in kg}}{\text{serum creatinine concentration } (\mu\text{mol/L})}.$$

Formal measurement of renal function should be reserved for patients in whom the latter is known to be significantly impaired.

- This is a potentially curative treatment, and it is important to maintain dose intensity. Dose delays should be avoided if at all possible. Therefore the use of haematopoietic growth factors (G-CSF/GM-CSF) to support neutrophil numbers may be justified. The dosage should be in accordance with local policy on haematopoietic growth factor use. Note that the use of G-CSF/GM-CSF should normally be avoided within 24 h of myelosuppressive chemotherapy (mitoxantrone, cyclophosphamide and etoposide), when it can exacerbate myelotoxicity, but it is generally considered acceptable to give these growth factors on the same day as vincristine and bleomycin, which are minimally myelosuppressive.
- Vincristine can cause peripheral neuropathy. The patient should be questioned about abnormal sensations, jaw pain or constipation, any of which may be indicative of neuropathy. Discuss such symptoms with a senior member of the medical team with a view to dose modification or possibly switching to vinblastine. The latter appears to be more myelosuppressive but less neurotoxic.
- To limit the potential for neurotoxicity, the dose of vincristine is capped at 2 mg.
- Lymphomas are very sensitive to chemotherapy, and massive tumour lysis is possible at the start of chemotherapy. This can result in the generation of large amounts of insoluble uric acid which are capable of precipitating in the kidneys, causing renal damage. To prevent this, oral allopurinol 300 mg (reduce the dose in cases of renal impairment) once daily should be commenced the day before starting cytotoxic therapy and continued for the first 4 weeks of treatment.
- Prophylactic H_2-antagonists or other gastroprotective agents may be justified during high-dose prednisolone courses, especially when platelet counts have been reduced as a consequence of chemotherapy.
- Prior to treatment, hair loss should be discussed with the patient. Extensive alopecia is fairly uncommon with PMitCEBO, but hair thinning is frequent. Scalp cooling is of limited benefit in preventing hair loss with PMitCEBO, because of the prolonged half-life of cyclophosphamide and etoposide. Liaise with the nurses with regard to referral to a wig-fitter at the start of treatment, before alopecia is evident, if the patient is particularly concerned about hair loss.
- If administering the drugs, *see* Administration section above for notes on the vesicant nature of vincristine and the associated problems with extravasation of etoposide and mitoxantrone.

- Although bleomycin can cause lung fibrosis, this is unlikely at the doses used in this regimen. However, any unexplained respiratory symptoms should be investigated thoroughly.

NOTES FOR NURSES

- Prior to treatment, hair loss should be discussed with the patient. Scalp cooling is unlikely to be of much benefit because of the prolonged circulation time of cyclophosphamide and etoposide. If appropriate, referral to a wig-fitter should be made at the start of treatment, before alopecia is evident. However, it should be noted that hair thinning is much more common than total alopecia with this regimen.
- If administering the drugs, *see* Administration section above for notes on the vesicant nature of vincristine and the problems associated with the extravasation of etoposide and mitoxantrone.
- The dose of cyclophosphamide is lower than that which is likely to cause haemorrhagic cystitis. Therefore prophylactic mesna, IV hydration and urine testing are not required. Any mild symptoms of dysuria may be treated by encouraging oral fluid intake and regular voiding of urine.
- Ensure that any diabetic patients are aware of the need to be extra vigilant about monitoring their blood sugar levels during treatment with prednisolone, and advise them to contact their doctor if they have problems with the control of their blood sugar levels.
- The dose of prednisolone changes from daily to alternate days after week 4 of treatment. This can be confusing to the patient. Therefore use every opportunity to remind them of the change.
- If you are involved in booking appointments for the patient, do not forget that this regimen requires *two* weekly appointments for chemotherapy.

NOTES FOR PHARMACISTS

- There are two alternating IV drug combinations used in this regimen. Make sure that you know which treatment week the patient is on.
- Check that the FBC has been determined and is within acceptable limits before issuing the chemotherapy. Because this is a potentially curative treatment, it is reasonable to treat on a somewhat lower neutrophil/platelet count than would be considered acceptable for a palliative regimen. In the main published trial with PMitCEBO,[1] on days when mitoxantrone, cyclophosphamide and etoposide were given, treatment was deferred for 7 days if the neutrophil count was $<0.5 \times 10^9$/L, and was reduced by 35% if the neutrophil count was between 0.5×10^9/L and 1.0×10^9/L. No reductions or dose delays were made for low neutrophil counts on days when only vincristine and bleomycin were due, nor were doses amended or delayed because of low platelet counts, although platelet support was recommended for patients with symptomatic thrombocytopenia and a platelet count of $<40 \times 10^9$/L, or a platelet count of $<10 \times 10^9$/L, even if asymptomatic. This dose reduction schedule was associated with acceptable toxicity.
- This is a potentially curative treatment, and it is important to maintain dose intensity. Dose delays should be avoided if at all possible. Therefore this is one

regimen where the use of haematopoietic growth factors (G-CSF/GM-CSF) may be justified. These should be used in accordance with local policies for haematopoietic growth factor use. Note that although there is no direct evidence for this, it is generally considered acceptable to give G-CSF/GM-CSF on days when bleomycin and vincristine are given, since the latter are minimally myelo-suppressive. Normally cytotoxic drugs should not be given within 24 h of cytotoxic chemotherapy, in order to avoid potentiation of myelotoxicity.

- Check the LFTs. If these show serious impairment, a reduction in mitoxantrone and vincristine doses may be required (*see* Appendix 1 for further guidance).
- Check the renal function. Reductions in etoposide and bleomycin doses should be considered in patients with a CrCl of <60 mL/min and <50 mL/min, respectively. A cyclophosphamide dose reduction should also be considered in cases of severe renal impairment (*see* Appendix 2 for further guidance).
- Check that the maximum dose of 2 mg for vincristine has not been exceeded.
- Check that anti-emetics appropriate to moderate (mitoxantrone, etoposide, cyclophosphamide days) or weakly (vincristine and bleomycin days) emetogenic chemotherapy have been prescribed. Note that the regimen incorporates significant doses of oral prednisolone, so additional steroids are unlikely to be appropriate.
- In the referenced trial for this regimen, prophylactic co-trimoxazole was prescribed. If co-trimoxazole is not prescribed, check with the prescriber whether it is required. If there is a reason for its omission, endorse any pharmacy patient record (*see* Appendix 3 for an example) to prevent inappropriate dispensing in the future.
- If the patient has a low platelet count, it may be appropriate to suggest the use of a gastroprotective agent (e.g an H_2-antagonist) during oral steroid therapy.
- Lymphomas are very sensitive to chemotherapy, and massive tumour lysis is possible at the start of chemotherapy. This can result in the generation of large amounts of insoluble uric acid which are capable of precipitating in the kidneys, causing renal damage. To prevent this, oral allopurinol 300 mg once daily (reduce the dose in cases of renal impairment) should be commenced the day before starting cytotoxic therapy and continued for the first 4 weeks of treatment.
- The dose of cyclophosphamide is below that which is likely to cause urothelial toxicity. Therefore prophylactic mesna, IV hydration and urine testing are not required.
- Make sure that the prednisolone dose is reduced to alternate daily dosing after the first 4 weeks of treatment. A note in any pharmacy patient record at the start of treatment may act as a suitable *aide-mémoire*. If you know that the patient is receiving their last dose of IV treatment, try to ensure that arrangements are in place to stop the prednisolone in order to avoid inadvertent continuation.

SOURCE MATERIAL

- Mainwaring PN, Cunningham D, Gregory W *et al.* (2001) Mitoxantrone is superior to doxorubicin in a multi-agent weekly regimen for patients older than 60 with high-grade lymphoma: results of a BNLI randomized trial of PAdriaCEBO versus PMitCEBO. *Blood.* **97**: 2991–7.

R-CHOP (rituximab, cyclophosphamide, doxorubicin [hydroxydaunorubicin], vincristine [Oncovin®], prednisolone)

USUAL INDICATION

High-grade non-Hodgkin's lymphoma.

DOSES

Rituximab 375 mg/m^2 IV on day 1
Doxorubicin 50 mg/m^2 IV on day 1
Cyclophosphamide 750 mg/m^2 IV on day 1
Vincristine 1.4 mg/m^2 (maximum 2 mg) IV on day 1
Prednisolone* 100 mg by mouth on days 1–5

ADMINISTRATION

Rituximab

As an intravenous infusion in 250 mL of 0.9% sodium chloride after premedication with an antihistamine (e.g. chlorpheniramine 10 mg IV) and paracetamol 1 g by mouth. At least the prednisolone part of day 1 of the CHOP part of the regimen should also be given prior to rituximab. The steroids have to be given in any case, so it makes sense to give them before the rituximab so that they can help to prevent infusion reactions to the antibody. If the patient has shown severe reactions to previous infusions, consideration should be given to doubling the chlorpheniramine dose.

First infusion
The infusion should start at a rate of 50 mg/h. After the first 30 min, the infusion rate can be escalated in 50 mg/h increments every 30 min up to a maximum of 400 mg/h. The infusion rate should only be increased if the patient is tolerating the existing rate well. In the event of infusion reactions, treatment should be temporarily suspended to allow their resolution.

If reactions are serious (especially if they involve severe dyspnoea, bronchospasm or hypoxia), evidence of resolution should include normalisation of laboratory tests and radiographic evidence of an absence of pulmonary infiltration. After severe reactions, infusions should be restarted at a rate not more than half of that at which the reactions occurred. If the same severe reaction occurs again, serious consideration should be given to stopping treatment permanently.

---

*In the original trial with this regimen, prednisone was used, but in the UK this is replaced by prednisolone at the same dose.

Subsequent infusions

The infusion can be commenced at an initial rate of 100 mg/h, and increased in 100 mg/h increments at 30-min intervals up to a maximum of 400 mg/h. Again the infusion rate should only be increased if treatment is being well tolerated.

Note: To calculate the infusion rate in mL/h, use the following formula:

$$\text{Infusion rate (mL/h)} = \frac{\text{infusion rate (mg/h)}}{(\text{dose [mg]/infusion volume [mL]})}.$$

Doxorubicin and vincristine

By slow IV injection into the side-arm of a free-running saline drip.

Doxorubicin and vincristine are powerful vesicants, and should be administered with appropriate precautions to prevent extravasation. If there is any possibility that extravasation has occurred, contact a senior member of the medical team immediately and follow local guidance on dealing with cytotoxic extravasation.

Cyclophosphamide

May be given as a slow IV bolus injection or short IV infusion (i.e. in 100 mL of 0.9% sodium chloride over 10–20 min).

Note: The order of administration of the IV drugs in this regimen is not critical.

ANTI-EMETICS

High emetogenic potential (follow local policy, although note that because of the high dose of prednisolone on days 1–5, no additional oral steroid is needed for anti-emetic purposes).

CYCLE LENGTH

21 days.

NUMBER OF CYCLES

8; the pivotal trial of R-CHOP compared 8 cycles of CHOP with 8 cycles of R-CHOP. Although 8 cycles of CHOP are more than is usually given in the UK, there can be no certainty that shorter courses of the combination will give the improvements in survival reported by Coiffier et al.[1]

---

[1] Coiffier B, Lepage E, Briere J et al. (2002) CHOP chemotherapy plus rituximab compared with CHOP alone in elderly patients with diffuse large-B-cell lymphoma. *NEJM.* **346**: 235–42.

SIDE-EFFECTS

Bone-marrow suppression, alopecia, nausea and vomiting, mucositis, cardiac arrhythmias, dilated cardiomyopathy (especially at cumulative doxorubicin doses in excess of 450 mg/m^2), peripheral neuropathy due to vincristine. Cyclophosphamide *can* cause haemorrhagic cystitis at high doses. However, the doses used in CHOP are not likely to cause this problem, so prophylactic mesna or hydration are not required.

The high doses of prednisolone used in this regimen can produce a variety of steroid side-effects, including euphoria/depression, epigastric discomfort, glucose intolerance, insomnia, psychosis, proximal myopathy, sodium and water retention, and potassium loss.

Rituximab is also associated with infusion reactions in more than 50% of patients, predominantly during the first 1–2 h of the first infusion. Infusion reactions may consist of a complex mixture of symptoms with features suggestive of tumour lysis syndrome, cytokine release syndrome and anaphylactoid reactions. Fever, chills and rigors are most common. Other symptoms include flushing, angioedema, nausea, urticaria/rash, fatigue, headache, throat irritation, rhinitis, vomiting and tumour pain, accompanied by hypotension and bronchospasm in about 10% of cases. Occasionally, pre-existing cardiac conditions can be exacerbated. Very occasionally, severe infusion reactions have had fatal outcomes, usually in patients with very high numbers of circulating malignant cells (>25 000/mm^3), pulmonary insufficiency or pulmonary tumour infiltration. Therefore special care should be exercised when treating such patients.

BLOOD NADIR

10 days.

TTOS REQUIRED

- Anti-emetics appropriate to highly emetogenic chemotherapy (according to local policy), although additional oral steroids are not required. The prednisolone in the regimen should be sufficient.
- Allopurinol 300 mg each morning (reduce the dose in cases of renal impairment) to prevent tumour lysis syndrome, especially early in treatment when there is a large tumour bulk.

NOTES FOR PRESCRIBERS

- Patients over 60 years of age or with a history of heart disease must have an echocardiogram or MUGA scan prior to treatment to ensure that there is adequate left ventricular function.
- Check the FBC prior to giving the go-ahead for chemotherapy. Seek advice if the neutrophil count is <1.5 × 10^9/L or the platelet count is <100 × 10^9/L. In the pivotal study with this regimen, patients with blood counts below these levels

on a scheduled treatment day had their treatment delayed by up to 2 weeks. If counts did not recover to these levels within 2 weeks, treatment was withdrawn. Patients who experienced grade 4 (severe) neutropenia or febrile neutropenia after any cycle of chemotherapy were given granulocyte-colony-stimulating factor. If grade 4 neutropenia persisted during the next cycle, the doses of cyclophosphamide and doxorubicin were reduced by 50%. For patients with grade 3 (moderate) or grade 4 thrombocytopenia, the doses of cyclophosphamide and doxorubicin were decreased by 50%.

Note that because rituximab has a minimal effect on bone-marrow function, doses of this drug do not normally require modification for haematological toxicity.

- Check the LFTs. If these show serious impairment, a reduction in doxorubicin and vincristine doses may be required (*see* Appendix 1 for further guidance).
- Check the renal function. A cyclophosphamide dose reduction is required in cases of severe renal impairment (*see* Appendix 2 for further guidance).
- Assuming that the schedule for escalation of infusion rates suggested above is followed with no interruptions, a typical first dose of rituximab can be infused over 3–4 h. However, first infusions often have to be interrupted or slowed down, and the total infusion time can be doubled. Therefore first doses should either be given on an inpatient basis or scheduled so that there is sufficient time to finish drug infusion during the working day of the outpatient clinic. Liaise with the nursing staff about this matter.
- This is a potentially curative treatment, and it is important to maintain dose intensity. Dose delays should be avoided if at all possible. Therefore the use of haematopoietic growth factors (G-CSF or GM-CSF) to support neutrophil numbers may be justified. The dosage should be in accordance with local policy on haematopoietic growth factor use.
- Vincristine can cause peripheral neuropathy. The patient should be questioned about abnormal sensations, jaw pain or constipation, any of which may be indicative of neuropathy. If such symptoms are reported, discuss them with an experienced prescriber with a view to dose modification or a switch to vinblastine. The latter appears to be more myelosuppressive but less neurotoxic.
- To limit the potential for neurotoxicity, the dose of vincristine is usually capped at 2 mg. This limit should be exceeded only with caution and after discussion with a senior member of the medical team. Some prescribers use a maximum dose of 1 mg in patients over 70 years of age, because of a perceived increased risk of peripheral neuropathy, although there is no evidence to support this.
- Lymphomas are very sensitive to chemotherapy, and massive tumour lysis is possible at the start of chemotherapy. This can result in the generation of large amounts of insoluble uric acid which are capable of precipitating in the kidneys, causing renal damage. To prevent this, allopurinol 300 mg once daily should be commenced the day before starting cytotoxic therapy, and continued for as long as a significant tumour bulk remains and cytotoxic therapy continues. Allopurinol doses should be reduced in patients with impaired renal function.
- Prophylactic H_2-antagonists or other gastroprotective agents may be justified during high-dose prednisolone courses, especially if platelet counts have been reduced as a consequence of chemotherapy.
- Prior to treatment, hair loss should be discussed with the patient. Scalp cooling is of limited benefit in preventing hair loss with R-CHOP because of the prolonged

half-life of cyclophosphamide. Liaise with the nurses with regard to referral to a wig-fitter at the start of treatment, before alopecia is evident, if this is required.

- If administering the drugs, *see* Administration section above for notes on the vesicant nature of doxorubicin and vincristine.
- Make sure that it is clearly stated on any prescription or in any communication with the patient's GP that the prednisolone is a short course of 5 days only. *Fatalities have resulted from the inadvertent continuation of short courses of steroids.*
- Premedication with paracetamol and an antihistamine (e.g. chlorpheniramine 10 mg IV) must be prescribed at the time of prescribing rituximab. It is also advisable to prescribe hydrocortisone (100 mg IV) on an 'as-needed' basis to treat serious infusion reactions without delay. In addition, consideration should be given to prescribing pethidine 50 mg IV as needed to treat rigors.
- Staff who are administering rituximab should be instructed on what action to take in the event of serious infusion reactions (*see* Administration section above).

NOTES FOR NURSES

- Prior to treatment, hair loss should be discussed with the patient. Scalp cooling is of limited value because of the prolonged circulation time of cyclophosphamide. If appropriate, referral to a wig-fitter should be made at the start of treatment, before alopecia is evident.
- If administering the drugs, *see* Administration section above for notes on the vesicant nature of doxorubicin and vincristine.
- The dose of cyclophosphamide is below that which is likely to cause haemorrhagic cystitis. Therefore prophylactic mesna, IV hydration and urine testing are not required. Any mild symptoms of dysuria may be treated by encouraging oral fluid intake and regular voiding of urine.
- Ensure that any diabetic patients are aware of the need to be extra vigilant about monitoring their blood sugar levels during treatment with prednisolone, and advise them to contact their doctor if they experience problems with the control of their blood sugar levels.
- If you are issuing prednisolone tablets to the patient, explain to them that these should be taken for 5 days only, and that they should not attempt to obtain further supplies from their GP. *Fatalities have resulted from the inadvertent continuation of short courses of steroids.*
- Assuming that the schedule for escalation of infusion rates suggested above is followed with no interruptions, a typical first dose of rituximab can be infused over a period of 3–4 h. However, first infusions often have to be interrupted or slowed down, and the total infusion time can be doubled. Therefore first doses should either be given on an inpatient basis or scheduled so that there is sufficient time to finish drug infusion during the working day of the outpatient clinic.
- Paracetamol and antihistamine premedication must be administered before rituximab infusion is started. Day 1 prednisolone should also be administered prior to rituximab infusion in order to minimise infusion reactions.
- Check that the prescription clearly states what schedule of dose escalation is to be used for rituximab (this is different for first and subsequent doses), and that the rate given is in mL/h not mg/h. If the rate is expressed in mg/h, *see* Administration section above for the formula for converting to mL/h.

- The patient should be counselled about the possibility of infusion reactions before rituximab infusion starts. These reactions affect more than 50% of patients to some degree, and are likely to be more alarming if they are unexpected. Patients who *do* experience infusion reactions should be reassured that they are likely to be considerably less severe after subsequent doses.
- If the patient develops infusion reactions during rituximab treatment (such reactions are much more common with the first infusion), treatment should be interrupted but the infusion left in place. It is normally possible to continue the infusion once the symptoms have resolved.

  If infusion reactions are serious (especially if they involve severe dyspnoea, bronchospasm or hypoxia), the infusion should be stopped immediately and a senior member of the medical team informed.
- For rituximab, use an infusion line separate to that which is being used for any other drugs or fluids.

NOTES FOR PHARMACISTS

- Check that the FBC has been determined and is within acceptable limits before issuing the chemotherapy. Because this is a potentially curative treatment, it is reasonable to treat on a somewhat lower neutrophil/platelet count than would be considered acceptable for a palliative regimen (*see* Notes for prescribers above). Note that rituximab has a minimal impact on bone-marrow function and the doses and scheduling of this drug do not need to be adjusted in the event of haematological toxicity.
- This is a potentially curative treatment, and it is important to maintain dose intensity. Dose delays should be avoided if at all possible. Therefore this is one regimen where the use of haematopoietic growth factors (G-CSF, GM-CSF) may be justified. This should be in accordance with the local policy for haematopoietic growth factor use.
- Check the LFTs. If these show serious impairment, a reduction in doxorubicin and vincristine doses may be required (*see* Appendix 1 for further guidance).
- Check the renal function. A cyclophosphamide dose reduction is required in cases of severe renal impairment (*see* Appendix 2 for further guidance).
- Check that the usual maximum dose for vincristine (i.e. 2 mg) has not been exceeded. If it has, confirm with the prescriber that this was intended. Some prescribers use a maximum dose of 1 mg in patients over 70 years of age because of a perceived increased risk of peripheral neuropathy, although there is no evidence to support this.
- Check that anti-emetics appropriate to highly emetogenic chemotherapy have been prescribed according to protocol. However, because R-CHOP incorporates 5 days of high-dose prednisolone, additional oral steroids are not required.
- Lymphomas are very sensitive to chemotherapy, and massive tumour lysis is possible at the start of chemotherapy. This can result in the generation of large amounts of insoluble uric acid which are capable of precipitating in the kidneys, causing renal damage. To prevent this, allopurinol 300 mg once daily should be commenced the day before starting cytotoxic therapy and continued for as long as there is significant tumour present and cytotoxic treatment continues. Allopurinol doses should be reduced in patients with renal impairment.

- Keep a close eye on the cumulative doxorubicin dose, and alert the prescriber if it exceeds 450 mg/m². It is especially important when a patient starts a course of treatment to check their medical notes and any pharmacy records to see whether they have received previous anthracycline therapy within your hospital or elsewhere.
- The dose of cyclophosphamide is below that which is likely to cause urothelial toxicity. Therefore prophylactic mesna, IV hydration and urine testing are not required.
- Make sure it is clearly stated on any prescription that is being sent elsewhere for dispensing that the prednisolone is a short course of 5 days only. It should not be continued by the GP, nor is routine tailing off of doses necessary. *Fatalities have resulted from the inadvertent continuation of short courses of steroids.*
- Check that paracetamol and chlorpheniramine premedication has been prescribed prior to rituximab. Day 1 prednisolone should also be given prior to starting rituximab infusion in order to reduce the likelihood and severity of infusion reactions. Also check that the prescription clearly states the schedule of rituximab infusion rate escalation. If the chart only gives infusion rates in mg/h, convert these to mL/h to assist those administering treatment. If such a conversion has already been made, check that it has been calculated correctly.
- Rituximab is not a conventional cytotoxic agent, so it can reasonably be manipulated in any aseptic dispensing facility. However, as it is being used for patients who are also receiving cytotoxic chemotherapy, it is also reasonable to handle it in any area that is set aside for cytotoxic drugs.

SOURCE MATERIAL

- Coiffier B, Lepage E, Briere J *et al.* (2002) CHOP chemotherapy plus rituximab compared with CHOP alone in elderly patients with diffuse large-B-cell lymphoma. *NEJM.* **346**: 235–42.

Rituximab (single-agent)

USUAL INDICATION

Relapsed follicular lymphoma.

DOSES

$375 \, \text{mg/m}^2$ by IV infusion on day 1

ADMINISTRATION

As an intravenous infusion in 250 mL of 0.9% sodium chloride after premedication with an antihistamine (e.g. chlorpheniramine 10 mg IV) and paracetamol 1 g by mouth. If the patient has shown severe reactions to previous infusions, consideration should be given to doubling the chlorpheniramine dose and adding hydrocortisone 100 mg IV to the premedication.

First infusion

The infusion should start at a rate of 50 mg/h. After the first 30 min, the infusion rate can be escalated in 50 mg/h increments every 30 min up to a maximum of 400 mg/h. The infusion rate should only be increased if the patient is tolerating the existing rate well. In the event of infusion reactions, treatment should be temporarily suspended to allow the resolution of these reactions.

If infusion reactions are serious (especially if they involve severe dyspnoea, bronchospasm or hypoxia), evidence of resolution should include normalisation of laboratory tests and radiographic evidence of the absence of pulmonary infiltration. After severe reactions, infusions should be restarted at a rate not more than half of that at which the reactions occurred. If the same severe reaction occurs again, serious consideration should be given to stopping treatment permanently.

Subsequent infusions

The infusion can be commenced at an initial rate of 100 mg/h, and increased in 100 mg/h increments at 30-min intervals up to a maximum of 400 mg/h. Again the infusion rate should only be increased if treatment is being well tolerated.

Note: To calculate the infusion rate in mL/h, use the following formula:

$$\text{infusion rate (mL/h)} = \frac{\text{infusion rate (mg/h)}}{(\text{dose [mg]/infusion volume [mL]})}.$$

ANTI-EMETICS

None required routinely (low emetogenic potential), although nausea and vomiting are sometimes an element of severe infusion reactions, and pretreatment may be appropriate before future infusions in patients who experience such reactions.

CYCLE LENGTH

7 days.

NUMBER OF CYCLES

4.

SIDE-EFFECTS

Infusion reactions are seen in more than 50% of patients, predominantly during the first 1–2 h of the first infusion. Infusion reactions may consist of a complex mixture of symptoms with features suggestive of tumour lysis syndrome, cytokine release syndrome and anaphylactoid reactions. Fever, chills and rigors are most common. Other symptoms include flushing, angioedema, nausea, urticaria/rash, fatigue, headache, throat irritation, rhinitis, vomiting and tumour pain accompanied by hypotension and bronchospasm in about 10% of cases. Occasionally, pre-existing cardiac conditions may be exacerbated. Very occasionally, severe infusion reactions have had fatal outcomes, usually in patients with very high numbers of circulating malignant cells ($>25\,000/\text{mm}^3$), pulmonary insufficiency or pulmonary tumour infiltration. Therefore special care should be exercised when treating such patients.

BLOOD NADIR

Rituximab selectively depletes B-lymphocytes. It is not myelosuppressive.

TTOS REQUIRED

• None required routinely.

NOTES FOR PRESCRIBERS

- Assuming that the schedule for escalation of infusion rates suggested above is followed with no interruptions, a typical first dose of rituximab can be infused over a period of 3–4 h. However, first infusions often have to be interrupted or slowed down, and the total infusion time can be doubled. Therefore first doses should either be given on an inpatient basis or scheduled so that there is sufficient time to finish drug infusion during the working day of the outpatient clinic. Liaise with the nursing staff about this matter.
- Rituximab is not myelotoxic, so dose reductions are not recommended for patients with low blood counts. In addition, there is no evidence that a dose reduction is needed in cases of renal or hepatic impairment.
- Premedication with paracetamol and an antihistamine (e.g. chlorpheniramine 10 mg IV) must be prescribed at the time of prescribing rituximab. It is also advisable to prescribe hydrocortisone (100 mg IV) on an 'as-needed' basis to treat serious infusion reactions without delay. In addition, consideration should be given to prescribing pethidine 50 mg IV as needed to treat rigors.
- Staff who are administering rituximab should be instructed on what action to take in the event of serious infusion reactions (see Administration section above).

NOTES FOR NURSES

- Assuming that the schedule for escalation of infusion rates suggested above is followed with no interruptions, a typical first dose of rituximab can be infused over a period of 3–4 h. However, first infusions often have to be interrupted or slowed down, and the total infusion time can be doubled. Therefore first doses should either be given on an inpatient basis or scheduled so that there is sufficient time to finish drug infusion during the working day of the outpatient clinic.
- Paracetamol and antihistamine premedication must be administered before treatment is started.
- Check that the prescription states clearly what schedule of dose escalation is to be used (this is different for first and subsequent doses), and that the rate given is in mL/h not mg/h. If the rate is expressed in mg/h, see Administration section above for the formula for converting to mL/h.
- The patient should be counselled about the possibility of infusion reactions before treatment starts. These reactions affect more than 50% of patients to some degree, and are likely to be more alarming if they are unexpected. Patients who do experience infusion reactions should be reassured that they are likely to be considerably less severe after subsequent doses.
- If the patient develops infusion reactions (which are much more common with the first infusion), treatment should be interrupted but the infusion left in place. It is normally possible to continue infusion once the symptoms have resolved. If infusion reactions are serious (especially if they involve severe dyspnoea, bronchospasm or hypoxia), the infusion should be stopped immediately and a senior member of the medical team informed.
- Use an infusion line separate to that which is being used for any other drugs or fluids.

NOTES FOR PHARMACISTS

- Rituximab is not myelotoxic, so dose reductions are not recommended for patients with low blood counts. In addition, there is no evidence that a dose reduction is needed in cases of renal or hepatic impairment.
- Check that paracetamol and chlorpheniramine premedication has been prescribed prior to rituximab, and that the prescription clearly states the schedule of infusion rate escalation. If the chart only gives infusion rates in mg/h, convert these values to mL/h to assist those administering treatment. If such a conversion has already been made, check that it has been calculated correctly.
- Rituximab is not a conventional cytotoxic agent, so it can reasonably be manipulated in any aseptic dispensing facility. However, as it is being used for patients with advanced malignancy who have received or are receiving chemotherapy, it is also reasonable to handle it in any area that is set aside for cytotoxic drugs.

SOURCE MATERIAL

- McLaughlin P, Grillo-Lopez AJ, Link B *et al.* (1998) Rituximab chimeric anti-CD20 monoclonal antibody therapy for relapsed indolent lymphoma: half of patients respond to a four-dose treatment program. *J Clin Oncol.* **16**: 2825–33.

Temozolomide (single-agent)

USUAL INDICATION:

Glioma that is recurring or progressing after standard therapy.

DOSES (adults and children 3 years of age or older)

Patients previously treated with chemotherapy

Temozolomide 150 mg/m^2/day by mouth on days 1–5

This dose can be escalated to 200 mg/m^2/day by mouth on days 1–5 in patients with a neutrophil count of 1.5×10^9/L and a platelet count of 100×10^9/L at the start of the next cycle

Patients *not* previously treated with chemotherapy

Temozolomide 200 mg/m^2/day by mouth on days 1–5

Note: Temozolomide is only available as oral capsules which cannot be crushed or broken. Therefore it is not a suitable treatment for patients who are unable to swallow capsules.

ADMINISTRATION

By mouth, swallowed whole as a single daily dose on an empty stomach with a glass of water.

ANTI-EMETICS

Weak to moderate emetogenic potential. It may be prudent to treat temozolomide as a moderately emetogenic drug, since vomiting soon after oral treatment will result in loss of drug.

CYCLE LENGTH

28 days.

NUMBER OF CYCLES

Treatment until disease progression.

SIDE-EFFECTS

Bone-marrow suppression (dose limiting), alopecia (infrequent), nausea and vomiting, fatigue, constipation.

BLOOD NADIR

Day 22.

TTOS REQUIRED

- Anti-emetics appropriate to mildly to moderately emetogenic chemotherapy according to local policy.

NOTES FOR PRESCRIBERS

- When prescribing the first course, check whether the patient has received previous chemotherapy, as this determines the starting dose.
- Check the FBC prior to giving the go-ahead for chemotherapy. The manufacturer of temozolomide recommends that treatment should be delayed if the neutrophil count is $<1.5 \times 10^9/L$ or the platelet count is $<100 \times 10^9/L$ on the day of treatment. In patients with unsatisfactory blood counts, the count should be repeated weekly until recovery to this level has occurred. Treatment (adjusted if necessary, for low nadir counts) (see below) can proceed once these blood counts are exceeded.
- Doses need to be adjusted for low nadir blood counts, which should be measured on day 22 ($\pm$48 h) of each cycle. If the neutrophil count falls to $<1.0 \times 10^9/L$ or the platelet count falls to $<50 \times 10^9/L$, doses should be reduced by 50 mg/m^2/day for the next cycle. If unacceptable myelotoxicity is still seen after doses of 100 mg/m^2/day, further treatment should not normally be attempted.
- Ensure that arrangements have been made for a nadir blood count to be measured on day 22 ($\pm$48 h) from the start of treatment.
- Dose modification is not recommended for cases of hepatic or renal impairment, although patients with severe impairment of either system should be treated with caution.
- Temozolomide is only available in 5, 20, 100 and 250 mg capsules. Therefore the smallest possible dose increment is 5 mg. However, some consideration should be given to dose rounding if this results in a more manageable combination of capsules.
- On any prescription and in any communication with GPs, etc., make it very clear that each course of temozolamide is for a fixed period of 5 days only and should

not be extended. On any inpatient drug chart, block out the administration spaces at either end of the course to prevent more than 5 days of treatment being given. *Fatalities have resulted from the inadvertent continuation of short courses of oral cytotoxic drugs.*

- Anti-emetics appropriate to moderately emetogenic chemotherapy should be prescribed according to local protocol.

NOTES FOR NURSES

- If you are counselling the patient about their treatment, make sure they understand that the capsules should be taken for 5 days only, and that they should not attempt to obtain further supplies from their GP, except as part of a formal shared-care arrangement. *Fatalities have resulted from the inadvertent continuation of short courses of oral cytotoxic drugs.*
- Ensure that the necessary arrangements have been made for a nadir blood count to be measured on day 22 (±48 h) from the start of treatment.
- The patient should be instructed to swallow their capsules whole, with plenty of water and on an empty stomach (e.g. first thing in the morning) after any anti-emetics.

NOTES FOR PHARMACISTS

- When you are checking the patient's first prescription, check the pharmacy records and the patient's notes to see whether they have received previous chemotherapy. This determines the starting dose.
- Check the FBC prior to giving the go-ahead for chemotherapy. The manufacturers recommend that treatment should be delayed if the neutrophil count is $<1.5 \times 10^9$/L or the platelet count is $<100 \times 10^9$/L on the day of treatment. In patients with unsatisfactory blood counts, the count should be repeated weekly until recovery to this level has occurred. Doses on the second and subsequent cycles should also be adjusted for low nadir blood counts performed on day 22 ± 48 h (*see* Notes for prescribers above for details of appropriate dose reductions). A check should be made that a nadir count was performed and acted upon before dispensing.
- On any prescription that is being endorsed for others to dispense, make it very clear that each course of temozolomide is for a fixed period of 5 days only and should not be extended. On any inpatient drug chart, block out the administration spaces at either end of the course to prevent more than 5 days of treatment being given. *Fatalities have resulted from the inadvertent continuation of short courses of oral cytotoxic drugs.*
- Dose modification is not recommended for cases of hepatic or renal impairment, although patients with severe impairment of either system should be treated with caution.
- The patient should be instructed to swallow their capsules whole, with plenty of water and on an empty stomach (e.g. first thing in the morning) after any anti-emetics.

- The range of capsule sizes available should allow a close approximation to any calculated dose to be delivered. However, if very small increments are required (e.g. in young children), consider giving unequal doses on successive days.

SOURCE MATERIAL

- Newlands ES, O'Reilly SM, Glaser MG *et al.* (1996) The Charing Cross Hospital experience with temozolomide in patients with gliomas. *Eur J Cancer.* **32A**: 2236–41.
- O'Reilly SM, Newlands ES, Glaser MG *et al.* (1993) Temozolomide: a new oral cytotoxic chemotherapeutic agent with promising activity against primary brain tumours. *Eur J Cancer.* **29A**: 940–42.

Topotecan (Hycamtin®) (single-agent)

USUAL INDICATION

Ovarian cancer resistant to platinum-based chemotherapy.

DOSES

1.5 mg/m^2/day by IV infusion on days 1–5

ADMINISTRATION

By IV infusion over a period of 30 min in 100 mL of 0.9% sodium chloride on 5 successive days.

ANTI-EMETICS

Moderate emetogenic potential. Because of the multiple-day schedule of moderately emetogenic drugs, this regimen does not fit well into standard anti-emetic regimens.

CYCLE LENGTH

21 days.

NUMBER OF CYCLES

6.

SIDE-EFFECTS

Bone-marrow suppression is very significant (all blood components are affected), alopecia (severe in around 50% of patients), nausea and vomiting, mucositis, diarrhoea, rash.

BLOOD NADIR

Around 12 days from the start of the treatment course. It is difficult to define precisely because treatment is spread over 5 days.

TTOS REQUIRED

Anti-emetics appropriate to moderately emetogenic chemotherapy (see above).

NOTES FOR PRESCRIBERS

- Check the FBC prior to giving the go-ahead for chemotherapy. Treatment should not be started (first cycle) if the neutrophil count is $<1.5 \times 10^9$/L or the platelet count is $<100 \times 10^9$/L. If counts are below these levels at the start of subsequent cycles, consult a senior member of the medical team before prescribing. Treatment should definitely be withheld (manufacturer's recommendation) if the neutrophil count is $<1 \times 10^9$/L, the platelet count is $<100 \times 10^9$/L or the haemo-globin concentration is <9 g/dL. Dose modifications are also required for patients who experience prolonged profound neutropenia (neutrophil count $<0.5 \times 10^9$/L for 7 days or more), neutropenia complicated by fever or infection, neutropenia requiring dose delay or a platelet count of $<25 \times 10^9$/L at any point after previous courses. Initially, a dose reduction to 1.25 mg/m^2/day is appropriate. A further reduction to 1 mg/m^2/day is acceptable, but if toxicity persists at this dose, treatment should be discontinued.

  Dose reductions that are made because of haematological toxicity should not be reversed. Although supporting the neutrophil count with haematopoietic growth factors may be considered, a dose reduction may be a more appropriate initial response to myelotoxicity. It should be remembered that G-CSF and GM-CSF will have no impact on anaemia or thrombocytopenia, and that treatment is being given with palliative intent, so reduced dose intensity is less important than with some other treatments.
- Check the LFTs prior to prescribing. Consideration should be given to dose reduction in patients with severely impaired hepatic function, including those with a serum bilirubin concentration of >170 µmol/L (*see* Appendix 1 for further guidance).
- Renal function should be assessed at the start of treatment. Estimation by the Cockcroft–Gault equation from serum creatinine levels is acceptable if the patient has a stable creatinine concentration and no confounding factors (e.g. catabolic states):

CrCl (mL/min)

$$= \frac{1.04 \text{ (females) or } 1.23 \text{ (males)} \times (140 - \text{age in years}) \times \text{weight in kg}}{\text{serum creatinine concentration (µmol/L)}}.$$

On subsequent cycles the renal function should be reassessed.

  Consideration should be given to dose reduction in patients with a CrCl of <40 mL/min (*see* Appendix 2 for further guidance).

- Hair loss should be discussed with the patient. Scalp cooling is unlikely to be particularly successful because of the prolonged serum half-life of topotecan and the multiple drug exposures during each cycle. Therefore it cannot be recommended. If appropriate, liaise with the nurses with regard to referral to a wig-fitter before hair loss becomes apparent.

NOTES FOR NURSES

- Hair loss should be discussed with the patient. Scalp cooling is unlikely to be particularly successful because of the prolonged half-life of topotecan and the multiple exposures to the drug during each cycle. Therefore it cannot be recommended. If appropriate, referral to a wig-fitter should be considered before hair loss becomes apparent.
- Ensure that the patient knows when to commence their oral anti-emetics.

NOTES FOR PHARMACISTS

- Topotecan is highly myelosuppressive. Check that the blood count is within acceptable limits before issuing chemotherapy. Note that the drug's manufacturer makes specific recommendations with regard to dose reductions and delays for myelotoxicity (*see* Notes for prescribers above).
- Check the LFTs prior to dispensing. Consideration should be given to dose reduction in patients with severely impaired hepatic function, including those with a serum bilirubin concentration of >170 μmol/L (*see* Appendix 1 for further guidance).
- Renal function should be assessed at the start of treatment. Estimation by the Cockcroft–Gault equation from the serum creatinine level is acceptable if the patient has a stable creatinine concentration and no confounding factors (e.g. catabolic states). Record the calculated CrCl and the corresponding serum creatinine concentration on any pharmacy patient record sheet (*see* Appendix 3 for an example).

  On subsequent cycles the renal function should be reassessed if the serum creatinine concentration has changed significantly.

  Consideration should be given to dose reduction in patients with a CrCl of <40 mL/min (*see* Appendix 2 for further guidance).

SOURCE MATERIAL

- Ten Bokkel Huinink W, Gore M, Carmichael J *et al.* (1997) Topotecan versus paclitaxel for the treatment of recurrent epithelial ovarian cancer. *J Clin Oncol.* **15**: 2183–93.

Trastuzumab (single-agent)

USUAL INDICATION

Metastatic breast cancer over-expressing HER2 at the 3+ level by immunohisto-chemistry (IHC) or exhibiting gene multiplication by fluorescence *in situ* hybridisation (FISH) testing.

DOSES

Loading dose: 4 mg/kg body weight IV on day 1
Subsequent treatment: 2 mg/kg body weight IV at weekly intervals

Note: A recent study[1] has suggested that an 8 mg/kg loading dose followed by 6 mg/kg every 3 weeks is as effective and more convenient than the weekly schedule.

ADMINISTRATION

As an IV infusion in 250 mL of 0.9% sodium chloride only (trastuzumab is incompatible with dextrose). The initial infusion should be administered over a period of 90 min. If the initial infusion is well tolerated, subsequent infusions can be administered over 30 min. The manufacturer recommends that the patient be kept under observation for 6 h from the start of the first infusion and 2 h from the start of subsequent infusions.

ANTI-EMETICS

Negligible emetogenic potential; no anti-emetics required.

CYCLE LENGTH

Weekly treatment (or 3-weekly treatment – unlicensed).

NUMBER OF CYCLES

Until disease progression.

---

[1] Verma S, Leyland-Jones B, Ayoub J-P *et al*. (2001) Efficacy and safety of three-weekly Herceptin with paclitaxel in women with HER2-positive metastatic breast cancer: preliminary results of a phase II trial. *Eur J Cancer*. **37 (Supplement 6)**: S146.

SIDE-EFFECTS

Infusion reactions including dyspnoea, hypotension, wheezing, bronchospasm, tachycardia, reduced oxygen saturation, anaphylaxis, respiratory distress, urticaria and angioedema. Infusion reactions are usually mild to moderate in intensity, and most occur within 2.5 h of starting the first infusion. Rarely they are severe or even life-threatening, and may develop up to 6 h or even longer after the start of infusion. Very rarely fatalities have been reported, which seem to be particularly associated with patients who are experiencing dyspnoea at rest as a result of advanced malignancy.

Other side-effects include cardiac failure (particularly when trastuzumab is administered in conjunction with anthracyclines), diarrhoea (not usually severe) and an increase in non-life-threatening infections.

BLOOD NADIR

Non-myelosuppressive.

TTOS REQUIRED

- None required routinely.

NOTES FOR PRESCRIBERS

- A prolonged 6-h observation period is required after the first dose, so treatment appointments should be made early enough in the day for this to be completed during the normal opening hours of the treatment area.
- Trastuzumab is not myelotoxic, so dose reductions are not recommended for patients with low blood counts. In addition, there is no evidence that a dose reduction is needed in cases of renal or hepatic impairment.
- Cardiac function should be assessed by means of history, physical examination, ECG, echocardiogram and/or MUGA scan in patients for whom trastuzumab therapy is being considered. In patients in whom there is evidence of compromised cardiac function, especially if they have a history of anthracycline therapy, a careful risk–benefit assessment should be performed before proceeding with treatment. In patients who are receiving trastuzumab, cardiac function should be monitored regularly (e.g. every 3 months), and even more frequently (e.g. every 6–8 weeks) in patients with asymptomatic cardiac impairment. Discuss any patient with symptomatic cardiac dysfunction or worsening asymptomatic dysfunction with a senior member of the medical team with a view to discontinuation of treatment.
- In the event of a hypersensitivity reaction, staff administering trastuzumab should be instructed to interrupt treatment until the symptoms have resolved, at which point infusion can be cautiously restarted.
- Antihistamines, paracetamol and hydrocortisone should be prescribed on an 'as-required' basis with trastuzumab in order to allow swift treatment of infusion

reactions. Even if these drugs are required with the first infusion, they should not be routinely administered on a prophylactic basis for subsequent infusions, since reactions are generally much less frequent and severe during subsequent infusions.

- Although 3-weekly treatment (*see* Doses section above) cannot yet be recommended for routine use, it may be appropriate for patients who will be unable to attend the hospital on a weekly basis because of holidays or similar commitments.
- If a patient misses a single dose, the next dose should be given without modification. If two or more doses are missed, a second loading dose of 4 mg/kg should be used.

NOTES FOR NURSES

- If the patient develops infusion reactions (which are much more common with the first infusion), treatment should be interrupted but the infusion left in place. It is normally possible to continue the infusion once the symptoms have resolved. Paracetamol and antihistamines are appropriate for treating most infusion-related symptoms.
- The prophylactic use of drugs to prevent infusion reactions cannot be recommended, even in patients who experienced such reactions with their first infusion, as they are much less likely to experience problems with their second treatment.
- A 6-h observation period is required from the start of treatment for the first infusion, and a 2-h period for subsequent infusions. Therefore treatments should be scheduled sufficiently early in the day to allow this. The observation period is recommended in case late infusion reactions occur, and the need for it should be explained to the patient, who may not understand why they are being kept waiting for such a long time.
- In-line filters should not be used with trastuzumab as there is insufficient information available about drug binding to such devices.

NOTES FOR PHARMACISTS

- Trastuzumab is not myelotoxic, so dose reductions are not recommended for patients with low blood counts. In addition, there is no evidence that a dose reduction is needed in cases of renal or hepatic impairment.
- Antihistamines, paracetamol and hydrocortisone should be prescribed on an 'as-required' basis with trastuzumab in order to allow swift treatment of infusion reactions. Even if these drugs are required with the first infusion, they should not be routinely administered on a prophylactic basis for subsequent infusions, since reactions are generally much less frequent and severe during subsequent infusions.
- Although 3-weekly treatment (*see* Doses section above) cannot yet be recommended for routine use, it may be appropriate for patients who will be unable to attend the hospital on a weekly basis because of holidays or similar commitments.
- If a patient misses a single dose, the next dose should be given without modification. If two or more doses are missed, a second loading dose of 4 mg/kg should be used.
- Trastuzumab is not a conventional cytotoxic agent, so it can reasonably be manipulated in any aseptic dispensing facility. However, as it is being used for patients

with advanced malignancy who have received or are receiving chemotherapy, it is also reasonable to handle it in any area that is set aside for cytotoxic drugs.

SOURCE MATERIAL

Weekly dosing

- Cobleigh MA, Vogel CL, Tripathy D *et al.* (1999) Multinational study of the efficacy and safety of humanized anti-HER2 monoclonal antibody in women who have HER2-over-expressing metastatic breast cancer that has progressed after chemotherapy for metastatic disease. *J Clin Oncol.* **17**: 2639–48.

Three-weekly dosing

- Verma S, Leyland-Jones B, Ayoub J-P *et al.* (2001) Efficacy and safety of three-weekly Herceptin with paclitaxel in women with HER2-positive metastatic breast cancer: preliminary results of a phase II trial. *Eur J Cancer.* **37** (**Supplement 6**): S146.

VAD (vincristine, doxorubicin ['Adriamycin'], dexamethasone)

USUAL INDICATION

Multiple myeloma.

DOSES

Doxorubicin 9 mg/m^2/day by continuous IV infusion on days 1–4
Vincristine 0.4 mg/day by continuous IV infusion on days 1–4

Note: This vincristine dose is the same for all patients regardless of body surface area.

Dexamethasone 40 mg by mouth on days 1–4, 9–12 and 17–20

ADMINISTRATION

Doxorubicin and vincristine

These are combined in the reservoir of a suitable infusion device and given by continuous infusion over a period of 96 h. These infusion devices are often small enough for the patient to carry around, so this regimen may be administered on an outpatient basis.

Doxorubicin and vincristine are powerful vesicants, and the doxorubicin/vincristine infusion should only be administered via a securely located central venous access.

Dexamethasone

This is administered by mouth as tablets. The strongest tablets available in the UK are 2 mg. For patients who are unable to swallow the 20 tablets each day that are required to make up the total dose, the tablets can readily be reduced to a slurry with water immediately before they are administered.

ANTI-EMETICS

Although doxorubicin is normally considered to be significantly emetogenic, the dose in this regimen is relatively low and is given over 4 days. In addition, the large doses of dexamethasone that are given with it reduce its impact. Therefore a dopamine antagonist (e.g. domperidone 20 mg three times a day by mouth for 5 days starting at the same time as the start of infusion) is usually appropriate. No anti-emetics are required on days when dexamethasone alone is given.

CYCLE LENGTH

28 days.

NUMBER OF CYCLES

Until the patient enters complete remission or paraprotein levels stabilise.

SIDE-EFFECTS

Bone-marrow suppression, alopecia, nausea and vomiting (not usually a significant problem), mucositis, cardiac arrhythmias (acute cardiac problems are rare with the low dose and prolonged infusion schedule used for doxorubicin in VAD), dilated cardio-myopathy (especially at cumulative doxorubicin doses in excess of $450\,mg/m^2$), peripheral neuropathy from vincristine.

The high doses of dexamethasone that are used in this regimen can produce a variety of steroid side-effects, including euphoria/depression, epigastric discomfort, insomnia, glucose intolerance and psychosis.

BLOOD NADIR

10–14 days.

TTOS REQUIRED

- It is sensible to prescribe all three pulses of dexamethasone on the first day of each cycle. This prevents it being forgotten at a subsequent date and also avoids the involvement of any other prescribers who may be unfamiliar with the patient and their potentially confusing intermittent steroid regimen. In addition, it allows the patient to get a fuller picture of the intended pattern of treatment at the time of initiation.
- Anti-emetics appropriate to moderately emetogenic chemotherapy (see above).
- Allopurinol 300 mg each morning (reduce the dose in cases of renal impairment) to prevent tumour lysis syndrome, especially early in treatment when there is a large tumour bulk.
- An H_2-antagonist (e.g. ranitidine) or other gastroprotective agent is appropriate to prevent mucosal irritation by dexamethasone. It may be given continuously while the patient is receiving VAD to avoid the complication of starting and stopping with each pulse of dexamethasone.
- Prophylactic anti-infective agents are not required routinely with this regimen.

NOTES FOR PRESCRIBERS

- If the VAD regimen is being used in ambulatory patients for home treatment, the recipient must be capable of looking after the pump and the associated venous access. This should be taken into account when treatment options are being considered.

- Patients over 60 years of age or with a history of heart disease must have an echo-cardiogram or MUGA scan prior to treatment to ensure that there is adequate left ventricular function.
- Check the FBC prior to giving the go-ahead for chemotherapy. Seek advice from a senior member of the medical team if the neutrophil count is $<1.5 \times 10^9$/L or the platelet count is $<100 \times 10^9$/L.
- Vincristine can cause peripheral neuropathy. The patient should be questioned about abnormal sensations, jaw pain or constipation, any of which may be indicative of neuropathy. If such symptoms are reported, discuss them with a senior member of the medical team with a view to dose modification or a switch to vinblastine, which appears to be more myelosuppressive but less neurotoxic.
- Myelomas are relatively sensitive to chemotherapy, and substantial tumour lysis is possible at the start of chemotherapy. This can generate large amounts of insoluble uric acid which are capable of precipitating in the kidneys, causing renal damage. To prevent this, allopurinol (300 mg once daily, reduced dose in cases of renal impairment) should be commenced the day before starting cytotoxic therapy and continued for as long as a significant tumour bulk remains and cytotoxic therapy continues.
- Care should be taken when prescribing dexamethasone, so that it is clearly understood by the pharmacy staff that this steroid is to be taken for three short pulses of 4 days during each cycle of VAD. It is sensible to prescribe the dexamethasone for all three pulses on the first day of each cycle, in order to prevent confusion. Communications with the patient's GP should emphasise that treatment with dexamethasone is discontinuous.
- Prophylactic H_2-antagonists or other gastroprotective agents may be justified during high-dose dexamethasone courses, especially if platelet counts have been reduced as a consequence of chemotherapy.
- Check the LFTs. If these show significant impairment, a reduction in doxorubicin and vincristine doses may be required (*see* Appendix 1 for further guidance).
- Prior to treatment, hair loss should be discussed with the patient. Hair thinning is more likely than total alopecia with this regimen. Scalp cooling is impractical with VAD because of the prolonged administration schedule that is used.
- If administering the drugs, *see* Administration section above for notes on the vesicant nature of doxorubicin and vincristine. The doxorubicin/vincristine combination should only be administered via a secure central venous access device.

NOTES FOR NURSES

- Prior to treatment, hair loss should be discussed with the patient. Hair thinning is more likely than total alopecia with this regimen. Therefore scalp cooling is unnecessary with VAD, as well as being impractical because of the prolonged administration schedule that is used.
- If administering the drugs, *see* Administration section above for notes on the vesicant nature of doxorubicin and vincristine. The doxorubicin/vincristine combination should only be administered via a secure central venous access device.
- The pulsed nature of dexamethasone treatment should be explained to the patient. It should be emphasised to them that they only take the steroid for three periods of 4 days during each cycle, and that if they have received sufficient

dexamethasone tablets for all three pulses from the hospital, they should not attempt to obtain further supplies from their GP.
- Ensure that any diabetic patients are aware of the need to be extra vigilant about monitoring their blood sugar levels during treatment with dexamethasone, and advise them to contact their doctor if they experience problems with the control of their blood sugar levels.

NOTES FOR PHARMACISTS

- Check that the FBC has been determined and is within acceptable limits before issuing the chemotherapy. Seek confirmation if the neutrophil count is $<1.5 \times 10^9$/L or the platelet count is $<100 \times 10^9$/L.
- If treatment is to be delivered at home via an ambulatory pump, the recipient must be capable of looking after the pump and the associated venous access. This should be taken into account when treatment options are being considered.
- Check the LFTs. If these show significant impairment, a reduction in doxorubicin and vincristine doses may be required (*see* Appendix 1 for further guidance).
- Remember that the vincristine dose is independent of body surface area – it is 0.4 mg/day for all patients.
- Check that appropriate anti-emetics have been prescribed (see above). The high doses of dexamethasone that are used in this regimen mean that additional steroids are not required for anti-emesis, and the infusion of doxorubicin over 4 days means that $5HT_3$-antagonists are not routinely required.
- Myelomas are fairly sensitive to chemotherapy, and substantial tumour lysis is possible at the start of chemotherapy. This can result in the generation of large amounts of insoluble uric acid which are capable of precipitating in the kidneys, causing renal damage. To prevent this, allopurinol 300 mg once daily (reduce the dose in cases of renal impairment) should be commenced the day before starting cytotoxic therapy and continued for as long as a significant tumour bulk remains and cytotoxic chemotherapy continues.
- Monitor the cumulative dose of doxorubicin, and alert the prescriber if this exceeds 450 mg/m². It is especially important when a patient starts a course of treatment to check the pharmacy records and the patient's medical notes to see whether they have received previous anthracycline therapy at your treatment centre or elsewhere.
- Make sure it is clearly stated on any TTO or prescription being sent elsewhere for dispensing that the dexamethasone is to be delivered as three short pulses of 4 days only during each course. The patient should have this explained to them and care should be taken to check that they understand, so that they do not try to obtain inappropriate continuation therapy via their GP. Tailing off of doses is not required with these short courses of steroids.

SOURCE MATERIAL

- Barlogie B, Smith L and Alexanian R (1984) Effective treatment of advanced multiple myeloma refractory to alkylating agents. *NEJM.* **310**: 1353–6.

Vinorelbine (single-agent)

USUAL INDICATION

Breast cancer relapsing after anthracycline-based treatment; first-line treatment of non-small-cell lung cancer.

DOSES

Vinorelbine IV 30 mg/m^2 (maximum dose 60 mg) weekly

ADMINISTRATION

Vinorelbine is administered as a slow IV bolus diluted to 20–50 mL with 0.9% sodium chloride and injected into a free-running saline drip. It should then be flushed in with 250 mL of 0.9% sodium chloride.

Vinorelbine is a vesicant and should be administered with appropriate precautions to prevent extravasation. If there is any possibility that extravasation has occurred, contact a senior member of the medical team immediately and follow local guidance on dealing with extravasation incidents.

ANTI-EMETICS

Low emetogenic potential (according to local policy).

CYCLE LENGTH

7 days.

NUMBER OF CYCLES

Usually until disease progression or unacceptable toxicity.

SIDE-EFFECTS

Bone-marrow suppression (neutropenia is dose limiting), alopecia (usually mild), nausea and vomiting, mucositis, phlebitis, peripheral and autonomic neuropathy leading to loss of deep tendon reflexes, parasthesiae, constipation and jaw pain.

BLOOD NADIR

Weekly treatment means that there is no clear-cut nadir. Recovery of low neutrophil counts is usually rapid (5–7 days), and because myelotoxicity is not cumulative, further treatment can normally be given at full dose after recovery.

TTOS REQUIRED

- Anti-emetics appropriate to weakly emetogenic chemotherapy (see local policy).

NOTES FOR PRESCRIBERS

- Ensure that it is clearly understood what dosage schedule is being used. Schedules other than that described above have been used.
- No single dose of vinorelbine should exceed 60 mg.
- Check the FBC prior to giving the go-ahead for chemotherapy. Seek advice if the neutrophil count is $<2.0 \times 10^9$/L or the platelet count is $<75 \times 10^9$/L (the manufacturer recommends withholding treatment until counts return to these levels).
- If administering vinorelbine, *see* Administration section above for notes about its vesicant properties. However, extravasation should be distinguished from phlebitis tracking along the vein that is used for injection. This can be minimised by liberal flushing of the vein during and after injection.
- Check the LFTs at the time of prescribing. A dose reduction should be considered in cases of significant hepatic impairment or very extensive metastatic liver disease (*see* Appendix 2 for further guidance).
- Check the serum creatinine concentration. The manufacturer of vinorelbine recommends that treatment should be suspended in patients with a serum creatinine level that is 2.6 or more times the normal value (*see* Appendix 2).

NOTES FOR NURSES

- If administering vinorelbine, *see* Administration section above for notes about its vesicant properties. However, extravasation should be distinguished from phlebitis tracking along the vein that is used for injection. This can be minimised by liberal flushing of the vein during and after injection.

NOTES FOR PHARMACISTS

- Ensure that it is clearly understood what dosage schedule is being used. Schedules other than that described above have been used.
- No single dose of vinorelbine should exceed 60 mg.
- Check the FBC and ensure that it is within an acceptable range before issuing the chemotherapy. The manufacturer recommends withholding vinorelbine if the neutrophil count is $<2.0 \times 10^9$/L or the platelet count is $<75 \times 10^9$/L.

- Check the LFTs. A dose reduction should be considered in cases of significant hepatic impairment or very extensive metastatic liver disease (*see* Appendix 1 for further guidance).
- Check the serum creatinine concentration. The manufacturer of vinorelbine recommends that treatment should be suspended in patients with a serum creatinine level that is 2.6 or more times the normal value (*see* Appendix 2).

SOURCE MATERIAL

Breast cancer

- Jones S, Winer E, Vogel C *et al.* (1995) Randomized comparison of vinorelbine and melphalan in anthracycline-refractory advanced breast cancer. *J Clin Oncol.* **13**: 2567–74.
- Tresca P, Fumoleau P, Roche H *et al.* (1990) Vinorelbine: a new active drug in breast carcinoma. Results of an Artac phase II trial. *Breast Cancer Res Treat.* **16**: 161 (abstract).
- Zelek L, Barthier S, Riofrio M *et al.* (2001) Weekly vinorelbine is an effective palliative regimen after failure with anthracyclines and taxanes in metastatic breast carcinoma. *Cancer.* **92**: 2267–72.

Non-small-cell lung cancer

- Le Chevalier T, Brisgand D, Douillard JY *et al.* (1994) Randomized study of vinorelbine and cisplatin versus vindesine and cisplatin versus vinorelbine alone in advanced non-small-cell lung cancer: results of a European multicenter trial including 612 patients. *J Clin Oncol.* **12**: 360–67.
- Malzyner A, Bruno S, Piris N *et al.* (1991) Randomized phase II trial of Navelbine (NVB) vs. NVB + CDDP (NP) in patients (PTS) with inoperable non-small-cell lung cancer (NSCLC). *Eur J Cancer.* **27** (**Supplement 2**): S172 (abstract).

VIP (etoposide [VP-16], ifosfamide, cisplatin)

USUAL INDICATION

Relapsed germ-cell tumours.

DOSES

Etoposide 75 mg/m^2 IV on days 1–5
Ifosfamide 1200 mg/m^2 IV on days 1–5
Mesna 400 mg IV bolus before first ifosfamide infusion, then 1200 mg/m^2/day
  as a continuous IV infusion for 5 days starting simultaneously with the first
  ifosfamide infusion
Cisplatin 20 mg/m^2 IV on days 1–5

Note: There are several variations on this regimen, and VIP has often been used with BOP as the hybrid BOP-VIP regimen. Make sure it is clearly understood exactly which regimen is required.

ADMINISTRATION

Ifosfamide and mesna

Mesna administration is mandatory with ifosfamide, to prevent the urothelial toxicity which can be caused by acrolein metabolites of the drug.

Both ifosfamide and mesna are infused in 0.9% sodium chloride. Each ifosfamide dose should be infused over a period of 1 h. Mesna is administered continuously as an IV infusion over a period of 5 days, starting at the time when the first ifosfamide infusion commences following the 400 mg bolus loading dose. Mesna administration must be continued for at least 8 h after completion of the final ifosfamide infusion. This scheduling is designed to ensure that there is adequate mesna in the bladder throughout the period when ifosfamide metabolites are appearing in the urine. If the final (day 5) mesna infusion is given more quickly to allow earlier patient discharge, it must still be continued for at least 8 h after the end of the last ifosfamide infusion.

Etoposide

By IV infusion in 1 L of 0.9% sodium chloride over a period of at least 1 h. More rapid infusion can cause hypotensive reactions.

Cisplatin

Hydration is necessary with cisplatin treatment in order to dilute the drug during its passage through the kidneys and thus minimise its nephrotoxicity. By administering each dose after that day's etoposide and ifosfamide doses, the need for additional pre-hydration can be avoided. Cisplatin is therefore typically given as an infusion in 1 L of 0.9% sodium chloride over a period of 4 h, followed by 1 L of 0.9% sodium chloride over a period of 6–8 h as post-hydration. The aim of hydration is to maintain a urine output of 100 mL/h during and for 6–8 h after cisplatin administration. Mannitol is sometimes given to ensure that urine output is brisk. Electrolytes are added to the hydration fluids to compensate for cisplatin-induced electrolyte wasting.

ANTI-EMETICS

High emetogenic potential (see local policy).

CYCLE LENGTH

21 days.

NUMBER OF CYCLES

Quite variable, especially as this regimen is often used as a hybrid regimen with BOP. Seek specialist advice.

SIDE-EFFECTS

Bone-marrow suppression (all blood components are affected), total alopecia, haemorrhagic cystitis leading to bladder fibrosis, encephalopathy during administration period, nephrotoxicity, vomiting (may be very severe), sensory and motor neuropathy (sometimes irreversible) including significant potential for ototoxicity, mucositis.

BLOOD NADIR

Around day 12.

TTOS REQUIRED

Anti-emetics appropriate to highly emetogenic chemotherapy (see local protocol).

NOTES FOR PRESCRIBERS

At the time of prescribing each course

- Make sure that this is the correct VIP protocol — there are others! Also ensure that it is clearly understood whether VIP is being used alone or as a hybrid with BOP.

- Check the FBC prior to giving the go-ahead for chemotherapy. Seek advice from a senior member of the medical team if the neutrophil count is $<1.5 \times 10^9$/L or the platelet count is $<100 \times 10^9$/L at the time of treatment. Note that this treatment is usually being given with curative intent, and therefore dose delays should be avoided if at all possible. Haematopoietic growth factor (G-CSF, GM-CSF) support may be appropriate if neutropenia is causing delays in treatment delivery, but not for asymptomatic low nadir counts.

  In a published trial of VIP,[1] doses of etoposide and ifosfamide were reduced in patients who developed neutropenic fever or thrombocytopenic bleeding between treatment cycles. For patients who showed severe myelosuppression on day 22, daily blood counts were taken. If the WBC and platelet counts did not increase to levels greater than 2.5×10^9/L and 100×10^9/L, respectively, then ifosfamide or ifosfamide and etoposide were omitted from day 5 of the next treatment cycle. It should be noted that this trial was conducted at a time when haematopoietic growth factors were not in routine use, and approaches to treatment on low blood counts were probably more conservative than they are today.

- Good renal function is important for all three cytotoxic components of VIP, and the creatinine clearance should be formally assessed at the start of treatment. Ideally this should be done by EDTA clearance, but estimation from serum creatinine levels using the Cockcroft–Gault equation is acceptable if the patient has a stable creatinine concentration and no confounding factors (e.g. catabolic states):

CrCl (mL/min)

$$= \frac{1.04 \text{ (females) or } 1.23 \text{ (males)} \times (140 - \text{age in years}) \times \text{weight in kg}}{\text{serum creatinine concentration } (\mu mol/L)}.$$

On subsequent cycles the renal function should be reassessed.

  Doses of cisplatin *must be reduced* if creatinine clearance drops to <60 mL/min, and doses of ifosfamide and etoposide should be reviewed if the creatinine clearance drops to <60 mL/min and <50 mL/min, respectively (*see* Appendix 2 for further guidance).

- Poor renal function is also (together with low serum albumin levels and a large pelvic tumour mass) a risk factor for ifosfamide encephalopathy. This is an insidious condition that can develop on any treatment course and presents in a variety of ways, although somnolence and confusion feature strongly in the early stages. It can be fatal. Therefore as well as keeping an eye on renal function, it is important to check the serum albumin concentration on each course. If a patient has two or more risk factors for encephalopathy, particularly if these have developed since a previous treatment cycle, discuss whether treatment should be continued with a senior member of the medical team.

- Check serum electrolytes for cisplatin-induced wasting, especially of magnesium, calcium and potassium. Additional supplementation may be required.

- Prescribe anti-emetics appropriate to highly emetogenic chemotherapy according to local policy.

---

[1] Loehrer PJ, Lauer R, Roth BJ *et al.* (1988) Salvage therapy in recurrent germ-cell cancer: ifosfamide and cisplatin plus either vinblastine or etoposide. *Ann Intern Med.* **109**: 540–46.

- Check the LFTs before prescribing. Consideration should be given to adjusting the doses of etoposide and ifosfamide in cases of significant hepatic impairment (*see* Appendix 1 for further guidance).
- Liaise with the nurses who are looking after the patient, who should be on a fluid-balance chart. The urine should be tested for blood (in case haemorrhagic cystitis develops), and the nurses should understand the significance of any changes in mental state which may be indicative of encephalopathy.
- If blood is reported in the urine, increasing the mesna dose may help. It is difficult to give precise dosage recommendations, but doubling the dose is not unreasonable. However, an experienced member of the medical team should be consulted in these circumstances. Note that currently available dipstick tests may be sensitive to very small amounts of blood, and the lowest level of positivity detectable using such tests may not require intervention.
- If a patient displays changes in mental state which suggest encephalopathy, liaise with a senior member of the medical team immediately. Suspension of treatment is strongly advised. Treatment with methylene blue (50 mg IV three times a day) should also be considered. This has been reported to reverse encephalopathy in these circumstances. Note that mesna has no ability to ameliorate CNS toxicity.

NOTES FOR NURSES

- The patient should be on a fluid-balance chart, and daily weights should be recorded during treatment. Intensive hydration is given with the aim of maintaining a urine output of 100 mL/h during and for 6–8 h after each day's cisplatin therapy. If the urine output is inadequate or the patient gains more than 1.5 L/kg from the start of hydration, the medical team should be contacted with a view to prescribing diuretics.
- Once the ifosfamide infusion has commenced, all urine should be tested for blood because of the possibility of ifosfamide-induced haemorrhagic cystitis. Note that currently available dipstick tests are very sensitive, and the lowest level of positivity detectable using such tests may be of little clinical significance. Haematuria should be reported promptly to the medical team responsible for the patient, as extra mesna may be indicated.
- Because of the possibility of ifosfamide-induced CNS toxicity, any excessive drowsiness or confusion should be reported promptly to the medical team.
- If there is a desire to speed up the final day's mesna infusion in order to facilitate early patient discharge, it is important to remember that it should still be administered sufficiently slowly to ensure that it continues for at least 8 h after the end of the final mesna infusion.

NOTES FOR PHARMACISTS

- Make sure that this is the correct VIP protocol – there are others! Also ensure that it is clearly understood whether VIP is being used alone or as a hybrid with BOP.
- Check that the FBC has been determined and is within acceptable limits before issuing the chemotherapy.

- As VIP is usually being given with curative intent, treatment is often continued despite a relatively low blood count. Moreover, if treatment is complicated by clinically significant myelotoxicity (i.e. symptomatic neutropenia or neutrophil counts too low for chemotherapy to be given on the date when it is due, but *not* asymptomatic low nadir blood counts), the use of haematopoietic growth factors (G-CSF, GM-CSF) to support the patient's neutrophil count may be justified (see local policy).

- Check that the renal function is acceptable at the start of treatment. If a formal measure of renal function is not available, calculate the CrCl from the serum creatinine levels using the Cockroft–Gault equation, and mark this value on any pharmacy patient record sheet (*see* Appendix 3 for an example), together with the corresponding creatinine concentration. On subsequent courses recalculate the CrCl if the serum creatinine concentration increases significantly. Poor renal function is a risk factor for ifosfamide encephalopathy, and both cisplatin and (to a lesser extent) ifosfamide are nephrotoxic. A reduction in the cisplatin dose is required if the CrCl is <60 mL/min, and should also be considered for ifosfamide and etoposide in the case of significant renal impairment (*see* Appendix 2 for further guidance).

- Check the serum albumin concentration at the start of treatment, as a low albumin concentration is another risk factor for ifosfamide encephalopathy. It should also be monitored on subsequent cycles, especially if the patient has other risk factors for encephalopathy (poor renal function or a large pelvic tumour mass). If the patient has multiple risk factors, especially if these include low albumin levels (which are often overlooked, as they are not usually checked for any other reason), point these out to the prescriber. Multiple risk factors are not an absolute contraindication to ifosfamide therapy, but where there is a choice of therapy they may point towards an alternative.

- Check the LFTs before prescribing. Consideration should be given to adjusting the doses of etoposide and ifosfamide in cases of significant hepatic impairment (*see* Appendix 1 for further guidance).

- Check that anti-emetics appropriate to highly emetogenic chemotherapy have been prescribed according to local policy.

- Check that mesna has been prescribed and that the dose is appropriate (i.e. if the dose of ifosfamide on the fluid chart has been altered, then the mesna dose should have been altered proportionally). Note that mesna is essentially non-toxic, and considerable rounding up of doses is acceptable to make treatment simpler.

- When you are visiting the ward, check that the patient is not in excessive positive fluid balance (i.e. has not gained more than 1.5 L/kg from the start of hydration) and that urine output is being maintained at a level above 100 mL/h during and for 6–8 h after cisplatin infusion. If excessive fluid retention is occurring, consult with the medical team about the possibility of extra diuretics being prescribed (e.g. furosemide 20–40 mg by mouth) (if this measure has not already been instituted).

  In addition, if any urine sample is described as containing blood, discuss with the prescriber the possibility of increasing the mesna dosage. It is difficult to give guidance on a suitable increase in the mesna dose, but it is not unreasonable to double it. However, note that modern dipstick tests for haematuria are very sensitive, and the lowest level of positivity detectable may not be clinically significant.

- Any reports of the patient being excessively drowsy or confused should be regarded as possible indicators of ifosfamide encephalopathy. As this is a progressive condition, liaise urgently with the prescriber with a view to halting treatment immediately and possibly instituting treatment with methylene blue (50 mg IV three times a day). This treatment has been reported to be beneficial but has not been rigorously assessed and should not be relied upon, particularly as a prophylactic measure. Note that mesna will not ameliorate ifosfamide-induced neurotoxicity, so encephalopathy is not an indication to increase the mesna dose.

SOURCE MATERIAL

Treatment of germ-cell tumours

- Loehrer PJ, Lauer R, Roth BJ *et al.* (1988) Salvage therapy in recurrent germ-cell cancer: ifosfamide and cisplatin plus either vinblastine or etoposide. *Ann Intern Med.* **109**: 540–46.

Methylene blue in ifosfamide encephalopathy

- Kupfer A, Aeschlimann C, Wermuth B *et al.* (1994) Prophylaxis and reversal of ifosfamide encephalopathy with methylene blue. *Lancet.* **343**: 763–4.
- Zulian GB, Tullen E and Maton B (1995) Methylene blue for ifosfamide-associated encephalopathy. *NEJM.* **332**: 1239–40.

XT (capecitabine [Xeloda®] plus docetaxel [Taxotere®]

USUAL INDICATION

Anthracycline-pretreated metastatic breast cancer.

DOSES

Docetaxel 75 mg/m^2 IV on day 1
Capecitabine 2500* mg/m^2 by mouth on days 1–14

ADMINISTRATION

Capecitabine

By mouth as two divided doses each day, taken with food.

Docetaxel

By IV infusion in 5% dextrose over a period of 1 h after the following pre-medication.

Dexamethasone 8 mg by mouth twice a day for 3 days starting the morning of the day prior to IV chemotherapy (i.e. day −1).

ANTI-EMETICS

Low emetogenic potential (see local policy, although note that the patient will be receiving dexamethasone in any case on days before, during and after docetaxel).

CYCLE LENGTH

21 days.

NUMBER OF CYCLES

Usually 6.

---

* 1900 mg/m^2/day for patients over 60 years of age who are receiving their first course of treatment. This may be cautiously increased to 2500 mg/m^2/day in patients who tolerate treatment well at the lower doses.

SIDE-EFFECTS

Bone-marrow suppression (mainly neutropenia, primarily as a result of docetaxel), total alopecia (mainly as a result of docetaxel), nausea and vomiting, myalgia/ arthralgia (due to docetaxel), fluid retention (due to docetaxel), allergic skin reactions (mostly due to docetaxel), sensory neuropathy (due to docetaxel), hypersensitivity (especially due to docetaxel), mucositis, diarrhoea, palmar-plantar erythrodysasthesia ('hand-and-foot' syndrome, primarily as a result of capecitabine).

BLOOD NADIR

Day 7, although it may be rather ill-defined because of the prolonged course of treatment with the moderately myelotoxic capecitabine component.

TTOS REQUIRED

- Anti-emetics appropriate to weakly emetogenic chemotherapy according to local policy.
- Dexamethasone 8 mg twice a day by mouth for 3 days (the day before, the day of and the day after docetaxel) to prevent fluid retention and hypersensitivity reactions. The prescription should direct the patient to 'Take 8 mg (4×2 mg tablets) twice daily for 2 days, including the day of docetaxel (Taxotere) treatment' and to 'Start taking again on the morning of the day before the next docetaxel (Taxotere) treatment'. The objective is 3 days of continuous dexamethasone (8 mg twice a day) treatment starting the day before each dose of docetaxel.

NOTES FOR PRESCRIBERS

- It should be remembered that the starting dose of capecitabine should be reduced in patients over 60 years of age. This suggested reduction should be observed. The capecitabine dose should be reassessed on subsequent cycles with a view to possibly escalating the capecitabine dose to the usual level in patients who tolerate the lower dose well.
- Check the FBC prior to giving the go-ahead for chemotherapy. Treatment should only be given if the neutrophil count is $>1.5 \times 10^9$/L, and an experienced prescriber should be consulted if the platelet count is $<100 \times 10^9$/L. The docetaxel doses should be reduced to 55 mg/m^2 in patients who experienced either febrile neutropenia or prolonged profound neutropenia (neutrophil count $<0.5 \times 10^9$/L for more than 7 days) on the previous course. If profound or febrile neutropenia recurs despite dose reduction, the docetaxel element of treatment should be discontinued.

  Note that docetaxel is by far the most myelotoxic part of this regimen, so measures for dealing with haematological toxicity emphasise docetaxel dose adjustments.

- Because this is a significantly myelotoxic regimen, strong consideration should be given to treating obese patients according to their ideal rather than their actual body weight, in order to minimise the risk of toxicity, especially with regard to docetaxel dosing.
- Check the patient's LFTs. Dose reductions of both capecitabine and docetaxel are mandatory in cases of significant hepatic impairment (*see* Appendix 1 or the manufacturer's SPCs for detailed advice).
- Renal function should be assessed before prescribing. Estimation from the serum creatinine levels using the Cockcroft–Gault equation is appropriate if the patient has a stable serum creatinine concentration and no confounding factors (e.g. catabolic states):

CrCl (mL/min)

$$= \frac{1.04 \text{ (females) or } 1.23 \text{ (males)} \times (140 - \text{age in years}) \times \text{weight in kg}}{\text{serum creatinine concentration (}\mu\text{mol/L)}}.$$

On subsequent cycles the renal function should be reassessed.

A capecitabine dose adjustment is necessary in cases of renal impairment (*see* Appendix 2 for further details).

- This regimen is an intensive one with potentially severe non-haematological toxicities. Serious problems can generally be prevented by careful monitoring of adverse effects (which should be recorded in order to guide future treatment) and adjusting treatment appropriately in response to problems. The manufacturer of capecitabine provides the following general advice on dose modification in response to treatment toxicity, which should be followed.

Toxicity (NCIC grades)	During a course of treatment	Dose adjustment for next cycle (% of starting dose)
Grade 1	Maintain dose level	Maintain dose level
Grade 2		
First appearance	Interrupt until resolved to grade 0–1	100
Second appearance	Interrupt until resolved to grade 0–1	75
Third appearance	Interrupt until resolved to grade 0–1	50
Fourth appearance	Discontinue treatment permanently	
Grade 3		
First appearance	Interrupt until resolved to grade 0–1	75
Second appearance	Interrupt until resolved to grade 0–1	50
Third appearance	Discontinue treatment permanently	
Grade 4		
First appearance	Discontinue permanently	
	or	
	If physician deems it to be in the patient's best interest to continue treatment, interrupt until resolved to grade 0–1	50

The grading of toxicity in the above table is that of the National Cancer Institute of Canada (NCIC) common toxicity criteria (version 1), except for hand-and-foot syndrome, for which the following scale was used.

Grade 1	Numbness, dysasthesia/parasthesia, tingling, painless swelling or erythema causing discomfort but no disruption of normal activity
Grade 2	Painful erythema and swelling of hands and/or feet and/or discomfort affecting the patient's activities of daily living
Grade 3	Moist desquamation, ulceration, blistering and severe pain of the hands and/or feet and/or severe discomfort that causes the patient to be unable to work or perform activities of daily living

- Question the patient about abnormal sensations, as these may indicate docetaxel-induced neuropathy that requires a dose modification. For neuropathy of grade 2 intensity the docetaxel dose should be reduced to $55\,mg/m^2$. For more severe neuropathy, docetaxel should be discontinued. This is in addition to dose modification of capecitabine according to the above schedule.
- Skin reactions may be due to either capecitabine or docetaxel. An experienced prescriber may be able to determine the more likely causative agent in a particular case. The manufacturer of docetaxel gives specific recommendations for dose adjustments for this problem in the Taxotere® SPC.
- Investigate weight gain on subsequent courses. This may be a result of docetaxel-induced fluid retention and therefore not an indication to increase doses.
- If severe fluid retention (pleural effusion, pericardial effusion, ascites) occurs, it is likely to be due to docetaxel, which should be discontinued. No capecitabine dose modification is required.
- The patient should be encouraged to contact an appropriate person at the treatment centre if they experience any of the following side-effects while at home: more than four bowel movements each day, or night-time diarrhoea; more than one vomit in any 24 h; nausea that is interfering with eating; hand-and-foot syndrome or mucositis that causes more than mild discomfort; fever or sore throat. When patients report these problems it is important to take the action dictated in the tables above. Timely treatment interruption and appropriate dose reductions are the key to preventing rare incidents of serious toxicity.
- Several of the toxicities of this regimen (diarrhoea, asthenia, anorexia, nausea and vomiting) predispose the patient to dehydration. Treatment should not be started in patients with uncorrected dehydration, and if grade 2 (or higher) dehydration develops during treatment, the latter should be interrupted and not restarted until the patient has been rehydrated and the underlying problem resolved.
- Capecitabine prescriptions should be for an entire 14-day cycle of treatment. Take care that, when prescribing, the total daily dose is divided into two to give the individual doses. Serious toxicity has occurred when the total daily dose was given twice a day. It should be made clear to the patient that the tablets should

be taken for 14 days only and then stopped, and that no attempt should be made to 'catch up' on any missed tablets. Any prescription should state the duration of treatment clearly, as should any communication with the patient's GPs. *Fatalities have resulted from the inadvertent continuation of short courses of oral chemotherapy.*

- Prescribed capecitabine doses should be multiples of 500 mg and 150 mg, as these are the available tablet strengths, and increments smaller than 150 mg are neither practicable nor necessary.
- Capecitabine tablets should not be crushed, and there is no liquid formulation available. Therefore capecitabine treatment is unsuitable for patients who cannot swallow tablets.
- Capecitabine may modify the action of warfarin and other coumarin anticoagulants and increase phenytoin levels in patients who are taking the drug. If a patient is taking these drugs concomitantly with capecitabine, arrangements should be made to monitor the PT/INR or phenytoin levels more closely than usual.
- Make sure that the patient has taken oral steroid premedication at home/in hospital before docetaxel administration, and ensure that steroids are prescribed to take home for use after this course and prior to the next one (see above). Steroids are needed to prevent acute hypersensitivity reactions. Correct steroid co-medication may also reduce skin reactions and fluid retention.

    The steroid regimen used is an unusual one. Make sure that any prescriptions state the dosage regimen clearly. In particular, ensure that any communication clearly states that the dexamethasone courses are of 3 days' duration only and should not be extended by the patient's GP. *Fatalities have resulted from the inadvertent continuation of short courses of oral steroids.*
- The patient should be observed reasonably closely during docetaxel treatment, especially during the first two treatment cycles, because acute hypersensitivity reactions have been reported.
- Prior to treatment, hair loss should be discussed with the patient. It will probably be extensive in most patients, and scalp cooling is unlikely to prevent it. Liaise with the nurses with regard to referral to a wig-fitter at the start of treatment, before alopecia is evident, if this is appropriate.

NOTES FOR NURSES

- Make sure that the patient has taken oral dexamethasone premedication at home/ on the ward. Docetaxel has been known to cause hypersensitivity reactions, and proper steroid co-medication will minimise the likelihood of this and also reduce the risk of fluid retention/skin reactions.
- The patient should be observed reasonably closely during docetaxel treatment, especially during the first two cycles, because acute hypersensitivity reactions have been reported.
- Inform the prescriber if the patient reports any abnormal sensations that may be indicative of drug-induced neuropathy.
- Ensure that any diabetic patients are aware of the need to be extra vigilant about monitoring their blood sugar levels during treatment with dexamethasone, and advise them to contact their doctor if they experience problems with the control of their blood sugar levels.

- Prior to treatment, hair loss should be discussed with the patient. It will probably be extensive in most patients, and scalp cooling is unlikely to prevent it. Refer the patient to a wig-fitter at the start of treatment, and before alopecia is evident, if this is appropriate.
- If you are counselling the patient about their treatment, check they understand that each cycle of capecitabine treatment should last for 14 days only, and that 14 days after starting treatment they should stop taking their tablets, *even if they have some left over.* Similarly, ensure that they understand how to take their take-home dexamethasone tablets, as these can be a little confusing.

    It is important that the patient does not seek continuation supplies of capecitabine or dexamethasone from their GP, except as part of a formal 'shared-care' arrangement. *Fatalities have resulted from the inadvertent continuation of short courses of oral chemotherapy.*
- The patient should have the likely side-effects of treatment explained to them. They should be encouraged to contact an appropriate person at the hospital if they experience any of the following: more than four bowel movements each day, or night-time diarrhoea; more than one vomit in any 24 h; nausea that is interfering with eating; hand-and-foot syndrome or mucositis that causes more than mild discomfort; fever, sore throat or other symptoms of possible neutropenic infection. Early identification of toxicity and dosage adjustment using the scheme described above are crucial for the prevention of severe toxicity during capecitabine treatment.
- Mucositis can be a problem with docetaxel and capecitabine, and the patient should be instructed on how to deal with this if it arises (i.e. use of soft toothbrushes, avoidance of spicy foods, etc.).

NOTES FOR PHARMACISTS

- For patients over 60 years of age, check that the reduced capecitabine starting dose has been applied (see above), and that on subsequent courses any dose escalation to full dose has been made deliberately after assessment of the patient's toleration of early treatment (i.e. not because the prescriber has failed to notice the patient's age).
- Check that the FBC has been determined prior to issuing chemotherapy. Seek confirmation of the prescription if the neutrophil count is $<1.5 \times 10^9$/L or the platelet count is $<100 \times 10^9$/L, as this is a highly myelosuppressive treatment. Treatment should not be given if the neutrophil count is $<1.5 \times 10^9$/L, and the docetaxel dose should be reduced from 75 mg/m^2 to 55 mg/m^2 in patients who experienced either febrile neutropenia or prolonged profound neutropenia (neutrophil count $<0.5 \times 10^9$/L for more than 7 days) on the previous course.
- Because this is an intensive regimen with potentially significant toxicity, strong consideration should be given to treating obese patients according to their ideal rather than their actual body weight, in order to minimise the risk of toxicity.
- If the patient experiences treatment toxicity, then the manufacturer's recommendations for dosage adjustment should be followed (*see* Notes for prescribers above).

- Check the patient's LFTs. Dose reductions are mandatory for both capecitabine and docetaxel in cases of significant hepatic impairment (*see* Appendix 1 or the manufacturer's SPC for detailed advice).
- Renal function should be checked before capecitabine is dispensed. In patients with no confounding factors (e.g. catabolic states), estimation from the serum creatinine concentration using the Cockcroft–Gault equation is appropriate. Record the calculated CrCl and the corresponding creatinine concentration in any pharmacy patient record (*see* Appendix 3 for an example), and recalculate the CrCl on future courses if the creatinine concentration changes significantly. For advice on dosage adjustment in renal impairment, *see* Appendix 2.
- Rounding off of capecitabine doses to the nearest 150 mg (i.e. the smallest whole tablet available) is appropriate. However, breaking or cutting of tablets is not appropriate.
- Capecitabine tablets should not be crushed, and there is no commercial liquid formulation available. Extemporaneous preparation of such a liquid product has not been reported, and in any case it would be expected to be unpalatable because of the bitter taste of capecitabine. Therefore capecitabine treatment is unsuitable for patients who cannot swallow tablets.
- If a dosage increase has been requested on the basis of significant weight gain since the previous course, check whether this is true weight gain or the result of docetaxel-induced fluid retention. The latter is not an indication to increase doses.
- If the patient is on their first course of treatment, make sure that they were previously prescribed oral dexamethasone premedication and have taken it prior to docetaxel treatment.
- Check that dexamethasone post-/premedication tablets are included among the patient's discharge medications. If oral steroid premedication is not given as part of the patient's discharge medication for any reason (e.g. because the patient is thought to be on their last treatment cycle), annotate any pharmacy patient record (*see* Appendix 3 for an example) clearly so that if the patient is retreated, care is taken to ensure that they receive premedication.
- If you are counselling the patient about their treatment, check they understand that each cycle of capecitabine treatment should last for 14 days only, and that 14 days after starting treatment they should stop taking their tablets, *even if they have some left over*. In addition, make sure that they understand how to take the short course of dexamethasone premedication that they should also have received. It is important that they do not seek continuation supplies of either of these drugs from their GP, unless a formal 'shared-care' agreement is in place. *Fatalities have resulted from the inadvertent continuation of short courses of oral chemotherapy.*
- If you are checking a prescription to be dispensed by others, make sure that it clearly indicates the dose schedules for capecitabine and dexamethasone and how to label the tablets. This is an unusual regimen and it can be difficult to interpret if one is not familiar with it.
- The patient should have the likely side-effects of treatment explained to them, and they should be encouraged to contact an appropriate person at the hospital if they experience any of the following: more than four bowel movements each day, or night-time diarrhoea; more than one vomit in any 24 h; nausea that is interfering with eating; hand-and-foot syndrome or mucositis that causes more than mild discomfort; fever, sore throat or other symptoms of possible neutropenic

infection. Early identification of toxicity and dosage adjustment using the scheme described above are crucial for the prevention of severe toxicity during capecitabine treatment.

- Capecitabine may modify the action of warfarin and other coumarin anticoagulants and increase phenytoin levels in patients who are taking the drug. In patients who are taking these drugs concomitantly with capecitabine, arrangements should be made to monitor the PT/INR or phenytoin levels more closely than usual. Alert the prescriber to this requirement if you are uncertain whether suitable arrangements have been made.
- Mucositis can be a problem with docetaxel and capecitabine, and the patient should be instructed on how to deal with this if it arises (i.e. use of soft toothbrushes, avoidance of spicy foods, etc.).

SOURCE MATERIAL

- O'Shaughnessy JA, Miles D, Vukelja S *et al.* (2002) Superior survival with capecitabine plus docetaxel combination therapy in anthracycline-pretreated patients with advanced breast cancer: phase III trial results. *J Clin Oncol.* **20**: 2812–23.

Z-DEX (oral idarubicin [Zavedos®] plus dexamethasone)

USUAL INDICATION

Multiple myeloma.

DOSES

Idarubicin ('Zavedos') 10 mg/m^2/day by mouth on days 1–4*
Dexamethasone 40 mg by mouth on days 1–4, 8–11 and 15–18

ADMINISTRATION

Both drugs are administered by mouth.

Idarubicin

As 5 mg or 10 mg capsules which should only be administered and swallowed whole with water.

Dexamethasone

Administered as tablets. The highest strength tablet available in the UK is 2 mg. For patients who are unable to swallow the 20 tablets each day that are required to make up the total dose, the tablets can readily be reduced to a slurry with water immediately before administration.

ANTI-EMETICS

Although idarubicin is normally considered to be significantly emetogenic, the daily dose in this regimen is relatively low. In addition, the large dose of dexamethasone reduces its impact. Therefore a dopamine antagonist (e.g. domperidone or meto-clopramide 20 mg by mouth three times a day), given for 5 days starting at the same time as cytotoxic treatment, is usually appropriate. No anti-emetics are required on days when dexamethasone is given alone.

---

*Idarubicin capsules are available in 5 mg and 10 mg strengths only. This gives very little flexibility for daily dose adjustment. To enable more accurate dosing, the total dose of 40 mg/m^2 may be given in four unequal instalments over a period of 4 days.

CYCLE LENGTH

21 days.

NUMBER OF CYCLES

Until the patient enters complete remission or paraprotein levels stabilise.

SIDE-EFFECTS

Bone-marrow suppression, alopecia, nausea and vomiting (not usually a significant problem), mucositis, oesophagitis, dilated cardiomyopathy (especially at cumulative idarubicin doses in excess of 400 mg/m^2), elevation of liver enzymes and bilirubin.

The high doses of dexamethasone used in this regimen can produce a variety of steroid side-effects, including euphoria/depression, epigastric discomfort, insomnia, psychosis, sodium and water retention, potassium loss, proximal myopathy and glucose intolerance.

BLOOD NADIR

10–14 days.

TTOS REQUIRED

- Dexamethasone as described above. It is sensible to prescribe all three pulses of dexamethasone on the first day of each cycle together with the idarubicin. This prevents it being forgotten at a later date and avoids the involvement of any other prescribers who may be unfamiliar with the patient and their potentially confusing intermittent steroid regimen. It also allows the patient to get a fuller picture of the intended pattern of treatment at the time of initiation.
- Idarubicin as described above. This agent is only available in 5 mg and 10 mg capsules, and each daily dose should be a multiple of 5 mg. However, different doses can be given on different days to ensure that the total idarubicin dose given over 4 days is close to the desired total of 40 mg/m^2.
- Allopurinol 300 mg (a dose reduction is needed in cases of renal impairment) each morning should be prescribed to prevent tumour lysis syndrome, especially early in treatment when there is a large tumour bulk.
- An H$_2$-antagonist (e.g. ranitidine) or other gastroprotective agent should be considered as a prophylactic against mucosal irritation caused by dexamethasone. It is often simpler to give this continuously while the patient is receiving Z-DEX in order to avoid the complication of starting and stopping with each pulse of dexamethasone.
- Suitable anti-emetics according to local policy (*see* Anti-emetics section above).

NOTES FOR PRESCRIBERS

- Patients over 60 years of age or with a history of heart disease or previous anthracycline therapy must have an echocardiogram or MUGA scan prior to treatment to ensure that there is adequate left ventricular function.

- Check that the FBC has been determined and is within acceptable limits prior to giving the go-ahead for chemotherapy. Seek advice from a senior member of the medical team if the neutrophil count is $<1.5 \times 10^9$/L or the platelet count is $<100 \times 10^9$/L.
- Myelomas are relatively sensitive to chemotherapy, and substantial tumour lysis is possible at the start of chemotherapy. This can generate large amounts of insoluble uric acid which are capable of precipitating in the kidneys, causing renal damage. To prevent this, allopurinol (300 mg once daily, reduced dose in patients with renal impairment) should be commenced the day before starting cytotoxic therapy and continued for as long as a significant tumour bulk remains and cyto-toxic therapy continues.
- Care should be taken when prescribing idarubicin, so that it is clearly understood by the pharmacy staff dispensing the drug that this is to be taken for 4 days *only* at the start of each cycle of Z-DEX. In addition, each daily dose should be a multiple of 5 mg (see above). All communications with the patient's GP should emphasise that treatment with idarubicin should not be continued beyond 4 days. Similar caution should be exercised when prescribing the short courses of dexamethasone that are used in this regimen. *Fatalities have resulted from the inadvertent continuation of short courses of oral cytotoxic drugs or steroids.*
- Prophylactic H_2-antagonists or other gastroprotective agents may be justified during dexamethasone courses, especially if platelet counts have been reduced as a consequence of chemotherapy.
- Check the LFTs. If these show serious impairment, a reduction in idarubicin dose may be required (*see* Appendix 1 for further guidance).
- Check the serum creatinine levels. If the serum creatinine concentration is >100 µmol/L, an idarubicin dose reduction should be considered (*see* Appendix 2 for further guidance).
- Prior to treatment, hair loss should be discussed with the patient. Hair thinning is more likely than total alopecia with this regimen. Scalp cooling is impractical with Z-DEX because of the prolonged administration schedule that is used.

NOTES FOR NURSES

- Prior to treatment, hair loss should be discussed with the patient. Hair thinning is more likely than total alopecia with this regimen. Therefore scalp cooling is unnecessary with Z-DEX, as well as being impractical because of the prolonged administration schedule that is used.
- The pulsed nature of dexamethasone treatment and the short course of idarubicin should be explained to the patient. It should be emphasised that they only take the steroid for three periods of 4 days during each cycle, and they only take the idarubicin for the first 4 days of each 3-week cycle. If you know that these drugs are all being supplied by the hospital, tell the patient not to try to obtain further supplies from their GP. *Fatalities have resulted from the inadvertent continuation of short courses of oral cytotoxic drugs or steroids.*
- Idarubicin capsules should be swallowed whole and not cut, crushed or dissolved before administration.
- Ensure that any diabetic patients are aware of the need to be extra vigilant about monitoring their blood sugar levels during treatment with dexamethasone, and

advise them to contact their doctor if they experience problems with the control of their blood sugar levels.

NOTES FOR PHARMACISTS

- Check that the FBC has been determined and is within acceptable limits before issuing the chemotherapy. Seek advice if the neutrophil count is $<1.5 \times 10^9$/L or the platelet count is $<100 \times 10^9$/L.
- Check the LFTs. If these show serious impairment, a reduction in the idarubicin dose may be required (*see* Appendix 1 for further guidance).
- Check the serum creatinine levels. If the serum creatinine concentration is $>100\,\mu$mol/L, an idarubicin dose reduction should be considered (*see* Appendix 2 for further guidance).
- Check that appropriate anti-emetics have been prescribed (see above). The high doses of dexamethasone that are used in this regimen ensure that additional steroids are not required for anti-emesis, and the delivery of idarubicin in low daily doses over a period of 4 days means that $5HT_3$-antagonists are not routinely required.
- Myelomas are fairly sensitive to chemotherapy, and substantial tumour lysis is possible at the start of chemotherapy. This can result in the generation of large amounts of insoluble uric acid which are capable of precipitating in the kidneys, causing renal damage. To prevent this, allopurinol 300 mg once daily (the dose should be reduced in cases of renal impairment) should be commenced the day before starting cytotoxic therapy and continued for as long as significant tumour bulk remains and cytotoxic chemotherapy continues.
- Monitor the cumulative dose of idarubicin and alert the prescriber if it exceeds $400\,$mg/m^2. Consideration must also be given to the contribution of other anthracyclines. It is especially important when a patient starts a course of treatment to check the pharmacy and patient records to see whether they have received previous anthracycline (idarubicin, doxorubicin, daunorubicin, epirubicin or aclarubicin) therapy elsewhere.
- Make sure that it is clearly stated on any TTO or prescription that is being sent elsewhere for dispensing that the dexamethasone is to be delivered as three short pulses of 4 days only during each course. The patient should have this explained to them, and it is important to check they understand that they should not try to obtain inappropriate continuation therapy via their GP. Tailing off of doses is not required with these short courses of steroids. Similarly, it should be made clear to the patient that idarubicin is given as a short course of 4 days once only in each 3-weekly cycle, *not* with each pulse of dexamethasone. *Fatalities have resulted from the inadvertent continuation of short courses of oral cytotoxic drugs or steroids.*
- Check that the patient has been prescribed ranitidine or another gastroprotective agent to take with their dexamethasone treatment. If this has not been done, check with the prescriber whether or not it is required.

SOURCE MATERIAL

- Cook G, Sharp RA, Tansey P *et al.* (1996) A phase I/II trial of Z-Dex (oral idarubicin and dexamethasone), an oral equivalent of VAD, as initial therapy at diagnosis or progression in multiple myeloma. *Br J Haematol.* **93**: 931–4.

Appendix 1 Dosage adjustment for cytotoxics in hepatic impairment

This table is a guide only. Pharmacokinetic data, summary of product characteristics (SPC), relevant pharmaceutical company data and various references have been reviewed for each drug. On the basis of this information, a recommendation has been suggested. The full clinical picture of the patient should always be taken into account.

The reference ranges for Guy's and St Thomas' NHS Trust are as follows:

- bilirubin: 0–22 µmol/L
- alkaline phosphatase (ALP):   31–116 IU/L
- alanine transaminase (ALT):   0–55 IU/L
- aspartate transaminase (AST):   0–35 IU/L.

Drug	Pharmacokinetics	Available information	Recommendation
Amsacrine	Amsacrine is extensively metabolised in the liver. The principal metabolites, via microsomal oxidation, are much more cytotoxic than the parent drug. Excretion is via the bile	SPC – for patients with impaired liver function, reduce dose by 20–30% (to 60–75 mg/m² per day) Goldshield – a 40% dose reduction is recommended in patients with bilirubin levels >34 μmol/L.	If bilirubin levels are >34 μmol/L, give 60% dose
Bleomycin	Rapid distribution to body tissues (highest concentration in skin, lungs, peritoneum and lymph). Inactivation takes place primarily in the liver. Around two-thirds of the drug is excreted unchanged in the urine, probably by glomerular filtration	SPC – no information Kyowa Hakko – patients with abnormal liver function tend to develop lung dysfunction	Clinical decision
Busulphan	The mean elimination half-life is 2.57 h. After low and high doses, 1 and 2%, respectively, of unchanged drug is excreted in the urine. The majority of an oral dose is excreted in the urine as methanesulfonic acid, an inactive metabolite	SPC – no information Glaxo-Wellcome – no information	Clinical decision
Capecitabine	Extensive absorption (c. 70%) after food intake. Metabolism is first in the liver and then in the tumour. Around 70% of the dose is recovered in the urine	SPC – insufficient safety and efficacy data are available in patients with hepatic impairment to allow a dose-adjustment recommendation. No information is available on hepatic impairment due to cirrhosis or hepatitis Roche – in a small study[1] it was concluded that mild to moderate hepatic dysfunction due to liver metastasis does not significantly affect the bioactivation of capecitabine. There is no need to reduce the dose in this group of patients	Lack of information available. In patients with mild to moderate hepatic dysfunction due to liver metastases, 100% dose is probably acceptable

Drug			
Carboplatin	Excretion is primarily by glomerular filtration in the urine, with most of the drug excreted in the first 6 h. Around 32% of the dose is excreted unchanged	*SPC* – no information. Transient increases in liver enzymes have been reported. ALP was increased in 30% of patients, AST increased in 15% of patients, and bilirubin increased in 4% of patients. *Faulding* – no further information	Probably no dose reduction is necessary
Carmustine	Partially metabolised to active species which have a long half-life by liver microsomal enzymes. It is thought that the antineoplastic activity may be due to metabolites. Around 60–70% of the total dose is excreted in the urine in 96 h and *c*. 10% as respiratory CO_2	*SPC* – when high doses have been used, a reversible type of hepatic toxicity manifested by increased transaminase, ALP and bilirubin levels has been reported in a small percentage of patients *BMS* – very little information	Clinical decision
Chlorambucil	Good oral absorption. The metabolic pathway is not fully elucidated, but is thought to be hepatic. Less than 1% is excreted unchanged in the urine	*SPC* – consider dose reduction in patients with gross hepatic dysfunction *Glaxo Wellcome* – experiments in mice have led to the hypothesis that hepatic cytochrome P450 is involved in the metabolism of this drug	Reduce dose in patients with gross hepatic dysfunction. Modify dose according to response
Cisplatin	There is good uptake of cisplatin in the kidneys, liver and intestine. The elimination of intact drug and metabolites is via the urine. In the first 24 h 20–80% of the drug is excreted	*SPC* – no information *Faulding* – no information	No dose reduction is necessary

Drug	Pharmacokinetics	Available information	Recommendation
Cladribine	Following administration, cladribine crosses the cell membrane and is phosphorylated. The nucleotide that is formed accumulates in the cell and is incorporated into the DNA. Around 20% is recovered unchanged in the urine	SPC – there is inadequate data on dosing of patients with hepatic insufficiency. Caution is advised in patients with hepatic insufficiency Janssen-Cilag – the role of the liver in cladribine clearance has not been determined. In a pharmacokinetic study it was found that the lowest cladribine clearance was in one patient with a bilirubin concentration of 39 μmol/L	Lack of information available. Clinical decision
Cyclophosphamide	Pro-drug – converted by hepatic microsomal enzymes to alkylating metabolites. Excretion is primarily renal. Around 30% is excreted as unchanged drug	SPC – not recommended in patients with a bilirubin concentration of >17 μmol/L or serum transaminases or ALP more than two to three times the upper normal limit Baxter – in patients with severely impaired hepatic function, there is a decrease in the peak plasma-alkylating activity, but the overall half-life is significantly increased and the total exposure to alkylating metabolites is the same as in patients with normal hepatic function. It has been reported that disorders of liver function without signs of jaundice may not be a contraindication, and that dosage adjustment may not be necessary	Consider SPC recommendations. However, exposure to active metabolites may not be increased, which suggests that dose reduction may not be necessary. Clinical decision
Cytarabine	Cytarabine is concentrated in the liver. A major fraction is inactivated by cytidine deaminase in the liver and other body tissues. After 24 h, 80% of the dose has been eliminated either as the inactive metabolite or as unchanged cytarabine, mostly in the urine, but some is eliminated in the bile	SPC – the human liver apparently detoxifies a substantial fraction of the administered dose. The drug should be used with caution and at a reduced dose if liver function is poor Faulding – limited guidance indicates that the drug should be started at 50% of the regular dose in patients with severe hepatic dysfunction (bilirubin concentration >34 μmol/L), and subsequent doses can be escalated in the absence of toxicity. The hepatotoxic properties of the drug have not been proven	If bilirubin concentration is >34 μmol/L, give 50% of dose Escalate doses in subsequent cycles in the absence of toxicity

Drug	Pharmacokinetics	Recommendations	Dose adjustment
Dacarbazine	Dacarbazine (DTIC) is assumed to be inactive. Microsomal metabolism in the liver produces the main metabolite, namely AIC. Around 50% of DTIC is renally cleared; half of this is unchanged DTIC and about half is AIC. DTIC is secreted in renal tubules rather than filtered in glomeruli	*SPC* – can be hepatotoxic: fatalities have been reported *Bayer* – no further information	Activated and metabolised in the liver. Can be hepatotoxic. Consider dose reduction
Dactinomycin	Minimal metabolism. Concentrated in nucleated cells and does not penetrate the blood–brain barrier. Around 30% of the dose was recovered in the urine and faeces within 1 week. The terminal plasma half-life is *c.* 36 h	*SPC* – no recommendations *MSD* – no further recommendations. Some correspondence on children with Wilms' tumour and hepatotoxicity.[2] Because of the sensitivity of Wilms' tumour to chemotherapy, lower doses may be appropriate (0.5–1 mg/m^2)	No dose changes are recommended
Daunorubicin	Daunorubicin is rapidly taken up by the tissues, especially by the kidneys, liver, spleen and heart. Subsequent release of both drug and metabolites is slow (half-life is *c.* 55 h). Rapidly metabolised in the liver, and the major metabolite, daunorubicinol, is also active. It is excreted slowly in the urine, mainly as metabolites, with 25% excreted within 5 days. Biliary excretion accounts for 40% of elimination	*SPC* – a dose reduction is recommended in patients with impaired hepatic or renal function. See recommendations *Aventis* – as SPC	*Bilirubin concentration (μmol/L)* / *Dose* <20 — 100% 20–50 — 75% >50 — 50%

Drug	Pharmacokinetics	Available information	Recommendation
Docetaxel	Cytochrome P450-mediated metabolism. Around 6% and 75% of the dose is excreted via the renal and faecal routes, respectively, within 7 days	SPC – ALT and/or AST > 1.5 × ULN and ALP > 2.5 × ULN – give 75 mg/m². If bilirubin concentration is >22 μmol/L and/or ALT/AST > 3.5 × ULN with ALP > 6 × ULN, docetaxel should not be used unless it is strictly indicated Aventis – as SPC	As SPC
Doxorubicin	Mainly metabolised in the liver by cytochrome P450 (also renal). Rapidly cleared from the plasma and slowly excreted in the urine and bile (50% of the drug is recoverable in the bile or faeces within 7 days)	SPC – for bilirubin concentration in the range 20–51 μmol/L, give 50% of dose for bilirubin concentration >51 μmol/L, give 25% of dose Pharmacia – Koren et al.[3] suggest the above, and if bilirubin concentration is >85 μmol/L, withhold. If AST is 2–3 × ULN, give 75% of dose	*Bilirubin concentration (μmol/L)* / *Dose* 20–51 — 50% 51–85 — 25% >85 — 0% If AST is 2–3 × ULN, give 75% of dose
Epirubicin	Mainly metabolised in the liver. Slow elimination through the liver is due to extensive tissue distribution. Around 27–40% is eliminated in the bile. Urinary excretion accounts for c. 10% of the dose in 48 h	SPC – for bilirubin concentration in the range 20–51 μmol/L, give 50% of dose for bilirubin concentration >51 μmol/L, give 25% of dose Pharmacia – No additional information	*Bilirubin concentration (μmol/L)* / *Dose* 24–51 — 50% >51 — 25%

Drug			

Etoposide	Metabolised by liver, yielding inactive metabolites. Around 45% of an administered dose is excreted in the urine, 29% being excreted unchanged in 72 h	SPC – etoposide reaches a high concentration in the liver and kidney. Etoposide use is contraindicated in patients with severe hepatic dysfunction
		BMS – creatinine clearance are the strongest predictor of etoposide clearance. There are conflicting data. Some studies indicate that toxicity, clearance and half-life are not altered in patients with impaired hepatic function
		Koren et al.[3] suggest the following:
		  Bilirubin 26–51 μmol/L or AST 60–180 units/L: 50% dose
		  Bilirubin >51 μmol/L or AST > 180 units/L: omit dose
			Arguments for and against dose reduction
			Bilirubin 26–51 μmol/L or AST 60–180 units/L: give 50% of dose
			Bilirubin >51 μmol/L or AST > 180 units/L: clinical decision

Fludarabine	Around 60% of an administered dose is excreted in the urine within 24 h	SPC – no information Schering – fludarabine is mainly eliminated by the renal route, so dose reductions are not necessary. However, there have been reports of liver dysfunction (<1 in 1000) – mainly elevated LFTs	No dose changes are recommended
Fluorouracil	Fluorouracil is distributed through the body water. Following a single IV dose, c. 15% of the dose is excreted unchanged in the urine. The remainder is mainly metabolised in the liver by the usual body mechanisms for uracil	SPC – fluorouracil should be used with caution in patients with reduced renal or liver function or jaundice Faulding – although c. 50% of fluorouracil is metabolised by the hepatic route, the clinical significance of this is unclear. Some studies of the plasma and tissue concentration of the drug and its derivatives in patients with hepatocellular carcinoma and liver cirrhosis or liver metastases detected no change in drug disposition relating to liver dysfunction, indicating that no dose reduction is required. However, a reduction of the initial dose by one-third to one-half is advised in cases of hepatic impairment. Koren et al.[3] suggest a 50% dose reduction, followed by an increase if there is no toxicity	Clinical decision For cases of moderate hepatic impairment, reduce initial dose by one-third. For cases of severe hepatic impairment, reduce initial dose by half. Increase dose if there is no toxicity

Drug	Pharmacokinetics	Available information	Recommendation
Gemcitabine	Rapid metabolism by cytidine deaminase in the liver, kidney, blood and other tissues. The active intracellular metabolites have not been detected in plasma or urine. Urinary excretion of parent drug and inactive metabolite (dFdU) accounts for 99% of the drug	*SPC* – use with caution in patients with hepatic insufficiency *Lilly* – very limited information is available. In a study of 8 patients with AST > 2 × ULN and 19 patients with bilirubin in the range 28–196 μmol/L, no dose-limiting toxicities were observed in patients with AST elevations, whereas half of the patients in the raised bilirubin group developed dose-limiting toxicities	Lack of information available AST elevations do not seem to cause dose-limiting toxicities. If bilirubin concentrations are elevated, it may be appropriate to reduce the dose. Clinical decision
Hydroxyurea	After oral administration, hydroxyurea is readily absorbed from the gastrointestinal tract. Peak plasma concentrations are reached by 2 h. Around 35% of the hydroxyurea dose is excreted via the kidneys as an active or toxic moiety[4]	*SPC* – no information *BMS* – no information	Lack of information available Probably no dose reduction is necessary. Clinical decision
Idarubicin	Extensive metabolism to idarubicinol, which has equipotent activity and a much longer half-life than idarubicin (50 vs. 18 h). Around 13% of the dose is recovered in the urine in 24 h. Elimination is via the hepatobiliary system	*SPC* – in a number of phase III clinical trials, treatment was not given if the bilirubin concentration was >34 μmol/L. For other anthracyclines, reduce dose by 50% if bilirubin is in the range 21–34 μmol/L. Contraindicated in cases of severe liver impairment *Pharmacia* – no further information. If bilirubin concentration is >85 μmol/L, then the drug should not be administered[5]	If bilirubin concentration is in the range 21–34 μmol/L, give a 50% dose reduction If bilirubin concentration is >85 μmol/L, then contraindicated

Drug	Pharmacokinetics	Recommendations	Comments
Ifosfamide	Pro-drug – converted by hepatic microsomal enzymes to alkylating metabolites. Excretion is primarily renal. Around 80% of the dose is excreted as parent compound. Serum half-life is in the range 4–8 h	*SPC* – not recommended in patients with a bilirubin concentration of >17 μmol/L or serum transaminases or ALP more than 2.5 × ULN. *Baxter* – good liver function is important for both activation and elimination of ifosfamide. Ifosfamide itself is not hepatotoxic, but concomitant hepatotoxic drug administration should be avoided	As SPC recommendations. Clinical decision
Irinotecan	The mean 24-h urinary excretion of irinotecan and SN-38 (its active metabolite) was 19.9% and 0.25%, respectively	*SPC* – in patients with a bilirubin concentration of <1.5 × ULN, give 350 mg/m². In patients with a bilirubin concentration of >1.5 × ULN, irinotecan is not recommended. *Aventis* – increased risk of developing febrile neutropenia if bilirubin concentration is >1.5 × ULN and ALT/AST is >5 × ULN	If bilirubin concentration is >1.5 × ULN and AST/ALT is >5 × ULN, irinotecan is not recommended, as there is an increased risk of febrile neutropenia
Liposomal daunorubicin	Pharmacokinetic profile significantly different to that of daunorubicin, with a longer half-life and a 200- to 400-fold reduction in volume of distribution. Metabolism did not appear to be significant at lower doses. Clearance of the liposomes may be mediated by the reticulo-endothelial cells, with selective enhancement of uptake in tumour cells. Anthracyclines are mainly excreted in the bile	*SPC* – no information. *Gilead Sciences* – no specific recommendations. Suggest extra caution and do not exceed 100 mg/m². Monitor toxicities, especially cardiotoxicity	Very little information. Use with caution – do not exceed 100 mg/m²

Drug	Pharmacokinetics	Available information	Recommendation
Liposomal doxorubicin (pegylated) (Caelyx®)	The plasma levels are 10- to 20-fold higher than equivalent doxorubicin doses. There is preferential retention of the drug in the reticulo-endothelial system, such as the liver, spleen and lungs. The liposomal preparation appears to serve as a slow-release preparation for free doxorubicin	SPC – in a small number of patients with bilirubin concentrations of up to 68 μmol/L, there appeared to be no change in the clearance and terminal half-life. However, until further experience with doxorubicin is gained, see Recommendations Schering-Plough – no further information	*Bilirubin concentration (μmol/L)* — *Dose* 20–51 — 50% >51 — 25%
Lomustine	Relatively rapid oral absorption followed by first-pass metabolism. Part of lomustine metabolism is mediated through hepatic microsomal enzymes	SPC – liver function should be assessed periodically Medac – no information	Lack of available information Consider dose reduction
Melphalan	Half-life is c. 1.5–2 h. There is spontaneous degradation rather than enzymatic metabolism. The proportion of the dose excreted in the urine as an active or toxic moiety is in the range 11–93%	SPC – no information Glaxo Wellcome – no information	No dose changes are recommended If there is excessive toxicity, consider dose reduction on subsequent cycles
Mercaptopurine	Absorption of an oral dose is incomplete, averaging around 50%. There is enormous inter-individual variability in absorption, which can result in fivefold variation in AUC.	SPC – mercaptopurine is hepatotoxic, and liver function tests should be monitored weekly during treatment. More frequent monitoring may be advisable in those who have pre-existing liver disease or are receiving other potentially hepatotoxic therapy Glaxo Wellcome – no information	Lack of available information. Clinical decision

Drug	Pharmacokinetics	SPC / Manufacturer information	Recommendation
(Mercaptopurine, cont.)	Mercaptopurine is extensively metabolised and excreted via the kidneys, and the active metabolites have a longer half-life than the parent drug		
Methotrexate	The drug is widely distributed throughout the body tissues, with the highest concentration in the kidneys, gall-bladder, spleen, liver and skin. It is retained for several weeks in the kidneys and for months in the liver. Methotrexate does not appear to be metabolised appreciably. The drug is excreted primarily by the kidneys (>90%), although small amounts are eliminated in the bile	SPC (*Faulding*) – contraindicated in cases of impaired hepatic function. Avoid concomitant use of other hepatotoxic agents, including alcohol SPC (*Wyeth*) – profound hepatic impairment is a contraindication *Faulding* – no further information *Wyeth* – no information It is eliminated mainly by the kidney. Methotrexate should be used with caution in patients with liver dysfunction because of its hepatotoxic potential, which may lead to fibrosis and cirrhosis. The clearance rate is not likely to alter in patients with liver dysfunction who have normal renal function. Conversely, liver disease is often associated with decreased protein-binding of drugs, and may therefore theoretically lead to increased toxicity of methotrexate[3]	Reduce dose, particularly in patients with concomitantly impaired renal function In cases of severe hepatic impairment, methotrexate is contraindicated
Mitomycin	Metabolism is predominantly by the liver. The rate of clearance is inversely proportional to the maximum serum concentration, due to saturation of the degradative pathways. Around 10% is excreted unchanged in the urine. Since metabolic pathways are saturated at low doses, the % dose excreted in the urine increases with increasing dose	SPC – no information *Kyowa Hakko* – no information *Faulding* – following metabolism at numerous sites, mitomycin is excreted in the urine and bile. Although sources have suggested that elevated AST levels may produce a prolonged plasma half-life, dosage adjustment may not be necessary	Consider dose reduction Clinical decision

Drug	Pharmacokinetics	Available information	Recommendation
Mitoxantrone	Extensive metabolism in the liver. Excretion is predominantly via the bile and faeces. Around 5–10% of the dose is excreted in the urine	SPC – careful supervision is recommended when treating patients with severe hepatic insufficiency. Wyeth – half-life is significantly longer in patients with abnormal LFTs (increased from 38 to 70h). A dose of 12 mg/m^2 in hepatocellular carcinoma has manageable toxicity. In some breast cancer trials, if bilirubin concentration is >50 µmol/L, then give 50% of dose. Chlebowski et al.[6] used a dose of 14 mg/m^2 in breast cancer patients with hepatic dysfunction, but haematological toxicity was more severe. Patients with bilirubin concentrations in the range 22–59 µmol/L tolerate the full dose, especially if they have good performance status (PS). Patients with bilirubin >60 µmol/L and good PS tolerate 8 mg/m^2. In patients with bilirubin >60 µmol/L and poor PS, mitoxantrone is not advised	Recommendations are based on breast cancer patients with single agent (14 mg/m^2). Clinical decision depending on bilirubin level and PS. As a guide, if bilirubin concentration is <59 µmol/L and there is good PS, give 100% of dose (i.e. 14 mg/m^2). If bilirubin is >60 µmol/L and there is good PS, give a maximum of 8 mg/m^2 (i.e. 40% dose reduction). If bilirubin is >60 µmol/L and there is poor PS, mitoxantrone is not recommended
Oxaliplatin	In vitro, there is no evidence of cytochrome P450 metabolism. Extensive biotransformation occurs. By day 5, c. 54% of the total dose was recovered in the urine and <3% was recovered in the faeces	SPC – not studied in patients with severe hepatic impairment. No increase in oxaliplatin acute toxicities was observed in the subset of patients with abnormal LFTs at baseline. No specific dose adjustment for patients with abnormal LFTs was performed during clinical development. Sanofi – no further information	Little information available. Probably no dose reduction is necessary. Clinical decision
Paclitaxel	Hepatic metabolism and biliary clearance may be the principal mechanism for elimination. Mean values for cumulative urinary recovery of unchanged drug ranged from 1.3% to 12.6% of the dose, indicating extensive non-renal clearance	SPC – 3-h infusion caused no increase in toxicity in mild abnormal LFTs. No data on severe baseline cholestasis. With longer infusions, severe impairment may see increased myelosuppression. Not recommended in cases of severely impaired hepatic function. BMS – clearance, especially metabolite clearance, was reduced in patients with impaired liver function. This effect was positively correlated with bilirubin, transaminase and ALP levels. When liver function improves during treatment, paclitaxel and metabolite levels normalise.	Limited information available. If bilirubin is <1.25 × normal value and transaminases are <10 × normal value, dose at 175 mg/m^2. If bilirubin is >1.25 × normal value, clinical decision

Drug		
Pentostatin	The metabolism of pentostatin has not been described, and most of a dose is apparently excreted intact in the urine	*SPC* – because of limited experience of treating patients with abnormal liver function, treat with caution *Wyeth* – no further information	Consider dose reduction, but no formal recommendations are available
Procarbazine	After oral absorption, the drug appears to be rapidly and completely absorbed. Procarbazine is metabolised by microsomal enzymes in the liver to an active alkylating agent. After 24 h, up to 70% of a dose is recovered in the urine	*SPC* – caution is advisable in patients with hepatic dysfunction *Cambridge Laboratories* – no further information. Koren et al.[3] suggest that if bilirubin concentration is >85 μmol/L or AST is >180 IU/L, dose should be omitted	If bilirubin concentration is >85 μmol/L or AST is >180 IU/L, then procarbazine is contraindicated
Raltitrexed	Not metabolised. Around 40–50% is excreted unchanged in the urine, and 15% of the dose is eliminated in the faeces over a 10-day period	*SPC* – no dose adjustment is necessary in cases of mild to moderate impairment. Due to some excretion via the faecal route, treatment is not recommended in patients with severe hepatic impairment *AstraZeneca* – studies included patients with mild to moderate impairment. Patients with severe impairment were excluded, and therefore no information is available about them. Liver metastases do not necessarily indicate impairment, as 80% of all trial patients had liver metastases and responded well to treatment. There is no need to reduce the dose in this group of patients unless AST/ALT is >5 ×ULN. In patients without liver metastases, treat if bilirubin is <1.5 × ULN or AST/ALT is <2.5 × ULN (patients outside these ranges were ineligible for trials)	If there are liver metastases, treat at full dose if AST/ALT is <5 × ULN; otherwise consider reducing the dose If there are no liver metastases, give full dose if bilirubin is <1.5 × ULN or AST/ALT is <2.5 × ULN; otherwise consider reducing the dose

If bilirubin is <1.25 × normal value and transaminase levels are <10 × normal value, a dose of 175 mg/m^2 seems to be safe, although more haematological toxicity is seen

Drug	Pharmacokinetics	Available information	Recommendation
Temozolomide	Temozolomide is rapidly absorbed. Half-life is c. 1.8 h. The major route of elimination is renal. Around 5–10% is excreted unchanged and the remainder is eliminated as metabolites	*SPC* – the pharmacokinetics of temozolomide were comparable in patients with normal hepatic function and in those with mild or moderate hepatic impairment. No data are available for severe hepatic impairment *Schering-Plough* – no further information. Around 38% of patients in clinical trials had grade I–IV raised LFTs, in particular ALP. A reduction in dose or discontinuation of the drug allowed LFTs to return to normal	Consider dose reductions for severe hepatic impairment. Clinical decision
Thioguanine	Extensive metabolism in the liver to several active and inactive metabolites. Around 24–46% of the dose is excreted in the urine	*SPC* – consideration should be given to reducing the dosage in patients with impaired hepatic or renal function. *Glaxo Wellcome* – very little information is available, but doses should be reduced in patients with hepatic impairment in order to avoid increased accumulation	Consider dose reduction, but no formal recommendations are available
Thiotepa	Only traces of unchanged thiotepa and triethylene phosphoramide are excreted in the urine, together with a large proportion of metabolites	*SPC* – no information *Wyeth* – no information	Consider dose reduction
Topotecan	The elimination of topotecan in humans has only been partially investigated. A major route of clearance is by hydrolysis. Around 20–60% is excreted in the urine as topotecan or the open-ring form	*SPC* – there is no experience of topotecan administration in patients with severely impaired hepatic function (bilirubin concentration >170 μmol/L). Plasma clearance in patients with a bilirubin concentration in the range 34–170 μmol/L decreased by c. 10%. Half-life was increased by c. 30% *SKB* – A total of 21 patients with hepatic dysfunction were studied. Toxicity and pharmacokinetic profiles were similar to those seen in patients without hepatic impairment. The clearance was also unaffected[7]	Lack of available information If bilirubin is <170 μmol/L, a dose of 100% can probably be given safely If bilirubin is >170 μmol/L – clinical decision

Drug	Pharmacokinetics	Manufacturer information	Recommendation
Treosulphan	Treosulphan is a pro-drug of a bifunctional alkylating agent. It has a high and relatively constant oral bioavailability. The mean urinary excretion of the parent compound is c. 15% over 24 h	SPC – no information Medac – no information	Lack of available information Clinical decision
UFT (tegafur–uracil)	Maximum absorption levels are reached within 1–2 h. Conversion of tegafur to 5-FU occurs via microsomal (CYP2A6) and cytosolic enzymes. The metabolism of 5-FU follows the natural pathways for uracil. Less than 20% of tegafur is excreted intact in the urine. The 3-hydroxy metabolites are excreted in the urine	BMS – UFT is contraindicated in patients who have severe hepatic impairment. Since hepatic disorders, including fulminant hepatitis, have been reported in patients receiving single-agent UFT, appropriate testing should be performed on any patient receiving the UFT/folinate combination who displays signs and symptoms of hepatic impairment	Clinical decision
Vinblastine	Vinblastine is extensively metabolised, primarily in the liver to desacetylvinblastine, which is more active than the parent compound. The drug is excreted slowly in the urine and also in the faeces via the bile	SPC (Faulding) – liver disease may alter the elimination of vinblastine in the bile, markedly increasing its toxicity to peripheral nerves and necessitating a dosage modification in affected patients SPC (Lilly) – as vinblastine is excreted mainly by the liver, it may be necessary to reduce initial doses in the presence of significantly impaired hepatic or biliary function. If bilirubin concentration is >51 µmol/L, a 50% dose reduction is recommended Faulding – no further information. It has been suggested that if bilirubin concentration is in the range 26–51 µmol/L or AST/ALT is 60–180 IU/L, a 50% dose reduction is needed. If the bilirubin is >51 µmol/L or AST/ALT is >180 IU/L, the drug should not be given[8]	Bilirubin concentration (µmol/L): AST/ALT (IU/L): Dose 26–51 or 60–180: 50% >51 and normal: 50% >51 and >180: Omit

Drug	Pharmacokinetics	Available information	Recommendation
Vincristine	Vincristine is metabolised by cytochrome P450 (in the CYP 3A subfamily). Elimination is primarily biliary (10% is excreted in the urine in 24 h)	SPC – an increase in the severity of side-effects may be seen in patients with liver disease sufficient to decrease biliary excretion. A 50% reduction is recommended for patients with a bilirubin concentration of >51 μmol/L Lilly – as SPC. It has been suggested that if the bilirubin concentration is in the range 26–51 μmol/L or AST/ALT is 60–180 IU/L, a 50% dose reduction is needed. If the bilirubin is >51 μmol/L or AST/ALT is >180 IU/L, the drug should not be given[8]	Bilirubin concentration (μmol/L) / AST/ALT (IU/L) / Dose: 26–52 or 60–180 normal: 50% >51 and normal: 50% >51 and >180: Omit
Vindesine	Metabolised by cytochrome P450 (in the CYP 3A subfamily). Elimination is primarily biliary (13% is excreted in the urine in 24 h)	SPC – Excreted principally by the liver. It may therefore be necessary to reduce initial doses in the presence of significantly impaired hepatic or biliary function Lilly – as SPC	Consider dose reduction of at least 50% in cases of severe hepatobiliary impairment
Vinorelbine	Metabolism appears to be hepatic. Half-life is more than 40 h. Excretion is mainly by the biliary route (18.5% appears in the urine)	SPC – vinorelbine metabolism and clearance are mainly hepatic. In breast cancer patients, clearance is not altered in the presence of moderate liver metastases (i.e. <75% of liver volume replaced by the tumour). In these patients there is no pharmacokinetic rationale for reducing doses. In patients with massive liver metastases (i.e. >75% of liver volume replaced by the tumour), it is suggested that the dose is reduced by one-third and the haematological toxicity is monitored Pierre Fabre – see recommendations	AST/ALT / Bilirubin / Dose: <5 × ULN <1.5 × ULN: 100% 1.5–20 × ULN 1.5–3 × ULN: Postpone and reassess 1 week later* >20 × ULN >3 × ULN: Discontinue *If liver toxicity persists for more than 3 weeks, discontinue treatment

1 Twelves C, Glynne-Jones R, Cassidy J et al. (1999) Effects of hepatic dysfunction due to liver metastases on the pharmacokinetics of capecitabine and its metabolites. Clin Cancer Res. **44**: 1696–702.
2 Pritchard J, Raine J and Wallendszus K (1989) Hepatotoxicity of actinomycin D. Lancet. **1**: 168.
3 Koren G, Beatty K, Seto A et al. (1992) The effects of impaired liver function on the elimination of antineoplastic agents. Ann Pharmacother. **26**: 363–74.
4 Kintzel PE and Dorr RT (1995) Anticancer drug renal toxicity and elimination: dosing guidelines for altered renal function. Cancer Treat. **21**: 33–64.
5 Dorr RT and Von Hoff DD (eds) (1994) Cancer Chemotherapy Handbook (2e). Appleton and Lange, Norwalk, CT.
6 Chlebowski RT, Bulcavage L, Henderson IC et al. (1989) Mitoxantrone use in breast cancer patients with elevated bilirubin. Breast Cancer Res Treat. **14**: 267–74.
7 O'Reilly S, Rowinsky E, Slichenmyer W et al. (1996) Phase I and pharmacologic studies of topotecan in patients with impaired hepatic function. J Natl Cancer Inst. **88**: 817–24.
8 Perry MC (1997) Hepatotoxicity of chemotherapeutic agents. In: MC Perry (ed.) The Chemotherapy Source Book (2e). Williams and Wilkin, Baltimore, MD.

Appendix 2 Dosage adjustment for cytotoxics in renal impairment

This table is a guide only. Pharmacokinetic data, summary of product characteristics (SPC), relevant pharmaceutical company data and various references have been reviewed for each drug. On the basis of this information, a recommendation has been suggested. The full clinical picture of the patient should always be taken into account.

The *British National Formulary* (40th edition) states the following:

- mild renal impairment: GFR 20–50 mL/min
- moderate renal impairment: GFR 10–20 mL/min
- severe renal impairment: GFR <10 mL/min.

Drug	Pharmacokinetics	Available information	Recommendation
Amsacrine	Amsacrine is extensively metabolised in the liver. The principal metabolites (via microsomal oxidation) are much more cytotoxic than the parent drug. Excretion is via the bile	SPC – for patients with impaired renal function, reduce dose by 20–30% (to 60–75 mg/m² per day) *Goldshield* – no information	If CrCl is <60 mL/min, reduce dose by 20–30%
Bleomycin	Rapid distribution to body tissues (highest concentration is in skin, lungs, peritoneum and lymph). Inactivation takes place primarily in the liver. Around two-thirds of the drug is excreted unchanged in the urine, probably by glomerular filtration	SPC – if creatinine concentration is in the range 177–354 µmol/L, give a 50% dose reduction. If creatinine is >354 µmol/L, a further reduction is necessary. The rate of excretion is strongly influenced by renal function; plasma concentrations are greatly elevated if usual doses are given to patients with renal impairment, with only up to 20% excreted in 24 h. Observations indicate that it is difficult to eliminate bleomycin by dialysis *Kyowa Hakko* – when GFR is <30mL/min, bleomycin excretion decreases rapidly, causing the blood concentration to rise. Patients with abnormal kidney function tend to develop lung dysfunction *Faulding* – suggested dose modification schedule is as follows: CrCl 10–50 mL/min, give 75% of dose; CrCl <10 mL/min, give 50% of dose	CrCl (mL/min) · Dose >50 · 100% 10–50 · 75% <10 · 50%
Busulphan	The mean elimination half-life is 2.57 h. After low and high doses, 1 and 2%, respectively, of unchanged drug is excreted in the urine. The majority of an oral dose is excreted in the urine as methanesulfonic acid, an inactive metabolite	SPC – no information *Glaxo Wellcome* – although very little unmetabolised drug is excreted in the urine, a complex range of metabolites is excreted via this route. The administration of high-dose busulphan has been evaluated in 15 patients with multiple myeloma (4 patients had CrCl < 30 mL/min), with no problems[1]	Very little information Consider a dose reduction in cases of severe renal impairment

Drug			

Capecitabine

There is extensive absorption (c. 70%) after food intake. Metabolism occurs first in the liver and then in the tumour. Around 70% of the dose is recovered in the urine

SPC – capecitabine is contraindicated in patients with severe renal impairment (CrCl < 30 mL/min). The incidence of grade 3–4 toxicities in patients with moderate renal impairment (CrCl of 30–50 mL/min) is increased. An initial dose of 75% is recommended. In patients with mild renal impairment (CrCl of 51–81 mL/min), no adjustment of the starting dose is recommended. Careful monitoring and prompt treatment interruption are recommended if the patient develops a grade 2, 3 or 4 adverse event, followed by the appropriate dose adjustment
Roche – as SPC

CrCl (mL/min)	Dose
51–81	100%
30–50	75%
<30	Contraindicated

Carboplatin

There is little if any true metabolism of carboplatin. Excretion is primarily by glomerular filtration in the urine, with most of the drug excreted in the first 6 h. Around 32% of the dose is excreted unchanged

SPC – reduce dose if there is renal impairment, and monitor haematological nadirs and renal function. Myelosuppression is closely related to renal clearance. Carboplatin is contraindicated if CrCl is <20 mL/min
Faulding – CrCl > 40 mL/min, maximum dose = 400 mg/m^2
CrCl 20–39 mL/min, maximum dose = 250 mg/m^2

Dose using Calvert equation: dose = AUC (25 + GFR)
Contraindicated if CrCl is <20 mL/min

Carmustine

Partially metabolised to active species by liver microsomal enzymes which have a long half-life. It is thought that the antineoplastic activity may be due to metabolites. Around 60–70% of the total dose is excreted in the urine within 96 h, and c. 10% is excreted as respiratory CO$_2$

SPC – no information
BMS – very little information. Clinical decision based on the haematological response to previous doses, with monitoring of blood counts. Kintzel et al.[2] suggest that for a CrCl of 60 mL/min, 80% of the dose should be used, and for a CrCl of 45 mL/min, 75% of the dose should be used. For a CrCl of 30 mL/min, carmustine is not recommended

CrCl (mL/min)	Dose
60	80%
45	75%
30	Not recommended

Chlorambucil

Good oral absorption. The metabolic pathway is not fully elucidated, but is thought to be hepatic. Less than 1% is excreted unchanged in the urine

SPC – monitor patients who show evidence of impaired renal function, as they are prone to additional myelosuppression associated with azotaemia
Glaxo Wellcome – very little information. Renal function does not appear to affect the elimination rate. Chlorambucil is unlikely to be dialysed

No dose reduction is necessary. However, monitor these patients carefully, as they are more prone to myelosuppression

Drug	Pharmacokinetics	Available information	Recommendation
Cisplatin	There is good uptake of cisplatin by the kidneys, liver and intestine. The elimination of intact drug and metabolites is via the urine. During the first 24 h 20–80% is excreted	SPC – cisplatin induces nephrotoxicity which is cumulative. It is therefore contraindicated in patients with renal impairment Faulding – Kintzel et al.[2] suggest that for a CrCl of 60 mL/min, 75% of the dose should be used, and for a CrCl of 45 mL/min, 50% of the dose should be used. For a CrCl of 30 mL/min, cisplatin is contraindicated Note: There is experience of using the same dose as the GFR (i.e. 1 mg per mL/min GFR). However, it should be noted that there is no evidence to support this practice	GFR (mL/min): Dose >60: 100% 50–60: 75% 40–50: 50% <40: Contraindicated Consider carboplatin if GFR is <40 mL/min
Cladribine	Following administration, cladribine crosses the cell membrane. It is then phosphorylated. The nucleotide that is formed accumulates in the cell and is incorporated into the DNA. Around 20% is recovered unchanged in the urine	SPC – acute renal insufficiency has developed in some patients who received high doses of cladribine. There is inadequate data on dosing of patients with renal insufficiency Janssen–Cilag – very limited information available. In a small study of 9 patients it was found that <30% of cladribine was excreted in the urine and <10% was excreted as metabolite	Lack of information available Clinical decision
Cyclophosphamide	Pro-drug – converted by hepatic microsomal enzymes to alkylating metabolites. Excretion is primarily renal. Around 30% is excreted as unchanged drug	SPC – not recommended in patients with a creatinine concentration of >120 µmol/L Baxter – patients with impaired renal function have been reported to show an increase in metabolite concentration. Therefore reduce dose in cases of renal impairment.[3] Cyclophosphamide and its metabolites can be eliminated by haemodialysis. The availability of mesna in the urinary tract depends on renal function	GFR (mL/min): Dose >50: 100% 10–50: 75% <10: 50%
Cytarabine	Cytarabine is concentrated in the liver. A major fraction of the dose is inactivated by cytidine deaminase in the liver and other body tissues. After 24 h, 80% of the dose has	SPC – dose reduction does not appear to be necessary in patients with impaired renal function. The human liver apparently detoxifies a substantial fraction of the administered dose Faulding – no further information	No dose reduction necessary

Drug			
	been eliminated either as the inactive metabolite or as unchanged cytarabine, mainly in the urine, although some is eliminated in the bile		
Dacarbazine	Dacarbazine (DTIC) is assumed to be inactive. Microsomal metabolism in the liver produces the main metabolite, namely AIC. Around 50% of DTIC is renally cleared. Half of this is unchanged DTIC and around half is AIC. DTIC is secreted in renal tubules, rather than filtered through glomeruli	SPC – no information Bayer – no information Faulding – as the drug is excreted 50% unchanged in the urine by tubular secretion, impairment of renal function is likely to necessitate a change in dosage. Kintzel et al.[2] suggest for a CrCl of 60mL/min that 80% of the dose should be used, and for a CrCl of 45 nL/min, 75% of the dose should be used. For a CrCl of 30mL/min, 70% of the dose should be used	CrCl (mL/min) / Dose 60 — 80% 45 — 75% 30 — 70%
Dactinomycin	Minimal metabolism. Concentrated in nucleated cells and does not penetrate the blood–brain barrier. Around 30% of the dose was recovered in the urine and faeces within 1 week. The terminal plasma half-life is c. 36 h	SPC – no information MSD – no information	Clinical decision
Daunorubicin	Daunorubicin is rapidly taken up by the tissues, especially by the kidneys, liver, spleen and heart. Subsequent release of drug and metabolites is slow (half-life is c. 55 h). Rapidly metabolised in the liver, and the major metabolite, daunorubicinol, is also	SPC – a dose reduction is recommended in patients with impaired hepatic or renal function. See recommendations Aventis – as SPC	Creatinine concentration (µmol/L) / Dose <105 — 100% 105–265 — 75% >265 — 50%

Drug	Pharmacokinetics	Available information	Recommendation
	active. It is excreted slowly in the urine, mainly as metabolites, 25% being excreted within 5 days. Biliary excretion accounts for 40% of elimination		
Docetaxel	Cytochrome P450-mediated metabolism. Around 6% and 75% of the dose is excreted via the renal and faecal routes, respectively, within 7 days	SPC – no information Aventis – no dose adjustment is necessary. One major and three minor metabolites have been identified, which are excreted in the faeces	No dose reduction is necessary
Doxorubicin	Mainly metabolised in the liver (also renal metabolism). Rapidly cleared from the plasma and slowly excreted in the urine and bile (50% of the drug is recoverable in the bile or faeces within 7 days)	SPC – no information Pharmacia – Yoshida et al.[4] have shown that the AUC of doxorubicin and doxorubicinol (active metabolite) is significantly higher in patients with renal failure	Reduce dose in cases of severe renal impairment
Epirubicin	Mainly metabolised in the liver. Slow elimination via the liver is due to extensive tissue distribution. Around 27–40% biliary excretion. Urinary excretion accounts for c. 10% of the dose in 48 h	SPC – moderate renal impairment does not appear to require a dose reduction, in view of the limited amount that is excreted via this route Pharmacia – little information available	Reduce dose in cases of severe impairment only. Clinical decision

Drug	Pharmacokinetics	Dosing in renal impairment
Etoposide	Metabolised in the liver, yielding inactive metabolites. Around 45% of an administered dose is excreted in the urine, 29% being excreted unchanged within 72 h	SPC – etoposide reaches a high concentration in the liver and kidney BMS – creatinine clearance is the strongest predictor of etoposide clearance. US prescribing information suggests a 25% dose reduction for GFR in the range 15–50 mL/min.[5] Subsequent dosing should be based on patient tolerance and clinical effect. A further dose reduction should be considered if GFR is <15 mL/min. Kintzel et al.[2] suggest for a CrCl of 60 mL/min that 85% of the dose is used, for a CrCl of 45 mL/min that 80% of the dose is used, and for a CrCl of 30 mL/min that 75% of the dose is used CrCl (mL/min): 60 = 85%; 45 = 80%; 30 = 75%. Subsequent doses should be based on clinical response
Fludarabine	Around 60% of an administered dose is excreted in the urine within 24 h	SPC – if CrCl is in the range 30–70 mL/min, give 50% of the dose, and use close haematological monitoring to assess toxicity. If CrCl is <30 mL/min fludarabine is contraindicated Schering – as SPC CrCl (mL/min): >70 = 100%; 30–70 = 50%; <30 = Contraindicated
Fluorouracil	Fluorouracil is distributed throughout the body water. Following a single IV dose, around 15% of the dose is excreted unchanged in the urine. The remainder is mainly metabolised in the liver by the usual body mechanisms for uracil	SPC – fluorouracil should be used with caution in patients with impaired renal or liver function or jaundice Faulding – Bennett et al. suggested that no dose adjustment is needed in cases of renal impairment[5] Only consider dose reduction in cases of severe renal impairment
Gemcitabine	Rapid metabolism by cytidine deaminase in the liver, kidney, blood and other tissues. The active intracellular metabolites have not been detected in plasma or urine. Urinary excretion of parent drug and inactive metabolite (dFdU) accounts for 99%	SPC – use with caution in patients with impaired renal function Lilly – since gemcitabine is extensively metabolised by various tissues, mild to moderate renal insufficiency would not be expected to affect its clearance significantly, although there is the possibility of accumulation of the inactive metabolite, dFdU. Lilly investigated the pharmacokinetics in 18 patients with renal insufficiency and found that there was no significant difference between patients on the basis of their GFR (GFR ranged from 30 mL/min upwards) CrCl >30 mL/min – standard dosing; CrCl <30 mL/min – consider dose reduction; clinical decision

Drug	Pharmacokinetics	Available information	Recommendation
Hydroxyurea	After oral administration, hydroxyurea is readily absorbed from the gastrointestinal tract. Peak plasma concentrations are reached by 2 h. Around 35% of the hydroxyurea dose is excreted via the kidneys as an active or toxic moiety[2]	SPC – use with caution in patients with marked renal dysfunction BMS – Kintzel et al.[2] suggest for a CrCl of 60 mL/min that 85% of the dose is used, for a CrCl of 45 mL/min that 80% is used and for a CrCl of 30 mL/min that 75% of the dose is used. Bennett et al.[6] suggest reducing the dose by 50% in patients with GFR < 10 mL/min	CrCl (monitor mL/min) / Dose 60 — 85% 45 — 80% 30 — 75% 10 — 50%
Idarubicin	Extensive metabolism to idarubicinol, which has equipotent activity and a much longer half-life than idarubicin (50 vs. 18 h). Around 13% of the dose is recovered in the urine in 24 h. Elimination is via the hepatobiliary system	SPC – in a number of phase III clinical trials, treatment was not given if creatinine level was > 177 µmol/L. For other anthracyclines, reduce dose by 50% if Cr is in the range 106–177 µmol/L. Contraindicated in cases of severe renal impairment Pharmacia – no further information	Creatinine concentration (µmol/L) / Dose <100 — 100% 100–175 — 50% >175 — Clinical decision
Ifosfamide	Pro-drug – converted by hepatic microsomal enzymes to alkylating metabolites. Excretion is primarily renal. Around 80% of the dose is excreted as parent compound. Serum half-life is in the range 4–8 h	SPC – not recommended in patients with a creatinine level of >120 µmol/L Baxter – dose-reduction schedules established for cyclophosphamide (which has similar metabolic pharmacokinetic parameters). Ifosfamide is known to be more nephrotoxic than cyclophosphamide, and it has CNS toxicity related to poor renal function. The availability of mesna in the urinary tract depends on renal function	GFR (mL/min) / Dose[3] >50 — 100% 10–50 — 75% <10 — 50% SPC states that if creatinine concentration is >120 µmol/L, ifosfamide is not recommended
Irinotecan	The mean 24-h urinary excretion of irinotecan and SN-38 (its active metabolite) was 19.9% and 0.25%, respectively	SPC – not recommended in patients with impaired renal function, as studies in this population have not been conducted Aventis – as above	No dose reduction is needed. However, use with caution, as there are no data on use in this setting

Drug	Pharmacokinetics	Comments	Recommendation
Liposomal daunorubicin	Pharmacokinetic profile is significantly different to that of daunorubicin, with a longer half-life and a 200- to 400-fold reduction in the volume of distribution. Metabolism did not appear to be significant at lower doses. Clearance of the liposomes may be mediated by the reticulo-endothelial cells, with selective enhancement of uptake by tumour cells. Anthracyclines are mainly excreted via the bile	SPC – no information. *Gilead Sciences* – no specific recommendations. Suggest extra caution and do not exceed 100 mg/m². Monitor toxicities, especially cardiotoxicity. As excretion is mainly via the bile, special care must be taken with hepatic dysfunction	Very little information. Use with caution – do not exceed 100mg/m²
Liposomal doxorubicin (pegylated)	The plasma levels are 10- to 20-fold higher than equivalent doxorubicin doses. There is preferential retention of the drug in the reticulo-endothelial system (e.g. liver, spleen and lungs). The liposomal preparation appears to serve as a slow-release preparation for free doxorubicin	SPC – as doxorubicin is metabolised by the liver and excreted in the bile, dose modifications should not be required for liposomal doxorubicin. *Schering-Plough* – no further information	No dose reduction is needed
Lomustine	Relatively rapid oral absorption followed by first-pass metabolism. Part of lomustine metabolism is mediated via hepatic microsomal enzymes	SPC – no information. *Medac* – no information. Kintzel *et al.*[2] suggest that for a CrCl of 60 mL/min, 75% of dose is used, for a CrCl of 45 mL/min, 70% of dose is used, and for a CrCl of 30 mL/min, lomustine is not recommended	*CrCl (mL/min)* / *Dose*: 60 — 75%; 45 — 70%; 30 — Not recommended

Drug	Pharmacokinetics	Available information	Recommendation
Melphalan	Half-life is *c.* 1.5–2 h. There is spontaneous degradation rather than enzymatic metabolism. Proportion of dose that is excreted in the urine as an active or toxic moiety is in the range 11–93%	SPC – clearance, although variable, is decreased in cases of renal impairment. For conventional IV doses (16–40 mg/m^2) and moderate to severe impairment, reduce the initial dose by 50%. Subsequent dosages are determined by haematological suppression. For high IV doses (100–240 mg/m^2) and a GFR in the range 30–50 mL/min, reduce the dose by 50%. Adequate hydration and forced diuresis are also necessary. High doses are not recommended in patients with a GFR of <30 mL/min *Glaxo Wellcome* – as above. Other authors have suggested that it may not be absolutely necessary to withhold high doses from patients with severe renal impairment, as the kidneys do not have a major influence on melphalan pharmacokinetics	For a GFR in the range 30–50 mL/min, give 50% of dose For a GFR of <30 mL/min, clinical decision, but not recommended
Mercaptopurine	Absorption of an oral dose is incomplete, averaging 50%. There is enormous inter-individual variability in absorption, which can result in fivefold variation in AUC. Mercaptopurine is extensively metabolised and excreted via the kidneys, and the active metabolites have a longer half-life than the parent drug	SPC – monitor renal function in the elderly *Glaxo Wellcome* – no information. For patients with renal impairment, use of the following dosing intervals has been suggested: 24–36 h for CrCl in the range 50–80 mL/min, and 48 h for CrCl in the range 10–50 mL/min[7]	Clinical decision Consider increasing the dosing interval as follows: CrCl in the range 50–80 mL/min, 24–36 h CrCl in the range 10–50 mL/min, 48 h
Methotrexate	The drug is widely distributed throughout the body tissues, with the highest concentration in the kidneys, gall-bladder, spleen, liver and skin. It is retained for several weeks in the kidneys and for	SPC (*Faulding*) – impaired renal function is usually a contraindication SPC (*Wyeth*) – profound renal impairment is a contraindication. Use with extreme caution in patients with renal impairment *Wyeth* – renal clearance correlates with CrCl. The half-life of methotrexate is inversely related to CrCl. Kintzel *et al.*[2] have made the following recommendations	CrCl (mL/min) Dose >80 100% 60 65% 45 50% <30 Contraindicated

	months in the liver. Methotrexate does not appear to be metabolised appreciably. The drug is excreted primarily by the kidneys (>90%), although small amounts are eliminated via the bile		
Mitomycin	Metabolism is predominantly via the liver. The rate of clearance is inversely proportional to the maximum serum concentration, due to saturation of the degradative pathways. Around 10% is excreted unchanged in the urine. Since metabolic pathways are saturated at low doses, the percentage of the dose that is excreted in the urine increases with increasing dose	SPC – no information is available on dose adjustment. Severe renal toxicity has occas.orally been reported after treatment, and renal function should be monitored before each course. Kyowa Hakko – no further information. Fisher et al.[3] suggest that for a GFR in the range 10–60 mL/min, 75% of the dose should be used, and for GFR <10 mL/min, 50% of the dose should be used	GFR (mL/min) Dose >60 100% 10–60 75% <10 50%
Mitoxantrone	Extensive metabolism in the liver. Excretion is predominantly via the bile and faeces. Around 5–10% of the dose is excreted in the urine	SPC – no information available. Wyeth – dose reductions appear to be unnecessary in patients with reduced renal function. The principal dose-limiting side-effect is myelosuppression, which should be monitored. Mitoxantrone does not appear to be eliminated by haemodialysis, and dose adjustments are not needed in such patients	No dose reductions are necessary
Oxaliplatin	In vitro, there is no evidence of cytochrome P450 metabolism. Extensive biotransformation occurs.	SPC – oxaliplatin has not been studied in patients with severe renal impairment (<30 mL/min). In patients with moderate renal impairment, treatment may be initiated at the normally recommended dose. Consider the risk–benefit ratio. There is no need to reduce the dose in patients with mild renal dysfunction	In cases of moderate renal impairment, treat at the normal dose, and monitor renal function. Adjust dose according to toxicity.

Drug	Pharmacokinetics	Available information	Recommendation
	By day 5, c. 54% of the total dose is recovered in the urine and <3% is recovered in the faeces	Sanofi – Massari et al.[9] looked at patients with normal and impaired (GFR 27–57 mL/min) renal function. Data showed the same plasma levels in the two groups, and the clearance of both total and free platinum as well as AUC correlated with the CrCl. Toxicities were similar in the two groups	If CrCl is <30 mL/min – not recommended
Paclitaxel	Hepatic metabolism and biliary clearance may be the principal mechanism for elimination. Mean values for cumulative urinary recovery of unchanged drug ranged from 1.3% to 12.6% of the dose, indicating that there is extensive non-renal clearance	SPC – no recommendations BMS – within 24–48 h after administration, <10% of the dose appears in the urine. In dialysis patients, a full dose has been given (on non-dialysis days) with a typical toxicity profile	No dose reductions are necessary
Pentostatin	The metabolism of pentostatin has not been described, and most of a dose is apparently excreted intact in the urine	SPC – two patients with impaired CrCl (50–60 mL/min) achieved complete response without unusual adverse events when treated with 2 mg/m² (50% of dose). Given the limited data, if CrCl is <60 mL/min, pentostatin is contraindicated Wyeth – no further information	CrCl > 60 mL/min, give 100% of dose CrCl 50–60 mL/min give 50% of dose CrCl < 50 mL/min, not recommended
Procarbazine	After oral absorption, the drug appears to be rapidly and completely absorbed. Procarbazine is metabolised by microsomal enzymes in the liver to an active alkylating agent. After 24 h up to 70% of a dose is recovered in the urine	SPC – caution is advisable in patients with renal dysfunction Cambridge Laboratories – no further information. With serum creatinine levels of >177 µmol/L, doses should be substantially reduced[7]	Lack of available information If serum creatinine concentration is >177 µmol/L, give 50% of dose. In cases of severe renal impairment – not recommended

Drug	Pharmacokinetics	Manufacturer/SPC information	Dose in renal impairment
Raltitrexed	Not metabolised. Around 40–50% is excreted unchanged in the urine; 15% of a dose is excreted in the faeces over a 10-day period	SPC – see recommendations AstraZeneca – as SPC	CrCl (mL/min): >65 — Dose 100%, Interval 3-weekly; 55–65 — Dose 75%, Interval 4-weekly; 25–54 — Dose 50%, Interval 4-weekly; <25 — Dose 0%, Interval —
Temozolomide	Temozolomide is rapidly absorbed. Half-life is c.1.8 h. The major route of elimination is renal. Around 5–10% is excreted unchanged, and the remainder is eliminated as metabolites	SPC – no data on use in patients with renal dysfunction. Analysis of population pharmacokinetic data revealed that plasma temozolomide clearance was independent of age and renal function. It is unlikely that dose reductions are required in patients with severe renal dysfunction Schering-Plough – no further information	Clinical decision
Thioguanine	Extensive metabolism in the liver to several active and inactive metabolites. Around 24–46% of the dose is excreted in the urine	SPC – consideration should be given to reducing the dosage in patients with impaired hepatic or renal function Glaxo Wellcome – very little information	Consider dose reduction, but no formal recommendations
Thiotepa	Only traces of unchanged thiotepa and triethylene phosphoramide are excreted in the urine, together with a large proportion of metabolites	SPC – no information Wyeth – no information	No of information available Clinical decision
Topotecan	The elimination of topotecan in humans has been only partially investigated. A major route of clearance is by hydrolysis. Around 20–60% is excreted in the urine as topotecan or the open-ring form	SPC – there is no experience of the use of topotecan in patients with CrCl <20 mL/min, and the drug is contraindicated in this group of patients. Plasma clearance in patients with CrCl in the range 41–60 mL/min decreased to c.67%. In cases of moderate renal impairment (CrCl in the range 20–39 mL/min), plasma clearance was reduced to c.34% SKB – dose-limiting toxicities, mainly neutropenia and thrombocytopenia, are seen in patients with impaired renal function. In patients with moderate renal impairment,	CrCl (mL/min): >60 — Dose 100%; 41–60 — Dose 75%; 20–39 — Dose 50%; <20 — Contraindicated

Drug	Pharmacokinetics	Available information	Recommendation
		a starting dose of 0.75 mg/m^2 is recommended. Further reductions are recommended in heavily pretreated patients Kintzel et al.[2] suggest that for a CrCl of 60 mL/min, use 80% of dose, for a CrCl of 45 mL/min, use 75% of dose, and for a CrCl of 30 mL/min, use 70% of dose	
Treosulphan	Treosulfan is a pro-drug of a bifunctional alkylating agent. It has high and relatively constant bioavailability. The mean urinary excretion of the parent compound is c. 15% over 24 h	SPC – no information Medac – no information	Lack of information available. Clinical decision
UFT (tegafur–uracil)	Maximum absorption levels are reached within 1–2 h. Conversion of tegafur to 5-FU occurs via microsomal (CYP2A6) and cytosolic enzymes. The metabolism of 5-FU follows the natural pathways for uracil. Less than 20% of tegafur is excreted intact in the urine. The 3-hydroxy metabolites are excreted in the urine	BMS – the effect of renal impairment on the excretion of UFT has not been assessed. Although the primary route of elimination of UFT is not renal, caution should be exercised in patients with impaired renal function. Monitor closely	Lack of information available. Probably no dose reduction is necessary. Monitor for toxicity
Vinblastine	Vinblastine is extensively metabolised, primarily in the liver to desacetyl-vinblastine, which is more active than the parent compound. The drug is excreted slowly in the urine and also in the faeces via the bile	SPC – no information Faulding – no dose reduction is necessary	No dose reduction is necessary

Vincristine	Metabolised by cytochrome P450 (in the CYP 3A subfamily). Elimination is primarily biliary (10% is excreted in the urine within 24 h)	SPC – no information Lilly – no dose reduction is necessary	No dose reduction is necessary
Vindesine	Metabolised by cytochrome P450 (in the CYP 3A subfamily). Elimination is primarily biliary (13% is excreted in the urine within 24 h)	SPC – no information Lilly – no dose reduction is necessary	No dose reduction is necessary
Vinorelbine	Metabolism appears to be hepatic. Half-life is more than 40 h. Excretion is mainly by the biliary route (18.5% appears in the urine)	SPC – 18.5% is excreted unchanged in the urine. There is no rationale for reducing the dose in patients with impaired kidney function Pierre-Fabre – dosage reduction is required in patients with severe renal impairment	If serum creatinine is >2.5 × ULN, postpone dosing and reassess 1 week later. If creatinine is still elevated by ≥2.6 × ULN, discontinue treatment

[1] Mansi J, da Costa F, Viner C et al. (1992) High-dose busulphan in patients with myeloma. *J Clin Oncol.* **10**: 1569–73.

[2] Kintzel PE and Dorr RT (1995) Anticancer drug renal toxicity and elimination: dosing guidelines for altered renal function. *Cancer Treat Rev.* **21**: 33–64.

[3] Joss R, Goldhirsch A and Brunner K (1980) Komplikationen im Bereich der Niere und der ableitenden Harnwege im Verlauf von Tumorkrankheiten. *Schweiz Med Wochenschr.* **110**: 390–404.

[4] Yoshida H, Goto M, Honda A et al. (1994) Pharmacokinetics of doxorubicin and its active metabolite in patients with normal renal function and in patients on hemodialysis. *Cancer Chemother Pharmacol.* **33**: 450–54.

[5] Anon. (2002) *The Physician's Desk Reference* (56e). Thomson Medical Economics, Montvale NJ.

[6] Bennett WM, Aronoff GR, Morrison G et al. (1983) Drug prescribing in renal failure: dosing guidelines for adults. *Am J Kidney Dis.* **3**: 155–93.

[7] Dorr RT and Von Hoff DD (eds) (1994) *Cancer Chemotherapy Handbook* (2e). Appleton and Lange, Norwalk, CT.

[8] Fisher DS, Tish Knobf M and Durivage HJ (1997) *The Cancer Chemotherapy Handbook* (5e). Mosby, St Louis, MO.

[9] Massari C, Brienza S, Rotarski M et al. (2000) Pharmacokinetics of oxaliplatin in patients with normal versus impaired renal function. *Cancer Chemother Pharmacol.* **45**: 157–64.

Appendix 3 Example of a pharmacy patient record

Name:							Sheet _ _ _ _ of _ _ _ _			
Hospital number:							Trial? Yes/No			
Date of birth:			Consultant:				Trial ID:			
Date				Diagnosis:			Treatment started on:			
Height										
Weight				Regimen:			Approval gained for expensive drug use (sign and date):			
BSA							REFERRAL FORM ☐ (Tick)			

Date	Course			Anti-emetics	Pharmacist clinical check	Date	Course			Anti-emetics	Pharmacist clinical check